Management of Cardiac Problems in Primary Care
Second Edition

Management of Cardiac Problems in Primary Care

Second Edition

CLIVE HANDLER
BSc, MD, MRCP, FACC, FESC
Consultant in Pulmonary Hypertension
The National Pulmonary Hypertension Service
Royal Free Hospital, London
Consultant Cardiologist
Hospital of St John and St Elizabeth, and Highgate Hospital, London
Honorary Senior Lecturer
Royal Free and University College Medical School, London

and

GERRY COGHLAN
MD, FRCP
Consultant Cardiologist and Director
The National Pulmonary Hypertension Unit, Royal Free Hospital, London

Foreword by
NICK BROWN
General Practitioner, Watford

Radcliffe Publishing
Oxford • New York

Radcliffe Publishing Ltd
18 Marcham Road
Abingdon
Oxon OX14 1AA
United Kingdom

www.radcliffe-oxford.com
Electronic catalogue and worldwide online ordering facility.

British Library Cataloguing in Publication Data

A catalogue record for this book is available from the British Library.

ISBN-13: 978 184619 144 2

Typeset by Pindar New Zealand (Egan Reid), Auckland, New Zealand
Printed and bound by Hobbs the Printers, Southampton, Hampshire, UK

Contents

Foreword

We have been rightly proud in this country of a National Health Service that has developed with primary care clinicians as generalists providing rapid access to a high-quality healthcare service. Medical care and therapies that are available now bear no relation to what could be done 10 years ago, let alone at the inception of the NHS in 1948.

The face of general practice in the UK has changed dramatically over my years in primary care, with recent NHS reorganisations bringing a set of new roles and responsibilities in commissioning health services for their patients. There are two fundamental elements that are essential to the successful implementation of recent organisational developments:

✧ team-working across the primary–secondary health provider divide
✧ improving knowledge and clinical skills among primary care clinicians.

Where these two elements coexist, it is clear that health service delivery is not only better for the patient, but it is also quicker, more efficient, less wasteful of resources and achieved at a lower cost. As cardiology drugs account for 30–35% of a GP's drug budget and the largest percentage of referral and intervention costs, this is a clinical area that any commissioner ignores at their peril.

What, I hear you ask, has all of this to do with this book?

Clive Handler and Gerry Coghlan have written a book that will become critical reading for the primary care physician managing cardiac problems in the new age of medical practice. In it the authors give clear, concise and readable information on diagnosis, management and treatment priorities in this most important field of medicine. The book uses current evidence and follows current guidelines to direct the clinician in treating conditions that are seen every day in general practice, and builds the reader's confidence in understanding their role and responsibility in commissioning cardiology specialist care. The narrative is peppered with real patient problems, as well as sections that give advice to patients in layman's language.

This is not just another textbook written by an academic from a large hospital. It has been born out of Dr Handler's work within our practice, where he has sought to bring high-quality cardiology into primary care, and we recognise our good fortune in this outreach. This co-operative, community-based team approach is a model for the future development of medicine in the UK and the wider world, where a mix of generalists and specialists working together is essential. This book will not only enhance the primary care physician's ability to manage problems in-house, but will also guide the commissioning clinician in putting in place appropriate and efficient specialist services.

I commend Clive Handler and Gerry Coghlan for their excellent text, which will be a valuable addition to the libraries of all general practices. Buy more than one copy – clinicians ranging from practice nurses, students and registrars to the most senior doctors will all find it essential reading.

Dr Nick Brown
General Practitioner, Watford
Ex Chair, Professional Executive Committee, Watford & Three Rivers PCT
Chair, West Herts Joint Prescribing Committee
Executive Member, Watford Locality Practice-Based Commissioning Group
April 2008

Preface

GPs and practice nurses have always been actively involved in the management of patients with cardiovascular conditions. The last few years have seen major changes in the management of cardiovascular disease. The next few years will see further blurring of the traditional boundaries with regard to how services are provided and who delivers them, due to the integration of primary and secondary care. Primary care clinicians will absorb some of the cardiac services that have traditionally been delivered in hospitals.

These developments prompted us to write this new book. The management of cardio-vascular risk factors is dealt with in the companion volume, *Preventing Cardiovascular Disease in Primary Care* (Radcliffe Publishing, Oxford, 2008). Both volumes are based on a previous book, *Cardiology in Primary Care*, written by Clive Handler (Radcliffe Publishing, Oxford, 2004).

Patients and their families expect the primary care team to answer questions about their heart condition, and to explain what they may have been told by a cardiologist or cardiac surgeon. Patients want to know what is wrong with them, why they have the problem, what they can do about it, what implications it has for their life, how they should live their life, what tests are necessary, what treatments are available, what these entail, and whether they should have these proposed treatments. Our aim is to provide primary care clinicians with the essential information that they require to manage common cardiovascular problems, and to be able to answer the questions that patients most commonly ask (although we believe patients appreciate that not all the questions they may have can be answered satisfactorily).

Interactions and discussions with colleagues working in primary care have taught us that busy primary care clinicians want a short, accessible reference book that they can dip into to help them decide whether they can manage the patient themselves or whether they should refer the patient for a specialist opinion. GPs also need to know what information their hospital colleagues like to see in the referral letter or mentioned on the telephone when discussing a case. GPs and nurses do not usually have the time to search the Internet or delve into large impenetrable textbooks for relevant practical clinical information. Our intention is to provide the principles and practice of clinical cardiology relevant to primary care clinicians. We have focused on what we think are the core pieces of information needed to make a diagnosis – namely the history and clinical examination, which tests to arrange in primary care or to request from hospital, and which treatments are most appropriate and when they should be started. We also advise when referral to a cardiologist is appropriate. Each chapter starts with clinical case histories. The chapters contain the information necessary to answer the questions, and we have provided answers at the end of each chapter, together with some suggestions for further reading. There are also sections on 'Advice to patients.' These are written in plain English without medical jargon, and can be read to patients and adapted accordingly.

Management guidelines are a major influence in clinical practice. There are guidelines for nearly every condition, and these appear to change just as we are getting familiar with them! We have incorporated national and international clinical guidelines from the UK, Europe and the USA. Although these are not identical, they are broadly in agreement. Clinicians in the developed world manage cardiac conditions in a similar way, whether they work in Dublin or Dunedin, or in London, England or London, Ontario. Clinicians should understand that guidelines should guide but not dictate management, which should be tailored to the patient sitting in your consulting room. This is particularly important for patients who do not fit neatly into an algorithm box, and for older patients.

We hope that this book fulfils our aims. We hope that our colleagues in primary care will enjoy reading and using the book, and that it will enhance the enjoyment of their practice of primary care cardiology. The subject is fascinating. There are always new things to learn that shape the way we think and work. There is a tremendous amount we can do to help our patients live a longer, more active, more productive and more enjoyable life. These are the main goals of medical practice.

Clive Handler
Gerry Coghlan
Royal Free Hospital
London
April 2008

About the authors

Dr Clive Handler BSc, MD, MRCP, FACC, FESC is Consultant in Pulmonary Hypertension in The National Pulmonary Hypertension Service at the Royal Free Hospital, London, Consultant Cardiologist at the Hospital of St John and St Elizabeth, and Highgate Hospital, London, and Honorary Senior Lecturer at the Royal Free and University College Medical School, London. He was previously Consultant Cardiologist at Northwick Park and St Mary's Hospitals, London. He trained at Guy's Hospital Medical School and at St Luke's Hospital, Milwaukee, University of Wisconsin. He edited *Guy's Hospital – 250 Years* in 1975, and his textbook *Cardiology in Primary Care* was published by Radcliffe Publishing in 2004. He is co-editor of *Classic Papers in Coronary Angioplasty* with Dr Michael Cleman from Yale University Medical School (Springer), and co-editor of *Vascular Complications in Human Disease: Mechanisms and Consequences* (Springer), and *Advances in Vascular Medicine* (Springer) with Professor David Abraham, Dr Mick Dashwood and Dr Gerry Coghlan. Together with Dr Gerry Coghlan, he wrote *Preventing Cardiovascular Disease in Primary Care* (Radcliffe Publishing, Oxford, 2008) and *Living with Coronary Disease* (Springer, 2007). He has also written numerous scientific papers.

Dr Gerry Coghlan MD, FRCP is Consultant Cardiologist and Director of the National Pulmonary Hypertension Unit at the Royal Free Hospital. He trained in Dublin and at Harefield and the Royal Free Hospitals. He is an international authority on pulmonary hypertension, and has wide interests in all aspects of the management of coronary heart disease and angioplasty. He also has an interest in service provision and policy in the NHS, and the organisation and integration of primary and secondary care services. He has written several books with Dr Clive Handler, as well as scientific papers on pulmonary hypertension and other aspects of cardiology.

Contributor

Dr Henrietta Hughes MA, MB BS, MRCGP, DRCOG, DFFP trained in medicine at Oxford University and St Bartholomew's Hospital, London. Her interests include women's health and postgraduate education. She works as a GP in West Hampstead, London.

Acknowledgements

We are grateful to our colleagues in primary care, and also to our colleagues at the Royal Free Hospital. We would also like to thank Dr Henrietta Hughes, who wrote Chapter 2 ('The patient's responsibilities in the NHS and around the world').

Dr Clive Handler would like to thank his wife, Caroline, and their three children, Charlotte, Sophie and Julius, for their support during the writing of this book. He would also like to acknowledge Professor Lawrence Cohen MD, Special Adviser to the Dean, Yale University Medical School, a great cardiologist and inspiring teacher.

Dr Gerry Coghlan would like to thank his wife, Eveleen, and their three sons, Niall, Cathal, and Eoin, for their support during the writing of this book.

Cardiovascular disease management in primary care

ONE

The changing role of primary care in cardiovascular disease

The past decade has seen a seismic shift in the management of cardiovascular conditions. As fundholding has moved to the primary care sector (managed by primary care trusts), so has responsibility for ensuring equal access to high-quality medical care throughout the patient's care pathway. This places an enormous burden on the primary care team, as they are responsible not only for the care that they deliver, but also for ensuring that they purchase quality services for secondary care. In addition, they must cater for the needs of the whole population, not merely those who come through the door of the primary care service or hospital. The primary care physician now lives in a world of targets relating to obesity, smoking, cholesterol, blood pressure, heart failure management and several other conditions.

The good (bad) old days

The obligations, duties and nature of the work of GPs and primary care nurses have changed considerably over the last 20 years. Home visits and out-of-hours duties have more or less disappeared from the routine work of GPs, except perhaps in isolated rural areas. Whether GPs will again take up these 'traditional' duties is unclear.

Until quite recently, GPs could essentially abandon all responsibility for the management of cardiovascular diseases to the specialist 'expert' if they wished, for several reasons, both professional and scientific. GPs were not expected to provide specialist services, and they were 'experts' on the 'best way' to treat patients. 'Experts' practised 'eminence-based' rather than evidence-based medicine. There were no nationally agreed management guidelines.

There was scant long-term epidemiological data to inform GPs about the relevance of individual risk factors. Some of the early large studies produced confusing information. Twenty years ago, there was controversy about the importance of what today are accepted as major risk factors. There was also less incentive to identify patients at high cardiovascular risk, because there were few available treatments. There was little information about the optimal levels of blood pressure, cholesterol and blood sugar. Where treatments were available (e.g. in type 2 diabetes), there were inadequate data to inform and persuade clinicians about which risk factors were important and should be treated. The same paucity of information applied to management of common cardiac conditions, including angina, myocardial infarction and heart failure. The major advances in cardiovascular disease prevention and management, which younger clinicians take for granted, occurred in the last 25 years.

Service provision

Rationing of healthcare could simply be managed through waiting lists. As there was no agreement on how to administer optimal cardiac care, the quality of and waiting times for services varied widely between hospitals just a few miles apart, depending on local 'expert' advice and management competence. Lapses in care were considered to be the responsibility of secondary care. There was therefore little incentive or expectation for GPs to try and improve the situation, and there were no levers available to those who recognised the limitations of care delivery.

Drivers for change: guidelines and audit

In the 1970s, politicians and the public became increasingly disgruntled about the apparent lack of mechanisms for ensuring that recognised standards of care could be delivered. Similar levels of funding appeared to produce very disparate levels of care in different areas of the country. By the mid-1990s, it was absolutely clear that the NHS was failing to deliver healthcare of First World quality. However, despite the shortcomings of the new system, compared with 10 years ago, high-quality care is now available to a much larger proportion of the population.

Throughout the 1980s and 1990s, large randomised controlled studies provided convincing evidence of the value of drug and other treatments in a variety of conditions. This led to a proliferation of guidelines on disease management. These allow clinicians and healthcare managers to evaluate whether treatments are justified and cost-effective, and whether service delivery is 'up to standard.' Questions such as the following are now addressed in several national and international practice guidelines:

✧ Does the patient need to be referred to a specialist?
✧ Does the patient need to be treated in a hospital by a specialist?
✧ What investigations should be performed?
✧ What is the most appropriate and cost-effective treatment?

Guidelines are now an integral part of all areas of clinical practice and the management mindset of clinicians in Europe and the USA.

Clinical audit was introduced a few years ago to allow healthcare professionals to measure and demonstrate their performance against agreed standards, to introduce measures to improve their performance, and then to re-check their performance in order to 'close the audit loop.' Audit is a difficult discipline, but it helps clinicians to think about how they can improve their clinical practice and service, and it provides objective information to help justify changes.

The NSF and all that

The National Service Framework (NSF) documents changed our world dramatically. Here, for the first time, the Government and medical experts agreed on the measurable standards of care that should be delivered. This contracted the Government to paying for a certain level of care, and the medical community to ensuring that this level of care would be delivered. Of course, the Government is committed to achieving this at the least possible cost, so there was a drive, largely based on cost, to deliver as much care as possible in primary care. This has been facilitated by the development of usually robust, evidence-based, clinical management guidelines and new service delivery (e.g. chest pain clinics and nurse-delivered domiciliary care for heart failure).

Preventative care in the community based on global risk estimation

The aims of prevention are to reduce the risk of heart attack or stroke, to reduce the need for revascularisation in all arterial territories, and to improve the quality and length of life. Chapter 2 of the NSF requires all primary care practices to assess the cardiovascular risk profile of their patients. Non-pharmacological or 'lifestyle' advice is recommended for all. Drugs to reduce thrombosis, blood pressure, lipids and glucose are used if non-pharmacological methods are inadequate.

Practices should audit the outcome of smoking cessation and the achievement of targets for blood pressure and lipids. Weight loss is easy to measure. Diet and exercise are less easy to measure, but important in prevention.

Global risk of cardiovascular disease

It is recommended that all adults aged over 40 years, who are not already on treatment and who have no history of cardiovascular disease or diabetes, should undergo global risk estimation. In addition, global cardiovascular risk should be estimated in people with a family history of premature cardiovascular disease, or with symptoms suggestive of cardiovascular disease. This should include ethnicity, smoking history, a family history of cardiovascular disease, weight and waist measurements, blood pressure, non-fasting lipids and non-fasting glucose. In the UK, the 10-year cardiovascular risk is estimated using the Joint British Societies' risk charts. In Europe, score tables are used. These provide an approximate estimated probability based on five risk factors, namely age–gender, smoking, systolic blood pressure and the ratio of total cholesterol to HDL-cholesterol (total cholesterol in mainland Europe).

The concept of global or total cardiovascular risk is sensible and practical. It has always, even subconsciously, underpinned clinical management decisions. In the same way that clinicians look at the 'whole patient' before recommending medical or surgical treatments when balancing the risk and benefit of any intervention – whether aspirin or an aortic valve replacement – global risk estimation helps clinicians and patients to make balanced decisions about preventative strategies and treatments.

Total risk based on all risk factors, rather than a single risk factor, is assessed. This is because cardiovascular disease is multifactorial, the presence of more than one risk factor is multiplicative and not additive, and risk factors tend to be associated or are clustered. Even if a target for one risk factor cannot be reached, a patient's global risk can still be reduced by treating other risk factors. Nevertheless, treatment of a high single-risk factor is necessary.

People with established cardiovascular disease, patients with diabetes, those with high levels of one or more risk factors, and apparently healthy individuals who are at high risk (> 20% risk over 10 years) of developing atherosclerotic disease should be treated equally. All of their risk factors should be treated. Initially, patients with a 10-year risk of more than 30% were to receive treatment. This has now been reduced to 20%.

Lifestyle advice for all

All people should be given lifestyle advice, irrespective of their global risk. Low-risk individuals should be reassessed annually depending on their age. Those at high risk should be given lifestyle advice and treatment of individual risk factors.

Lipids

Statins have revolutionised the management of hypercholesterolaemia, and have made a considerable difference to the prognosis of patients with vascular disease, and the clinical outcomes in all age groups.

Patients with a ratio of total cholesterol to HDL-cholesterol of > 6.0 mmol/l should be treated with lifestyle and dietary advice and a statin. People with familial hyperlipidaemia should be treated with a statin. An LDL-cholesterol target of < 2.5 mmol/l (or < 2.0 mmol/l in the USA and some parts of Europe) for those with vascular disease and < 3 mmol/l for primary prevention have provided simple, auditable targets.

Hypertension

Stepped therapy for hypertension (calcium-channel blockers, ACE inhibitors and diuretics) has provided a logical sequence of drugs to be prescribed before patients are referred to secondary care.

Simple guidelines for therapy (all patients with a persistent blood pressure level above 160/100 mmHg, and those with a level above 140/90 mmHg who have end-organ damage, or a greater than 20% 10-year risk) identify the population to treat.

Treatment targets (< 140/85 mmHg for most patients and < 130/80 mmHg for diabetics) have simplified and standardised management. Lower treatment targets in high-risk patients reinforce the concept of global risk and more aggressive intervention to achieve more stringent targets in high-risk patients.

Service organisation and delivery of care

Service delivery for cardiovascular prevention has required major reorganisation of primary care services. As most of this care is protocol driven, nurse-led clinics have been set up throughout the country. Computerisation of practices has allowed live database entry to simplify audit. Regular audit meetings are held by most practices to ensure that standards are being met. Limited resources have forced clinicians and healthcare managers to question the merits of and necessity for traditional practices, which sometimes makes life uncomfortable and uneasy for patients, doctors and nurses.

GPs with a special interest in cardiology

The Department of Health advocates the use of GPs with a special interest in cardiology to improve access to cardiology services in the community. A national training and accreditation programme is being developed. The scheme has been endorsed by the British Cardiovascular Society, the Royal College of General Practitioners, the Royal College of Physicians, the Royal College of Nursing, the Primary Care Cardiovascular Society and the British Society of Echocardiography. It is not yet known whether this service will be popular with GPs or what the cost-effectiveness and clinical outcomes will be.

Specialist advice for dyslipidaemia, hypertension and diabetes

Secondary care is now recommended only for individuals with complex lipid abnormalities (familial hyperlipidaemia, some endocrine-associated dyslipidaemia), and for the more complex hypertensive patients – that is, those with unsatisfactory control despite three or more different medications, secondary hypertension (e.g. hypertension during pregnancy) and young patients (below the age of 25 years).

> Diabetes is a powerful risk factor for cardiovascular disease. There are lower prevention treatment thresholds for diabetics.

The NSF for diabetes has also cleared the way for most diabetics to be managed in the community, setting simple strategies for regular assessment of complications and simple goals for therapy (HbA$_{1c}$ < 6.5%). Specialist referral is now only necessary for the minority of patients with diabetes that is difficult to control or where there are complications.

Chronic care in the community

Recognition that secondary care centres were delivering inadequate, unsatisfactory and inefficient care for chronic conditions has led to primary care clinicians taking on this increasingly important role. Conditions such as coronary heart disease and heart failure are punctuated by acute episodes that necessitate hospital admission or augmented care. However, for most patients who are living with these conditions, hospital visits are an inconvenience; only those requiring specialist evaluation, complex investigations or a fundamental change to their treatment need to be referred to hospital.

Angina and acute coronary syndromes

The precise diagnosis of these conditions remains essentially the preserve of secondary care. Rapid-access chest pain clinic assessments exclude angina in most patients within a single hospital visit. Those with probable angina can be stratified as low or high risk based on their clinical profile and exercise test results, and arrangements for intervention planned. Once a patient has a firm diagnosis, and any necessary intervention has been undertaken, one moves to a more chronic phase of disease management, where optimisation of risk factors, and simple therapies (aspirin, β-blockers, nitrates, calcium-channel blockers and/or nicorandil) are all that are required. Secondary care facilities are then required only for acute episodes (unstable angina and myocardial infarction), and for the relatively small group of patients in whom conventional therapies fail to deliver an adequate quality of life because of poorly controlled angina.

Heart failure

The availability of a blood test for heart failure brain natriuretic peptide (BNP) or the more stable analogue, N-terminal brain natriuretic peptide (N-TproBNP), which can be requested in primary care, has revolutionised the assessment of breathless patients. However, heart failure clinics remain an essential part of secondary care services. Echocardiography is currently performed mainly in secondary care, but should be widely available in primary care. Establishing whether a patient has heart failure and, if so, identifying the cause – whether it be poor pump function (systolic failure), impaired pump relaxation (diastolic failure) or another underlying heart problem (e.g. valvar heart disease) – has implications for both immediate and long-term management. These problems can be managed, with remote secondary care input or outreach services, in primary care.

The expanding role of implantable cardioverter defibrillators (ICDs) for the prevention of sudden death, and biventricular pacing for advanced heart failure (cardiac resynchronisation therapy), as well as the recognition of familial forms of dilated cardiomyopathy and the role of revascularisation for some patients with ischaemic heart failure, means that precise diagnosis is important for most patients once heart failure is established as a diagnosis. However, as with angina, for the majority of patients, once secondary care has finished playing with its 'toys', chronic care is best delivered in the community. Ensuring that patients with heart failure are on angiotensin-converting enzyme (ACE) inhibitors and β-blockers has become an important target for primary care clinicians.

For patients with advanced heart failure, the community heart failure nurse has a pivotal role in ensuring that spironolactone is used safely in these individuals, performing and checking blood test results for possible haematological and biochemical abnormalities, ensuring that low-sodium diets are adhered to, and advising and supervising patients with regard to weighing themselves daily, exercising regularly and modifying their diuretic dosage according to weight changes.

Atrial fibrillation

Most arrhythmias have become firmly the province of secondary care, but this is not the case for atrial fibrillation. Atrial flutter and supraventricular tachycardia can be cured by ablation, bradyarrhythmias are treated with pacing, and ICDs are used to treat serious ventricular arrhythmias. Years ago cardioversion was widely practised for the management of atrial fibrillation, but it has now been recognised that such efforts are in vain, as rate control and anticoagulation give the same quality of life and prognosis for the majority of patients.

In cases that require a more aggressive approach, radio-frequency ablation is generally a better option. However, ablation for atrial fibrillation is a tedious and frequently unsuccessful undertaking, and as the left atrium must be entered, these procedures are associated with a modest risk of stroke. Therefore, ablation of atrial fibrillation remains a procedure for patients whose symptoms are not satisfactorily controlled with one or a combination of the following: digoxin, verapamil, β-blockers and amiodarone.

The role of anticoagulation for atrial fibrillation probably does necessitate some secondary care involvement. While many GP surgeries can monitor warfarin, the decision to start long-term warfarin to reduce the risk of thromboembolic complications has to be individualised, but patients should have a risk factor assessment. In essence, low-risk patients (< 1% per annum stroke risk: age under 65 years, normotensive, with a normal-sized and normally functioning heart on echocardiography, no thyroid dysfunction and no history of embolic phenomena) should not be anticoagulated. High-risk patients (> 5% per annum stroke risk: those with embolic phenomena, especially within the previous 12 months, those with poor left ventricular systolic function, and those with significant valvular lesions, especially mitral stenosis), should be anticoagulated unless there are significant risks of bleeding, or major logistic problems with monitoring. However, the majority of patients fit into the intermediate group, where rules become fuzzy (such as age over 70 years, a normal left ventricle and no significant valve lesion). Yet once the decision has been made, secondary care has little to add to the management of these patients, and patients can be appropriately monitored in primary care and referred back for a specialist review when necessary.

Murmurs and valvular heart disease

Hospital consultants have a long history of collecting 'valve' patients for the purposes of teaching medical students and providing examination fodder. This has been justified on the basis that such conditions may deteriorate asymptomatically to a point beyond which surgery is safe. This is clearly true for regurgitant lesions, and there is a growing body of evidence to support the belief that aortic stenosis, too, may cause symptoms that are not noted by the patient, but which are elucidated during exercise testing. Therefore, in the setting of significant valve disease, the involvement of secondary care is justified unless a primary care group has a general practitioner with special interest (GPSI) who has been specifically trained in the management of valvular heart disease patients, and who is competent to manage these patients.

In general, patients with heart murmurs are increasingly the preserve of primary care. In most cases, an 'open-access' echocardiogram to demonstrate either that there is no valve lesion, or that the degree of abnormality is minor, will reassure the patient and the referring GP that the patient does not need to be either referred or followed up in hospital. However, some patients should be carefully flagged and followed up in primary care and referred for serial echocardiography, depending on their symptoms. Patients with aortic stenosis may need follow-up, depending on their valve area and aortic valve gradient. Similarly, patients with important mitral stenosis and/or mitral regurgitation and aortic regurgitation should be followed up jointly by both the GP and a cardiologist.

Open-access echocardiography is available to most primary care physicians. So long as reporting is sufficiently detailed and includes management advice and guidelines for referral, secondary care need not be involved in a large proportion of patients with valvular heart disease. An adequate report should comment on the following:

- any valvular abnormalities detected
- whether these are within the range of normality (e.g. 70% of people have mild tricuspid regurgitation) or considered abnormal
- if abnormal, whether this abnormality requires antibiotic prophylaxis during future potentially septic procedures
- what, if any, follow-up is necessary (e.g. a repeat echo in five years' time for a patient with aortic sclerosis).

Rare conditions and tertiary care

Rare conditions such as hypertrophic cardiomyopathy, Marfan's syndrome, most congenital cardiac lesions, familial risk of sudden cardiac death and pulmonary arterial hypertension should almost always be the preserve of tertiary care.

The brave new world

The clarification of the roles of primary versus secondary and tertiary care in the management of cardiovascular disease should lead to a much higher quality service. Care that needs to be delivered to the entire population (risk assessment and management) can be delivered only by primary care. Chronic disease management for common conditions, such as the 10% of the older population with atrial fibrillation, coronary heart disease and heart failure, is best delivered close to the patient's home. In return, secondary care must concentrate on delivering efficiently those aspects of care that require either a high level of expertise (echocardiography, angioplasty, cardiac surgery and electrophysiology), or management that is not easily delivered by prescribed protocol-driven care.

An obvious consequence of the paradigm shift from medicine as an art form (with unquantifiable benefits) to medicine as a business model (delivering 'x' amount of care to 'y' people in 'z' time frame) is that we can now plan care delivery, and explore and refine models of care. This has already led to a substantial expansion of nurse-led clinics both in primary care and in hospitals, and it has changed the nature of the doctor–patient relationship for ever.

In the following chapters we shall deal with the specific cardiac conditions in more detail. As one works through the care delivery package, and the relationships among the various professionals involved, it will become apparent that although the model starts off with clear lines of responsibility, the role of professional judgement has not diminished but merely moved to more defined decision points. The patient now has expectations in terms of waiting times, courteousness and standards of care, but still relies on our judgement and humanity.

The patient's responsibilities in the NHS and around the world *Henrietta Hughes*

TWO

Modern medicine is continually evolving in every aspect, including that of the clinician–patient relationship. The stereotype of a doctor behaving in a paternalistic way, with a patient meekly submitting to their instructions, has long gone. Patients are now more knowlegeable, have higher expectations of the healthcare that they receive, and are more likely to participate in their healthcare decisions. The advent of patients' rights has become more widespread worldwide. There has been recent debate that patients have both rights and responsibilities, although it is not clear whether sanctions could be imposed on patients who 'breach' their responsibilities.

There are clear benefits in setting out what is expected of patients, not least because it establishes that healthcare is a reciprocal and mutual relationship. This implies that both the patient and the healthcare professional are involved in improving the individual's health, and that they have a shared interest in doing so. This chapter aims to describe the approaches of the situation in the NHS and to compare it with other healthcare providers worldwide, to establish whether a consensus exists, and whether other factors such as the methods of healthcare delivery impose their own restraints.

The Patient's Charter

The NHS is funded by UK taxpayers who are entitled to treatment first set out in the Patient's Charter. Originally published in October 1991, the Patient's Charter aimed to improve the quality of health service delivery to patients.[1] The Charter set out patients' rights in the NHS and the standards of service that they could expect to receive with regard to, among other areas, waiting times, information about services and treatment, and privacy and dignity of the patient.

The Wanless Report

The Patient's Charter was abolished as part of changes to the NHS implemented in the year 2000 under the 10-year 'NHS Plan.'[2] In 2002, the Wanless Report[3] on the future of health services argued that significant improvements in life expectancy and health status will require the public to be 'fully engaged' with their own healthcare, leading healthy lifestyles and being confident in, and demanding of, the health service. Derek Wanless set out the rights and responsibilities of patients in the NHS, suggesting that:

> a more effective partnership is recommended, based on the twin planks of public and patient rights and responsibilities. This partnership should be focused on a new relationship between health professionals and the public, driven by Government and arising from the patient-focused service set out in this report.

The key messages were as follows:
- the setting of standards for the service, to help to give people a clearer understanding of what the health service will, and will not, provide for them
- the development of improved health information to help people to engage with their care in an informed way
- encouraging a reduction in key health risk factors
- enabling patients to become more engaged in the health service.

The patient's responsibilities

It was also proposed that patients have responsibilities that go alongside such rights. In particular, they should seek to use health services responsibly and ensure that their actions do not add unnecessarily to the costs of the service. For example, missed appointments impact seriously on the health service's ability to plan and deliver timely care. In 2000, 1.56 million out of a total of 12.5 million outpatient appointments were missed, equivalent to a rate of 12.5%. Data are not available for missed GP appointments. By way of illustration, a rate of 12.5% would equate to over 30 million missed GP appointments each year – or around 600 000 a week.

The public are encouraged to co-operate and comply with the Government's health-promotion policies – for example, with regard to smoking, weight reduction, a healthy diet and exercise.

Scotland

The Scottish Executive recently developed a draft set of proposed patient responsibilities to sit alongside proposed patient rights.[4] It acknowledged that the rights to treatment in the NHS in Scotland are balanced by responsibilities that can help the health service to work more efficiently. Patients are exhorted to:

✦ be on time
✦ treat healthcare staff politely and with respect
✦ follow the advice and treatment that they receive
✦ maintain up-to-date contact information
✦ take and dispose of their medicines correctly
✦ pass on their comments to healthcare staff
✦ use emergency services appropriately
✦ provide self-care.

Wales

The Bevan Foundation Think Tank has recently proposed that the Welsh Assembly should introduce a contract setting out the rights and responsibilities of NHS patients, and that it should consider imposing 'sanctions' on patients who do not comply.

The report, entitled *Setting the Agenda: Priorities for Public Policy 2007–2012*,[5] states that:

> it is now well established that rights are accompanied by responsibilities, and this should be no less so in healthcare than in other areas.

However, few healthcare organisations set out what they expect of patients, and there are questions about whether defining patient responsibilities is meaningful if it is not accompanied by sanctions.

Patients' responsibilities to their NHS GP

In the UK, individual providers such as GP surgeries have produced information on the rights and responsibilities of patients registered with their practices.[6,7] These mainly focus on time-keeping and cancelling appointments, but also include appropriately managing resources such as home visits and use of out-of-hours services. Patients are also reminded of their responsibilities to treat all surgery staff with respect and courtesy at all times, in keeping with the 'zero tolerance' policy across the NHS with regard to the protection of all its staff, and to inform the practice if their contact details change.

In countries where healthcare is not provided free at the point of delivery, a subtle difference in patient responsibilities can be observed.

South Africa

In South Africa, the 10 responsibilities of patients are displayed alongside the Patient's Rights Charter.[8] They include the responsibility to:

✧ live a healthy lifestyle
✧ care for and protect the environment
✧ respect the rights of other patients and healthcare staff
✧ utilise the health system optimally without abuse
✧ be aware of the health services available locally and what they offer
✧ provide healthcare staff with accurate information for diagnosis, treatment, counselling and rehabilitation purposes
✧ advise healthcare staff on the patient's wishes with regard to death
✧ comply with the prescribed treatment and rehabilitation procedures
✧ ask about management costs and arrange for payment
✧ take care of the patient-carried health cards and records.

USA

In the USA, patients at the University of Michigan Hospital are responsible for providing a complete and accurate medical history, following the suggestions and advice prescribed by the healthcare providers, and making it known whether they clearly understand their plan of care. In addition, they are responsible for providing the healthcare provider with correct information about sources of payments and their ability to pay their bill.[9]

The American Medical Association (AMA) advises that:

> patients generally have a responsibility to meet their financial obligations with regard to medical care or to discuss financial hardships with their physicians. Patients should be cognizant of the costs associated with using a limited resource like healthcare, and try to use medical resources judiciously.[10]

In addition, the AMA suggests that patients have a responsibility to communicate with their healthcare providers. This also includes discussing end-of-life decisions and organ donation. Patients should be committed to health maintenance through health-enhancing behaviour. Illness can often be prevented by a healthy lifestyle, and patients should take personal responsibility when they are able to avert the development of disease.

Australia

The health funding in Australia is by patient insurance to reimburse health costs. In the state of Victoria, the Public Hospital Patient Charter outlines the rights and responsibilities of patients while attending a public hospital in Victoria. It aims to support a partnership between patients and their healthcare providers by providing a clear statement of expectations that is understood by both patients and providers. The responsibilities of patients are to provide relevant information about their health and circumstances that may influence their treatment, recovery or stay in hospital.[11]

Conclusions

The issue of patient responsibilities is controversial. It may be 'perceived to be paternalistic, a direct threat to patient autonomy and driven by a desire to contain costs.'[12] It may also appear to focus unjustly on one particular lay group, making it unreasonable to use public policy to enforce the responsibilities of certain types of patients. As a consequence, medical ethics still 'dwells on the ethical obligations of doctors to the exclusion of those of patients.'[13] Nevertheless, a concerted and explicit effort has been made internationally to specify and promote patient responsibilities in healthcare. Patient responsibilities have been suggested to include the following:[14]

◇ promotion of self health
◇ respect for others, including behaviour in good faith
◇ appropriate use of health resources in the public sector
◇ sharing of relevant information
◇ serious consideration of offered advice
◇ adherence to agreed treatment plans.

REFERENCES

1 Department of Health. *The Patient's Charter.* London: The Stationery Office; 1991.
2 Department of Health. *The NHS Plan.* London: The Stationery Office; 2000.
3 Department of Health. *The Wanless Report.* London: The Stationery Office; 2004.
4 Scottish Executive. Patient Rights and Responsibilities. A draft for consultation 2003. Available at www.scotland.gov.uk/Publications/2003/03/16740/19888.
5 The Bevan Foundation. *Setting the Agenda for Public Policy 2007–2012.* Tredegar, Gwent: The Bevan Foundation; 2006. p. 41.
6 Available at www.yorkmedicalgroup.nhs.uk.
7 Available at www.e-mpowerdemosite.co.uk.
8 Department of Health. *The Patients' Rights Charter.* Pretoria, South Africa: Department of Health; 2003.
9 University of Michigan Health System. *Patient and Visitor Guide.* Ann Arbor, MI: University of Michigan; 2001.
10 American Medical Association Council on Ethical and Judicial Affairs. *Code of Medical Ethics.* Chicago, IL: American Medical Association; 2006. p. 320.
11 State Government of Victoria, Australia. *Public Hospital Patient Charter.* Victoria, Australia: State Government; 1995.
12 Buetow S. The scope for patient involvement in doctor/patient consultations in primary care: the rights, responsibilities and preferences of patients. *J Med Ethics.* 1998; **24:** 243–7.
13 Draper H, Sorell T. Patients' responsibilities in medical ethics. *Bioethics.* 2002; **16:** 335–52.
14 Ibid.

History

THREE

Clinical cases
1. A 43-year-old woman who is going through a divorce comes to see you complaining of 'palpitation' and chest pain. What do you do?
2. A 92-year-old man with occasional episodes of angina during the last 20 years comes to see you complaining of chest pain while gardening. What do you do?
3. A 70-year-old man complains of breathlessness. What do you do?
4. A 31-year-old woman complains of fluttering in her chest with stress. What do you do?
5. A 60-year-old businessman with a previous history of coronary artery bypass surgery notices increasing breathlessness when walking upstairs. What do you do?
6. A 78-year-old woman with a history of breast cancer consults you about three recent episodes of feeling faint, each episode lasting for a few seconds, without any other symptoms. What do you do?

The history
Why the history is crucial to patient management
Try to get as good a history as possible at the first consultation. This provides the essential data for diagnosis and background information for any other subsequent consultations. A comprehensive history saves time, confusion and unnecessary investigations.

> The history often provides the diagnosis, is therapeutic and forms the basis for management. It is the foundation of the doctor–patient relationship.

A sympathetic and productive consultation will form the foundation of a long-lasting bond of trust, friendship and respect, which are key components of the doctor–patient relationship. Patients may forgive medical mistakes but do not forget an abrupt, uncaring manner, and this may make them angry and litigious if they or a relative feel that something has gone wrong at any stage.

With the increasing use of protocol-driven, nurse-delivered clinical services in primary care, and the availability of open-access investigations, the history is essential for clinical management. Information from the history points to which investigations should be undertaken and how the results should be used for clinical management.

What is the patient worried about?
It is very important to understand and record accurately (in the patient's own words when appropriate) the patient's main symptoms and how they affect their life. If the patient uses a medical word – for example, 'palpitation' – ask them what they mean. For example, a patient who complains of 'palpitation' may feel the regular forceful beat of sinus rhythm associated with stress or exercise, or ectopic beats, or atrial fibrillation. 'Dizzy turns' may mean vertigo or episodes of feeling light-headed.

Patients present with symptoms. It is essential for clinicians to understand precisely what the patient is concerned about.

Assessing cardiovascular risk

The history provides essential information for assessing cardiovascular risk, the probability of an individual having vascular disease and its prognosis, which in turn determines management. Age, previous cardiovascular events or interventions, smoking, hypertension, hyperlipidaemia, diabetes, a family history of premature coronary heart disease, diet, weight, lifestyle and less well established risk factors are important components of the history. Their presence or absence assist in risk stratification – helping to identify those at high and low risk of having cardiovascular disease. For example, coronary artery disease is unlikely in a young patient with no risk factors, but almost certain in a patient with exertional chest pain and more than one risk factor.

Vascular disease is common. All adult patients should be questioned about risk factors so that they can be given advice to reduce their cardiovascular risk and improve their prognosis. Nearly all adult members of your practice and most young people understand the importance of lifestyle and cardiovascular risk factors. Asking them about these important parts of the history is a useful way to emphasise to them the crucial role that only they can play in reducing their cardiovascular risk.

When can the history provide the diagnosis?

A diagnosis can often be made from the history. For example, patients may give a clear history of angina. Ectopic beats may be the most likely cause of a patient's unpleasant palpitation, although this diagnosis usually needs ECG confirmation. Episodes of syncope may be due to heart block or ventricular tachycardia. A diagnosis of heart failure is difficult to make from the history alone, and investigations are required to assess cardiac function and establish the cause.

Symptom severity determines management

It is essential to gain a clear understanding of the frequency and severity of the patient's symptoms and their effect on the patient's day-to-day activities and what lifestyle changes the patient has had to make. For example, the management of a patient with unstable angina and rest pain is very different from that of an elderly patient who has occasional episodes of mild angina only with severe exertion. Patients with acute coronary syndromes and infarction should be referred as an emergency for inpatient assessment and treatment. Patients with infrequent, predictable angina may be suitably treated in primary care with aspirin, prophylactic glyceryl trinitrate (GTN), anti-anginal medication and statins, and may not need a specialist opinion unless the symptoms become unstable.

It is helpful to grade the symptoms of angina and breathlessness according to severity, using internationally accepted classifications. The Canadian Cardiovascular Society classification for grading angina and the World Health Organization or New York Heart Association classification of heart failure and functional ability aid the assessment of severity and prognosis, and help to guide management. However, in many patients a clear description of the symptom and how it impacts on the patient's day-to-day activities provides a more memorable, relevant and vivid record of their problem.

Patients with cardiac disorders may have symptoms only when they exert themselves, and may therefore reduce their activities. It is important to document a patient's exercise tolerance. They may not volunteer this information, so should be asked whether they can exercise or walk quickly on the flat, how far they can walk, whether they can walk upstairs and how many stairs they can walk, whether they have had to slow down and over what time period this has been occurring.

Taking the history

There is no 'best' way to do this. Patients should be encouraged to tell their story in their own time. Taking a good history is an art. The patient should be allowed to describe how they feel, what they are most concerned about, when the problem started and whether their symptom(s) have progressed or are intermittent. The chronological sequence of all the medical and surgical history is important. This is particularly relevant in, for example, patients who present with unstable angina or acute heart failure. A history of hypertension and other cardiovascular risk factors, or a history of previous myocardial infarction and revascularisation, will help to explain the pathology of the condition and guide management.

Pro formas

Structured history pro formas filled in by nurses may be helpful and time saving in recording details of family and personal history, including details of medication and past illnesses. On their own, however, they are no substitute for a carefully taken history and do not provide the same therapeutic impact. Patients may not understand the value of pro formas and may feel that their symptoms are not being taken seriously.

The patient's story

Despite time restrictions in general practice, the patient should be allowed to talk about their symptoms and concerns. As with formal psychotherapy, they feel better as soon as they start doing so, and feel that they are being helped. Knowing when to interrupt the patient's narrative to ask direct questions or encourage them to expand or contract on part of their history is a difficult art.

The importance of the primary care record

It is important for the GP to provide all the relevant history in referral letters. Even with modern information technology, hospital medical records are less than perfect, so the primary care records are very important and may be the most complete and readily accessible patient record. The advent of community polyclinics will test the ability of the NHS to provide all the documentation of a patient's history, which may be on a GP's surgery computer database and in a number of different hospitals. Ultimately, it may be the responsibility of the patient to carry their updated medical record on a 'smart card' that can be read by any clinician they see.

History possibly relevant to the presenting complaint

Angina may occasionally be precipitated by severe anaemia and hypothyroidism. Patients with usually well controlled heart failure may decompensate as a result of an intercurrent chest infection or myocardial infarction. They may simply forget to take or not like taking diuretics. Recent-onset atrial fibrillation may precipitate heart failure. Coexisting relevant medical or social conditions should be recorded.

Drug history

Ensure that the patient is taking their prescribed drugs in the prescribed doses at the pre-scribed times. Ask them whether they take any non-prescription tablets. It is important to be aware of potential side-effects of commonly used cardiac medication. Eye drops containing β-blockers are relevant to patients with heart failure, bradycardia, asthma or fatigue and may make these conditions worse. Non-steroidal anti-inflammatory drugs may cause renal failure, gastrointestinal bleeding and anaemia. Homeopathic drugs have a variety of actions. Cocaine and opiates have major cardiovascular side-effects. Young, otherwise healthy patients with chest pain or breathlessness should be asked about substance abuse, particularly cocaine and other sympathomimetic drugs.

Possible drug-related symptoms

More patients are using more drugs, and patients are often worried that their symptoms are drug side-effects. It is sometimes necessary to test this possibility. Suspected drugs may need to be stopped to see whether the symptoms resolve, and then restarted to see whether the symptoms recur.

Alcohol

Patients should be asked about alcohol consumption. Alcohol has a variety of cardio-vascular side-effects, but it is not clear how much an individual can take without adverse effects. Adverse effects include arrhythmia (excess alcohol in young people is recognised as a common cause of atrial fibrillation and ectopic beats). Chronic heavy alcohol consumption may lead to dilated cardiomyopathy. Good-quality red wine in moderation may be beneficial in reducing cardiovascular risk.

Cardiovascular risk factors

These should be on the patient's database. Adults need to be checked and monitored for cardiovascular risk factors. Children should be advised to reduce their future risk of developing cardiovascular disease by having a healthy diet, not smoking and taking regular exercise. Obesity in people of all ages is a major health problem.

All patients who smoke should be helped as much as possible and strongly advised to stop.

Family history

A patient with a close family relative who had a definite myocardial infarct or who had angioplasty or coronary artery surgery before 50 years of age is at high risk of developing coronary artery disease.

Hypertrophic cardiomyopathy also has a genetic and familial basis. Screening children and young adults of affected individuals aged less than 50 years is recommended.

The most common and important cardiac symptoms are:
✧ chest pain, tightness or discomfort
✧ shortness of breath
✧ palpitation
✧ loss of consciousness (syncope) or dizziness.

Patients do not usually describe their symptoms in these words.
Related vascular symptoms include:
✧ transient ischaemic attacks
✧ claudication
✧ leg swelling
✧ impotence (erectile dysfunction).

Chest discomfort, chest pain and breathlessness

Patients may present either to primary care or directly to the hospital emergency department.

The most important causes of chest pain are angina, myocardial infarction or other acute coronary syndromes.

The diagnosis must be made from the history. Physical examination is usually

unremarkable, but heart failure, arrhythmia and hypertension should be looked for.
The differential diagnosis of chest pain is listed in Table 3.1.

TABLE 3.1: Differential diagnosis of chest pain

Cause	History
Angina	Lasts a few minutes, precipitated by exertion and stress, and relieved by rest and GTN
Myocardial infarct	Intense pain, autonomic symptoms, lasts more than 20 minutes
Aortic dissection	Severe back pain, most patients have had hypertension
Oesophageal pain	Epigastric, related to food, position, sometimes exertion, nausea, relieved by antacids and H_2 blockers
Pleuritic	Sharp chest pain aggravated by breathing or coughing, caused by pneumonia, pulmonary embolus, pneumothorax
Gall bladder	Nausea, fever, possible obstructive biliary features
Chest wall pain	Costochondritis or trauma, localised tenderness, positional, long lasting
Anxiety	Personality problems, stress, previous history of anxiety, features not compatible with angina
Acute pericarditis	Sharp, worse with inspiration, positional – relieved by leaning forward, recent flu-like illness, fever
Acute pancreatitis	Epigastric, continuous, fever, abdominal symptoms, nausea, vomiting
Shingles	Skin rash, unilateral rash in dermatome distribution

Angina

The diagnosis of angina is made from the history and not from a test result. Virtually all patients with angina have coronary heart disease. Patients may have angina but normal non-invasive test results. Patients may have abnormal test results and coronary artery disease but may not have angina. A 'positive' exercise test result may indicate ischaemia, but this alone, in the absence of symptoms, does not mean that the patient has angina.

> Angina is a clinical diagnosis made from the history. Patients only have angina if they have compatible symptoms.

Angina is likely if:
- the patient has cardiovascular risk factors
- chest discomfort/breathlessness is related to exercise/emotion
- symptoms are relieved promptly by rest/GTN
- there are one or more risk factors for coronary artery disease.

Character of anginal symptoms

Angina is usually described as chest discomfort, tightness, pressure, burning or breathlessness lasting seconds or a few minutes in the chest, radiating to the arms and/or neck. It is often more noticeable in cold weather (which increases blood pressure through peripheral vasoconstriction, and increases cardiac work and oxygen demand) or after heavy meals when blood is diverted to the gut decreasing the amount to the heart. Angina may be felt only in the jaw or arms. Patients occasionally present to their dentist with jaw ache in cold weather. The location of the symptom is less important than the relationship to precipitating situations.

Localised 'pin-pricking' pain felt under the left breast is very rarely angina. Angina is very unlikely in patients under 35 years of age. Patients rarely describe 'pain' unless they are experiencing a heart attack or infarct, when the pain is more intense, lasts longer and is associated with autonomic symptoms of sweating and nausea. It is preferable to ask them about chest discomfort or heaviness, rather than pain.

It is important to recognise that breathlessness may be the only symptom of coronary artery disease. It is an 'anginal equivalent.' In patients at risk of having coronary artery disease, it should always be considered to represent myocardial ischaemia rather than a respiratory symptom.

Angina or indigestion?

This is a common clinical question. It is often very difficult to distinguish between angina and oesophageal pain, which may also be precipitated by exertion and relieved by GTN. The two conditions are common and may coexist. The important practical management point is to exclude coronary artery disease before investigating a gastro-oesophageal problem in patients with cardiovascular risk factors. Oesophageal pain responds to antacids, H_2 blockers and proton pump inhibitors, but angina does not.

The Canadian Cardiovascular Society classification of severity of angina

Angina is graded according to its severity and its impact on the daily activities of the patient. Cardiologists use this classification to describe a patient's symptoms. However, it is equally important to record the patient's description of their symptoms in the notes, and to relay these in a referral letter.

Class	Canadian Cardiovascular Society classification of angina
I	'No limitation to ordinary physical activity' – for example, walking and running up stairs, jogging, gardening. Angina only with strenuous physical activity.
II	'Slight limitation of ordinary activity' – patients can perform all of the above activities, but may experience angina when exercising in cold weather, after eating heavy meals, or when performing ordinary activities quickly (e.g. running up stairs).
III	'Marked limitation of ordinary physical activity' – for example, angina when walking 100 metres, or when walking up one flight of stairs at a normal pace under normal conditions.
IV	'Inability to carry out any physical activity without discomfort' – that is, angina at rest.

Breathlessness (dyspnoea)

This is an unpleasant and uncomfortable awareness of breathing. It is described using the New York Heart Association classification. The causes are listed in Table 3.2.

It is important to know:

⬥ how long the patient has been breathless

- what level of activities the patient was able to do previously and what they are now able to do
- if the condition is primarily a heart or lung disorder, or due to anaemia, obesity or being unfit
- orthopnoea suggests left heart failure, whereas ankle swelling suggests right heart failure
- past medical history – rheumatic heart disease, lung disease
- any associated symptoms:
  — chest pain/discomfort – angina
  — palpitation – arrhythmia, cardiomyopathy
  — cough/wheeze – asthma/chronic airways disease, angiotensin-converting-enzyme inhibitor
  — ankle swelling – congestive heart failure or right heart failure due to chronic obstructive lung disease.

Class	New York Heart Association functional classification to grade severity of heart failure
I	No symptoms with ordinary physical activity. Symptoms only with severe physical exertion.
II	Slight limitation of physical activity, but none at rest. Ordinary physical activity results in any or all of the following: fatigue, angina, palpitation, breathlessness.
III	Comfortable at rest, but slight physical activity results in symptoms.
IV	Discomfort with any physical activity, and breathlessness at rest.

TABLE 3.2: Causes of breathlessness

Cause	Clinical and investigative clues
Angina	Exercise or stress-related chest tightness or breathlessness
Heart failure	Myocardial infarct – ECG, echocardiogram
	Cardiomyopathy – echocardiogram
	Valve abnormality – examination, echocardiogram and Doppler
Arrhythmia	ECG, 24-hour ECG
COAD	Bronchitis – productive cough, chest X-ray
	Emphysema – lung function, chest X-ray
Asthma	Lung function
Pregnancy	Usually after the second trimester
Obesity	Snoring or phasic breathing (sleep apnoea) at night
Pneumothorax	Chest X-ray
Pulmonary emboli	Ventilation/perfusion lung scan, CT pulmonary angiogram
Pleural effusion	Examination, chest X-ray
Severe anaemia	Blood count
Unfit	History and examination, exercise test
Anxiety	History and examination, exercise test

Sudden severe breathlessness
Pulmonary oedema
Acute pulmonary oedema is usually due to left heart failure resulting from myocardial infarction. It causes breathlessness, cough or wheeze, usually while lying flat, and is relieved after a few minutes when the patient stands or sits up. It can be confused with asthma and is sometimes confusingly termed 'cardiac asthma.'

Pulmonary oedema may be caused by any condition that increases the pulmonary venous pressure. This includes left heart failure due to any cause (hypertension, aortic valve disease, mitral valve disease, cardiomyopathy, and rarely a left atrial myxoma).

A prolonged arrhythmia (e.g. atrial fibrillation or ventricular tachycardia) may, in patients with impaired left ventricular function, result in pulmonary oedema.

'Flash' pulmonary oedema is occasionally seen in patients with bilateral renal artery stenosis.

Palpitation
This is an unpleasant awareness of the heartbeat. The history is important, but the diagnosis is made by recording the electrocardiogram or an ambulatory ECG during symptoms.

Regular palpitation
Sinus tachycardia is very common, and is precipitated by exercise, stress or visiting the surgery. Patients may describe a fast forceful pounding in the chest. It is important to capture this on the ECG and explain it to the patient so that reassurance can be given rather than further tests ordered.

Supraventricular tachycardia
This is less common and may be due to abnormal electrical pathways in:
⬦   the atrioventricular node (atrioventricular node re-entry)
⬦   the atrioventricular bypass tracts (Wolff–Parkinson–White syndrome).

With fast heart rates, patients may feel light-headed or faint. Patients with underlying coronary heart disease may experience angina or breathlessness.

Both conditions are generally benign and, importantly, can be cured by radio-frequency ablation. Patients with symptoms of palpitation should be referred to an electrophysiologist to decide whether investigation and ablation are indicated.

Irregular palpitation
Atrial and ventricular ectopic beats are the most common cause of 'extra beats', a thump in the chest or 'missed beats.' Some patients worry that their heart might stop or that they may have a heart attack. These symptoms are due to the compensatory pause initiated by an ectopic beat occurring after a normal sinus beat. The sinus beat delayed by the compensatory pause may be felt as a forceful thud in the chest. This is because the heart has longer to fill during the prolonged diastole induced by the ectopic beat. The sinus beat feels stronger because the heart contains more blood.

Patients like to see proof that their symptoms are understood and are being taken seriously. Showing them and explaining the ECG recording is very effective, and they are usually fully reassured when told that ectopic beats are always benign if the heart muscle and blood supply are normal.

Treatment is not needed unless the patient is very symptomatic despite reassurance.

Antiarrhythmic drugs are proarrhythmic and can induce arrhythmias. Ectopic beats due to bradycardia may become more frequent if treated with β-blockers.

Atrial fibrillation

The incidence of atrial fibrillation increases with age, and the condition is common in patients aged over 70 years. Patients may experience 'flutters' in the chest. Paroxysmal atrial fibrillation may be detected on a 24-hour ECG recording, and patients may be symptom free.

Syncope

This word derives from the Greek word meaning 'to cut short.' There are cardiac and neurological causes. Sudden loss of consciousness, due to inadequate blood supply to the brain, is frightening for the patient and the witnesses. It is also termed 'failed sudden death.'

> Cardiac causes should be investigated first, so patients should be referred initially to a cardiologist.

Cardiac causes of syncope

These are listed in Table 3.3. The presence of coronary artery disease, impaired ventricular function, congestive heart failure and congenital heart disease identify patients who may have cardiac syncope and who may have a serious ventricular arrhythmia.

Ventricular tachycardia and bradycardia are the most common causes of cardiac syncope and usually occur in patients with structural heart disease. These patients have a six-month mortality of more than 10%. Therefore, patients with known or suspected cardiovascular or structural heart disease who present with syncope should initially be referred to a cardiologist. Syncope due to structural heart disease and ventricular tachycardia is treated with an automatic implantable cardioverter defibrillator (AICD). Syncope due to bradycardia is treated with a pacemaker.

A cardiac cause for syncope should be suspected in patients who have coronary heart disease, have had a myocardial infarction or myocardial revascularisation, or who have left ventricular hypertrophy due to hypertension or aortic valve stenosis. Ventricular muscle cell abnormalities due to hypertrophy or ischaemia may cause abnormal electrical activity with increased electrical automaticity and self-generating electrical circuits in the scarred heart muscle. Syncope may also be due to pulmonary embolism.

The history in a patient with syncope provides the diagnosis in around 40% of cases. Examination may reveal underlying heart failure, hypertension, signs of hypertrophic cardiomyopathy, a ventricular aneurysm or important valve disease. An ECG and 24-hour ambulatory ECG recording may show ventricular arrhythmias. Echocardiography will show structural abnormalities and cardiac function. Recording the heart rhythm during an attack or a symptom of near syncope, is the only certain way to identify or exclude an arrhythmia as the cause of syncope. This may be difficult in patients with occasional symptoms. A continuous loop recorder or a small device implanted under the skin is used to track and record a patient's heart rhythm for several weeks when a cardiac arrhythmia is suspected but has not been shown on a shorter ECG recording.

Exertional syncope suggests aortic stenosis, hypertrophic cardiomyopathy, coronary artery disease or Wolff–Parkinson–White syndrome.

Long QT syndrome is a prolonged repolarisation duration of the heart muscle cells predisposing to a form of ventricular tachycardia called Torsade de Pointes and syncope.

There are inherited forms where genetic defects have been identified. The condition is rare. There are abnormalities in the flow of electrolytes across heart muscle cells – several of these rare syndromes. They are diagnosed from the ECG showing a long QT interval corrected for heart rate (QTc) greater than 660 ms. Family history of sudden death suggests the inherited form of long QT syndrome (most commonly, Romano Ward, an autosomal dominant condition) or the Brugada syndrome, which is diagnosed by ST elevation in leads V_1 to V_3 and is eight times more common in males. Hypokalaemia, hypomagnesiaemia and hypocalcaemia predispose to long QT syndrome in susceptible individuals.

A careful drug history should be taken in patients with syncope. A long QT syndrome has been described with:

✧ antiarrhythmics (quinidine, procainamide, disopyramide, flecainide, propafenone, sotalol, amiodarone and dofetilide)
✧ antimicrobials (erythromycin, clarithromycin, trimethoprim, ketoconazole and chloroquine)
✧ antihistamines (terfenadine); amitriptyline, chlorpromazine, cisapride and glibenclamide.

Examination in patients with syncope may show hypertension, a heart murmur of aortic or mitral valve disease or, less commonly, signs of heart failure. These should be investigated with echocardiography. Look for orthostatic hypotension by measuring the blood pressure three minutes after the patient stands up following a five-minute supine period.

The ECG may show signs of myocardial infarction, bundle branch block, bradycardia or complete heart block (which necessitate urgent pacemaker implantation), or a long QT interval. Rarely, arrhythmogenic right ventricular dysplasia may cause syncope and is often diagnosed by T-wave inversion in leads V_1, V_2 and V_3. Tall QRS complexes and T-wave inversion suggests hypertrophic cardiomyopathy. A short PR interval indicates pre-excitation. These patients should be referred to a cardiologist.

Exercise testing is useful in the evaluation of suspected coronary artery disease, exercise-related syncope (which may be due to chronotropic incompetence or exertional arrhythmia) and hypertrophic cardiomyopathy, when an arrhythmia or an abnormal blood pressure response to exercise identifies patients at risk who should be referred. Severe aortic stenosis as a cause of exertional syncope should be excluded by clinical examination and echocardiography because exercise testing may induce collapse.

Blood tests may show hypokalaemia or hyperkalaemia, or hyponatraemia, but are usually normal. Check also for hypomagnesaemia and hypocalcaemia.

Treatment of cardiac syncope

Patients with suspected arrhythmia should be referred to a cardiologist for investigation, which may include ambulatory ECG monitoring, exercise testing, echocardiography, and invasive electrophysiological testing. Coronary angiography is indicated for patients with known or suspected coronary heart disease (the most common cause of ventricular tachycardia). Both myocardial revascularisation and an implantable cardioverter defibrillator (ICD) may be necessary for patients with reversible ischaemia and those with impaired left ventricular function. Permanent pacing is indicated for patients with complete heart block and symptomatic bradycardia.

Neurally mediated syncope

Around 50% of cases of syncope are neurally mediated. This mechanism accounts for emotional fainting, fainting after prolonged standing, situational syncope (cough, micturition, defecation syncope), vasovagal syncope, exercise-related syncope in fit people and carotid sinus syncope.

> Young patients without structural heart disease who have a history consistent with the presence of vasovagal, orthostatic or medication-induced syncope have a good prognosis.

Investigation of neurally mediated syncope

Tilt testing is used to provoke vasovagal syncope. It has a sensitivity of 66% and specificity of 90%, so is useful for excluding neurally mediated syncope. Both false positives and false negatives are common. Patients are tilted head up while their blood pressure and pulse rate are recorded. Patients with neurally mediated syncope have an impaired heart rate and blood pressure response, and may benefit from implantation of a pacemaker.

Treatment of neurally mediated syncope

There is little evidence from trials to guide treatment. No drug has been shown to result in long-term significant benefit.

Dual-chamber pacemaker implantation reduces symptoms by 85% in selected patients.

Orthostatic hypotension

Orthostatic hypotension occurs when a person stands up quickly. It is common in patients taking hypotensive agents or β-blockers, which blunt the compensatory tachycardia of a reduced blood pressure. Orthostatic hypotension may be due to volume depletion, medications (hypotensive drugs and β-blockers) or autonomic dysfunction (Parkinson's disease and diabetes). Treatment includes volume replacement and a detailed review of the patient's drugs.

TABLE 3.3: Causes of syncope

Cause	Diagnosis	Treatment
Arrhythmias		
Complete heart block and asystole	ECG/24-hour ECG	Pacemaker
Ventricular tachycardia and/or fibrillation (CHD/DCM/HOCM)	ECG/24-hour ECG EPS	Revascularisation Cardioverter/defibrillator
Mechanical outflow obstruction of the left ventricle		
Severe aortic stenosis	Echocardiogram	Valve replacement
Severe obstructive cardiomyopathy	Echocardiogram	Medical ± ICD
Non-cardiac causes		
Cough syncope	History	Education
Postural hypotension	History	Education
Malignant vasovagal syndrome	Tilt test	Pacemaker

ECG, electrocardiogram; 24-hour ECG, 24-hour electrocardiography; CHD, coronary heart disease; DCM, dilated cardiomyopathy; HOCM, hypertrophic obstructive cardiomyopathy; ICD, implantable cardioverter defibrillator; EPS, electrophysiological study.

Around 20% of cases of syncope are due to panic disorders, anxiety, depression, and alcohol and substance abuse. The remainder include cardiac arrhythmias and other cardiac conditions, but it is important to exclude these early in the investigation of syncope.

Differential diagnosis of syncope

Syncope must be distinguished from vertigo, which is associated with a sense of motion or rotation. Syncope may be precipitated by pain, exercise, micturition, defecation or stress, and may be associated with nausea and sweating.

Seizures due to epilepsy may be associated with disorientation, an aura, slowness in returning to consciousness after the attack, and tonic and clonic movements.

Unexplained syncope

This is a diagnosis of exclusion and, except in patients with undiagnosed cardiac syncope, it has a benign prognosis.

Transient ischaemic attacks

A transient ischaemic attack is defined as an episode of cerebral ischaemia lasting for less than 24 hours and manifested as any one of the following:

✧ brain dysfunction
✧ dysphasia, dysarthria
✧ weakness or sensory disturbance in the face and/or arm and/or leg
✧ visual disturbance in either one eye or a hemianopia.

Full investigation is required. Transient ischaemic attacks must be distinguished from migraine, other cerebral problems, local eye problems and vascular problems. Patients should be referred to a neurologist or physician with expertise in this field.

Leg pain

TABLE 3.4: Causes of leg pain

Cause	Clinical features	Investigations
Claudication	Related to walking, relieved by rest diminished or absent foot pulses	Duplex ultrasound
	Diabetes	
	Signs of vascular disease elsewhere	
Deep vein thrombosis	Swelling, tenderness	Duplex ultrasound
	Recent immobility/surgery	D-dimer
	Obesity, previous DVT	Venography
	Cancer	
Nerve root pain	Shock-like pain	MRI scan of spine
	Relieved by sitting	
Rheumatological	Joint disorders – arthritis	Blood tests
		X-ray
		MRI scan
		Examination of fluid

Leg swelling

TABLE 3.5: Causes of leg swelling

Cause	Clinical features	Investigations
Venous hypertension	Varicose veins	Exclude other causes
	Phlebitis/cellulitis	
	History of childbirth	
	Prolonged standing	
Deep vein thrombosis	See above	See above
Heart failure	Right or congestive heart failure	ECG
	Raised venous pressure	Chest X-ray
	Liver enlargement	Echocardiogram
	Mitral valve murmur	
	Added heart sounds	
	Arrhythmia	

Advice to patients

✧ The most important and common heart problems are due to furring up of the heart arteries. The probability that you have this depends on a number of risk factors.

✧ The character of your symptoms often provides the diagnosis. Tell the doctor or nurse as precisely as you can what you feel and how it affects you.

✧ If you are over 40 years old and have chest or arm pain or tightness, sweating, nausea or shortness of breath, go to your local accident and emergency department immediately to make sure that these symptoms are not due to your heart. Heart attack symptoms can occur at rest or during exercise. If you are young and otherwise fit and do not have risk factors for vascular disease, the symptoms are less likely to be due to your heart.

✧ A smoker aged over 60 years who also has high blood pressure and a high cholesterol level and who is overweight is more likely to have vascular disease than a young person.

✧ There are many causes of chest pain. Chest pain may arise from any structure in the chest, including the gullet, stomach, upper gut, gall bladder, chest wall, aorta and the outer membrane of the heart.

✧ If the symptoms get worse with exercise and improve with rest, they may be related to your heart. If not, they are less likely to be related to your heart.

✧ A lot of people can hear or feel pulsation in their head or ears when they lie in bed. This may be normal, but it should be assessed.

✧ Breathlessness, giddiness or loss of consciousness should always be investigated. There are several possible causes.

✧ Palpitation is an awareness of your heartbeat. It does not mean that you are having or are about to have a heart attack. It is often harmless and usually nothing to worry about. If it is unpleasant or happens frequently, come to see us and we may need to do some tests.

✧ There are many causes of tiredness, and heart disease is usually not the cause, except in people who have a very weak heart.

Answers to questions about clinical cases

1. It is essential to find out what this patient means by 'palpitation' and chest pain. Patients use the term 'palpitation', which is an awareness of their heart beat, to describe a regular forceful heart beat associated with stress, anxiety or exercise, as well as an irregular heart rhythm, most commonly ectopic beats. Palpitation may be caused by any arrhythmia as well as sinus rhythm. It is important to understand what causes this patient's palpitation, when it started, how long the attacks last and whether there are associated symptoms. If this condition is troublesome and persistent, an ECG and 24-hour ECG recording may be necessary to identify the rhythm. The chest pain must also be elucidated and the history should provide the diagnosis. Tests (e.g. exercise testing) may be necessary if coronary heart disease is suspected. If the patient is very anxious and stressed about her divorce (and this is to be expected), treatment and counselling for this should be offered.

2. The differential diagnosis includes reflux oesophagitis (gastro-oesophageal reflux disease) and other disorders. Underlying malignancy in this age group should not be overlooked. These and other possibilities may need further investigation. If this patient has nocturnal angina (angina decubitus), it may indicate deterioration in previously stable angina. All of his medication should be reviewed. He should be on aspirin, a statin and full prophylactic anti-anginal medication, and all of his risk factors should be evaluated and treated. Check his blood tests for anaemia, diabetes, infection, lipid profile and renal function. If medical treatment is insufficient to control his symptoms, and his life is intolerable, he should be referred for further investigation, but this should first be discussed with the patient and his family.

3. All causes of breathlessness should be considered. Find out whether this is new or whether it is a progressive problem, possibly due to chronic obstructive lung disease, asthma, lung cancer or heart failure. Angina may present as breathlessness. Underlying systemic illness, including anaemia, obesity, liver and renal failure, should be investigated. Sometimes patients complain of breathlessness due to pain. A full history and examination is essential, followed by a chest X-ray, ECG, haematology and biochemistry and, if necessary, an exercise test, echocardiogram and lung function tests. These can be organised from primary care, and this approach should identify most causes of breathlessness.

4. A full history and examination should be undertaken. Ectopic beats or forceful sinus rhythm are the most likely causes. If captured on an ECG or 24-hour ECG recording, this can be shown to the patient and an explanation may be all that is required. If her heart is clinically normal, echocardiography is not usually necessary and she can be reassured, because ectopic beats are usually not dangerous in a structurally normal heart.

5. We need to find out why this patient is breathless. Is it due to heart failure, recurrent angina or another cause? Ask about symptoms of orthopnoea, nocturnal dyspnoea, chest infection, leg swelling and chest pain. Look for relevant signs on examination. He will need referral and investigation. A chest X-ray will exclude pneumonia, lung cancer and heart failure. An ECG might show signs of new infarction or an arrhythmia.

6. The differential diagnosis includes cerebral metastases and epilepsy, transient ischaemic attacks and a cardiac arrhythmia. Anxiety is a possibility, but other causes must be excluded before this is proposed. Ask the patient about symptoms related to a space-occupying lesion(s) in the brain (mental acuity, memory, localised limb weakness or sensory disturbances). From the cardiac standpoint, palpitation, chest pain or breathlessness are relevant. Look for papilloedema, assess focal neurology and check her walking and balance. With regard to the heart, feel the pulse, check for murmurs, particularly of aortic valve disease, check for carotid bruits, feel all of

the peripheral pulses, and check the blood pressure in both arms, with the patient lying and standing. Record the ECG. If there are no abnormalities, arrange a 24-hour ECG to look for a paroxysmal arrhythmia. Check the haematology and biochemistry. Request a chest X-ray to look for metastatic disease.

FURTHER READING

The Canadian Cardiovascular Society classification of angina and the New York Heart Association functional classification are both adapted from the following:

Goldman L, Cook EF, Loscalzo A. Comparative reproducibility and validity of systems for assessing cardiovascular functional class: advantages of a new specific activity scale. *Circulation*. 1981; **64:** 1227–34.

Kapoor WN. Syncope. *NEJM*. 2000; **343:** 1856–62.

Examination

FOUR

Clinical cases

1. You hear a murmur in a 23-year-old pregnant woman. What characteristics of the murmur and other findings on examination are important for management?
2. You feel an irregular pulse and hear a heart murmur in a 71-year-old woman who had 'scarlet fever' as a child. What do you do?
3. A 76-year-old man with chronic airways disease and a recent chest infection comes to see you, and you hear lung crackles. What other physical signs do you specifically look for?
4. A fit 38-year-old marathon runner comes for a check-up. You hear a systolic murmur. What other aspects of the murmur do you record and how do you decide whether it is necessary to refer him?
5. A 68-year-old diabetic woman comes to see you with aching legs, tiredness, breathlessness and a history suggestive of a transient ischaemic attack. What physical signs do you look for and why?
6. A 69-year-old woman complains of leg swelling for several weeks. What do you do?

Diagnostic benefits of physical examination

Modern cardiac investigations provide important diagnostic and prognostic information, but they have not made physical examination redundant. Although time restraints on consultations may make it difficult to examine patients in primary care, physical examination remains an essential and diagnostically useful part of the consultation. A gentle and focused systematic physical examination has an incalculable therapeutic effect for patients who can be reassured that their symptoms have been taken seriously. A thorough examination need not take more than a few minutes, is highly cost-effective, and contributes to professional satisfaction and education. Recording relevant clinical findings is an important part of the consultation.

The finding of hypertension, an irregular pulse, signs of heart failure, heart murmurs, a dilated pulsating abdominal aorta, leg swelling, absent leg pulses and femoral artery or carotid artery bruits provides important diagnostic information. Investigations may be requested, treatment can be started and specialist referral considered depending on the diagnosis, the patient's wishes and their response to treatment.

Requesting investigations

The request form should provide relevant clinical details and ask the clinical question.

> Investigations should only be requested if the result would influence management.

Professional benefits of physical examination

Patients without cardiac disease are grateful and reassured when told after the examination that they have nothing to worry about. If abnormalities are found, this can be explained to the patient and further tests and specialist referral arranged if necessary.

An informed and comprehensive clinical evaluation improves the quality of referral letters and the validity of requests for open-access investigations.

With new specialist training programmes, junior doctors are often less clinically experienced than GPs. Overbooked and rushed hospital outpatient clinics are not conducive to careful, comprehensive clinical examinations. The examination in primary care is therefore very important. It is not unusual for GPs to find clinical abnormalities that may be missed by a specialist. With the advent of polyclinics, GPs and hospital specialists may examine patients together, and this can have major educational advantages for both parties.

Examining patients

Ask the patient's permission to examine them. A chaperone may be required for some patients. Patients should be examined on an examination couch in a good light. They should be comfortable, warm and relaxed.

Questions to be answered by cardiac examination

It is very helpful to have a system of examination. It would be perfectly reasonable for primary care clinicians to request the opportunity to refresh their clinical skills by sitting in at hospital cardiology clinics.

- ✧ Does the patient look well?
- ✧ Are there xanthelasma or xanthomata of dyslipidaemia?
- ✧ Is there a sternotomy scar of coronary artery surgery or any chest scars of minimal-access surgery?
- ✧ Is the patient breathless after undressing?
- ✧ Are there features of infective endocarditis?
- ✧ Is the patient in sinus rhythm? If not, is the pulse completely irregular (atrial fibrillation), or regular with occasional extra beats (ectopic beats)?
- ✧ Does the patient have a normal heart?
- ✧ Are there heart murmurs? If so, which valve(s) is affected?
- ✧ Is the blood pressure normal?
- ✧ Are there any signs of heart failure? If so, what is the cause? Is the jugular venous pulse raised? Are the lungs clear? Is there peripheral or sacral oedema? Are there added heart sounds?
- ✧ Are there signs of peripheral vascular disease or carotid artery disease?
- ✧ Does the abdominal aorta feel normal?
- ✧ What investigations are necessary?

Useful and reliable physical signs: high predictive accuracy

Several cardiac conditions can be diagnosed in primary care after a systematic physical examination and attention to discriminatory signs (*see* Table 4.1). The cause of each physical sign must be investigated and established.

Physical signs that should be interpreted with caution

Some physical signs have a low predictive accuracy for diagnosis (*see* Table 4.2) because they are not specific or sensitive for cardiac disease. They may be caused by non-cardiac conditions.

TABLE 4.1: Physical signs, their possible causes and investigations

Sign	Possible diagnosis	Investigations
Xanthelasma	Hyperlipidaemia	Lipid profile
Irregular pulse	Ectopic beats	ECG
	Atrial fibrillation	24-hour ECG if arrhythmia is not captured on ECG
Slow pulse rate < 40 bpm	Complete heart block	ECG
Raised venous pressure	Right heart failure	Echocardiogram
	?cause	Chest X-ray
Systolic waves in venous pulse	Tricuspid regurgitation	Echocardiogram
Visible carotid artery pulsation	Aortic regurgitation	Echocardiogram
	Kinked carotid artery	Carotid ultrasound
Slow carotid upstroke	Aortic stenosis	Echocardiogram
Jerky carotid upstroke	HOCM	Echocardiogram
Dyskinetic apex beat	Left ventricular aneurysm	Echocardiogram
Left ventricular heave	Hypertension	Check blood pressure
	Aortic stenosis	Echocardiogram
Pansystolic murmur (S1 and S2 inaudible)	Mitral regurgitation	Echocardiogram
	Ventricular septal defect	
Midsystolic click + late systolic murmur	Mitral valve prolapse	Echocardiogram
Ejection murmur	Normal	Echocardiogram
	Aortic stenosis	
	Thickened aortic valve	
	HOCM	
Diastolic murmur	Aortic regurgitation	Echocardiogram
Carotid artery pulsation	Always abnormal	
Loud first heart sound + diastolic murmur	Mitral stenosis	Echocardiogram
	Always abnormal	
Absent or reduced leg/ foot pulses	Peripheral vascular disease	Doppler examination
		Consider vascular disease elsewhere
Abdominal aortic pulsation	Aortic aneurysm	Ultrasound

HOCM, hypertrophic obstructive cardiomyopathy.

TABLE 4.2: Physical signs that should be interpreted with caution

Sign	Implication	Confounder	Test
Splinter haemorrhages	Infective endocarditis	Trauma	Clinical picture
			Blood tests
Lung crackles	Heart failure	Lung disease	Chest X-ray
	Lung fibrosis	Normal	Lung function
External jugular vein distension	Right heart failure	Kinked vein	Ultrasound
Visible carotid artery pulsation	Aortic regurgitation	Anxiety	History
		Hyperthyroidism	TFTs
			Ultrasound
High blood pressure	Hypertension	Anxiety/white coat syndrome	24-hour BP
Systolic murmur	Valve disease	Normal	Echocardiogram

TFTs, thyroid function tests.

Inspection

Occasionally, the possibility of a cardiac abnormality is suggested by the patient's physical appearance (*see* Table 4.3).

TABLE 4.3: Abnormal physical features and their possible related cardiac abnormality

Physical feature	Cardiac abnormality
Tall stature	Marfan's syndrome, aortic regurgitation, mitral valve prolapse, mitral valve regurgitation, aortic dissection
Dwarfism	Septal defects
Down's syndrome	Septal defects
Obesity	Hypertension, dyslipidaemia, diabetes, sleep apnoea
Skin pigmentation	Addison's disease
Kyphoscoliosis	Spurious cardiac enlargement on chest X-ray
Depressed sternum	Spurious cardiac enlargement on chest X-ray
Breathless at rest	Heart failure
Foot and leg oedema	Heart failure
Varicose veins	Venous hypertension, foot oedema, implications for coronary artery surgery and vein harvesting
Earlobe crease	Premature coronary heart disease
Arcus	Dyslipidaemia
Xanthomata	Vascular disease
Xanthelasma	Dyslipidaemia

Systematic examination of the cardiovascular system
The hands

Warm dry hands with a low venous tone (dilated veins) indicate a good peripheral circulation and cardiac output. Cold hands with a high venous tone are a sign of circulatory impairment and low cardiac output. Hand veins may be less prominent in young female patients. People with normal circulation may have cold hands and peripheral cyanosis if they are cold.

The pulse
Radial pulse

Measure rate and rhythm. The normal heart rate is in the range 50–100 bpm. An absent radial pulse may be truly absent following occlusion of the brachial artery after using the radial or brachial artery for cardiac catheterisation, or it may be aberrant and difficult to feel. An irregular pulse may be due to ectopic beats or atrial fibrillation. A hard artery is a sign of atheroma and hypertension.

Carotid artery

Look for the vigorous outward pulsation of aortic regurgitation. Feel the pulse for its rate of rise and amplitude. A slow rate of rise and amplitude suggests aortic stenosis. A jerky upstroke suggests hypertrophic obstructive cardiomyopathy. Listen for bruits, which suggest widespread atheroma and the possibility of other risk factors.

Femoral arteries

A bruit and decreased amplitude suggests local atheromatous disease. Feel the radial and femoral arteries together. A delay in the femoral pulse suggests coarctation of the aorta, which is a cause of hypertension.

Foot arteries

Absent foot artery pulses indicate peripheral vascular disease. Record the presence or absence of all pulses in the legs. The absence of leg pulses increases the probability of associated renal artery stenosis and aortic disease. Occasionally patients may lose a pulse in their leg following cardiac catheterisation or angioplasty – this is due to cholesterol emboli or damage to the femoral artery. The GP record of the arterial state of the leg may be very helpful in the management of this complication.

The internal jugular venous pulse

It is important to measure the height and characterise the jugular venous pulse. It is a difficult clinical skill. Examine the patient in a good light. The external jugular venous pulse is easier to see but may not provide accurate information about the right heart filling pressure and right atrial pressure, due to kinking of the vessel in the neck fascia. Make sure that the patient is lying at approximately 45° with the neck relaxed and with the head turned to one side. Venous pulsation causes both an outward and inward movement of the skin, whereas arterial pulsation causes a single outward movement. The height of the venous pulse is measured from the sternal angle. It should normally be 4 cm, and is low or invisible in patients who are dehydrated.

Normal venous pulse

There should be a soft double pulsation medial to the clavicular head of the sternocleidomastoid muscle. The pulsation radiates up to the jaw and to the ears. A normal jugular pulsation is seen as a 'flicker' above the clavicle, which can be compressed by one finger at the base of the neck.

Abnormal venous pulse

The height of the pulse is raised in right heart failure. A raised fixed pulse is found in superior vena caval obstruction due to malignant disease. Large systolic waves are seen in tricuspid regurgitation.

Auscultation

Non-specialists may find auscultation difficult and intimidating, but practice with a cardiologist will improve this important and productive clinical skill. Record your findings and differential diagnosis in your referral letter. Your opinion may well be proven correct by investigations! From a personal development and educational point of view, this is important, enjoyable and takes very little extra time.

Echocardiography and Doppler examination have shown that although auscultation is a useful diagnostic part of the examination, it is imperfect even with the best and most experienced ears.

Objectives of auscultation in primary care

The priority in primary care is to listen for and record heart murmurs and added heart sounds, and to refer patients for a specialist opinion and further investigation. The commonly occurring conditions encountered in primary care are listed in Table 4.1. Auscultation may be difficult in primary care, due to the background noise of other patients and children.

Characterising a murmur

Evaluation of a cardiac murmur usually includes the location of maximum loudness, radiation, timing (systolic or diastolic) and duration. High-pitched sounds are most easily heard with the diaphragm of the stethoscope, and low-pitched sounds with the bell.

> If you think the heart sounds are normal, record this.

Record and report abnormalities, and suggest a diagnosis. The information from a subsequent echocardiogram and Doppler examination will be educational. Try to grade and record the loudness or intensity of the murmur (quiet, moderately loud or very loud). Some cardiologists grade the loudness of murmurs from 1 to 6, and the duration from 1 to 4. This will provide a useful clinical baseline.

Positioning the patient to maximise the murmur

> Mitral murmurs are most easily heard with the patient lying on the left side. The murmur of mitral stenosis may be missed unless patients are routinely examined lying on their left side.
> Aortic murmurs are most easily heard with the patient sitting forward.

Tricuspid regurgitation can usually be diagnosed by seeing systolic (V) waves in the venous pulse. The murmur is quiet because the pressure gradients on the right side of the heart are lower than those on the left side.

The ejection systolic murmur of aortic stenosis can be heard all over the chest, and radiates to the neck. Diastolic murmurs are quieter. Aortic regurgitation is heard most easily with the patient sitting forward with their breath held in expiration.

Order of examination for auscultation

It is useful to use a system for auscultation. Murmurs originating from the left side of the heart are louder than those originating from the right side because the pressure differences are greater on the left.

1. *Listen to the first and second heart sounds separately.*

The first heart sound: closure of the mitral and tricuspid valves

⋄ Loud:
  — mitral stenosis
  — tachycardia
  — short PR interval
⋄ Quiet:
  — aortic stenosis
  — long PR interval (first-degree heart block)

The second heart sound: closure of the aortic and pulmonary valves

⋄ Loud A2 – hypertension
⋄ Loud P2 – pulmonary hypertension
⋄ *Quiet A2 – aortic stenosis*
⋄ *Quiet P2 – pulmonary stenosis*
⋄ Fixed split of second heart sound – atrial septal defect

2. *Listen for added sounds.* These include the ejection click of congenital aortic stenosis, the mid-systolic click of mitral valve prolapse, and the diastolic opening snap of mitral stenosis.
3. *Listen for systolic murmurs.* These can be normal (physiological) in anxious people, and after exercise or during pregnancy, and may be heard in patients with thyrotoxicosis and anaemia. The first and second heart sounds are heard normally and remain audible in a patient with a purely ejection systolic murmur. The first and second heart sounds may be obliterated by a pansystolic (throughout systole) murmur, typical of mitral regurgitation (although this may also cause an ejection murmur) and a ventricular septal defect.

   Causes of systolic murmurs include:
   ⋄ normal or physiological causes
   ⋄ structural heart disease
   ⋄ aortic stenosis
   ⋄ mitral regurgitation
   ⋄ hypertrophic obstructive cardiomyopathy
   ⋄ coarctation of the aorta
   ⋄ atrial septal defect (increased flow across the pulmonary valve due to left to right shunting of blood).

4. *Listen for diastolic murmurs.* The murmur of aortic regurgitation is most easily heard with the patient leaning forward and holding their breath in expiration. Mitral regurgitation tends to be most easily heard with the patient lying on their left side.
5. *Measure and record the blood pressure.*
6. *Diagnosis.* Analyse your findings and make a diagnosis and management plan.

Advice for patients

✧ If you want to check your blood pressure yourself, come to see our practice nurse or one of the doctors and we will advise you about what machine to buy and teach you how to use it.

✧ Weighing yourself once or twice a week makes you mindful of your diet and weight, and is important for patients with heart failure or swollen legs.

✧ We use your weight measurements to help decide the dose of your water tablets.

✧ Checking your pulse can be difficult, and we will teach you how to do it properly. It is helpful to know how to do this if you live or care for someone who has dizzy turns or palpitation. A normal pulse at the time makes a heart cause unlikely.

✧ If you feel a pulsation in your tummy, come to see us. This may be important if you have a high blood pressure.

Answers to questions about clinical cases

1. Short ejection systolic murmurs are almost universal during pregnancy, due to the increase in plasma volume and the increased cardiac output. It is important to distinguish this benign murmur from previously undiagnosed rheumatic heart disease (consisting of mitral valve stenosis, mitral regurgitation and less commonly aortic valve disease) or the mid-systolic click and late-systolic murmur of mitral valve prolapse. Both a pregnancy-related tachycardia and mitral stenosis may cause a loud first heart sound, but an opening snap may be heard with a pliable stenosed mitral valve. A slow carotid upstroke distinguishes the ejection systolic murmur of important aortic valve stenosis from the increased blood flow and turbulence that are heard during pregnancy or tachycardia. You should request an echocardiogram, which is completely safe during pregnancy, will provide the diagnosis and, if normal, will reassure the patient. If she has structural heart disease (this is more likely in a patient from Asia, India, Pakistan or Africa), she should be referred. Patients with mitral valve prolapse and mitral regurgitation should have antibiotic prophylaxis during labour and delivery.

2. One possibility is atrial fibrillation and mitral valve disease. Listen for the loud first heart sound, opening snap and diastolic murmur of mitral stenosis and the pansystolic murmur of mitral regurgitation. Probably more common is the combination of ectopic beats and an aortic ejection murmur. Arrange an echocardiogram and perform an ECG. Refer the patient if there is significant aortic or mitral valve disease.

3. You should look for signs of heart failure – a raised jugular venous pressure, an enlarged liver and peripheral oedema. Signs of left heart failure include a tachycardia and a third and/or fourth heart sound (if the patient is in sinus rhythm). The lung crackles may be due to his airways disease and chest infection, and less likely may be due to lung fibrosis rather than pulmonary oedema. Arrange a chest X-ray and spirometry, and request an echocardiogram.

4. The murmur may be benign, due to the hypertrophic heart, slow heart rate and increased stroke volume of an athlete. It could also be due to undiagnosed structural heart disease, including mitral valve prolapse, aortic valve disease, or hypertrophic obstructive or non-obstructive cardiomyopathy. Feel the carotid upstroke, which may be 'jerky' in HOCM. An ECG and echocardiogram will provide the diagnosis and the information necessary to differentiate these conditions.

5. This patient may have heart failure and widespread vascular disease. Examine her carotid arteries for bruits, and her leg and foot arteries. Listen over her renal arteries for bruits. She may have a dilated abdominal aorta, too. Look for signs of heart failure and localised chest signs. This patient will need echocardiography, a chest X-ray and

leg Doppler studies. She may also need brain scanning (CT or preferably MRI). Check her renal and thyroid function, glucose, lipids and blood count.

6. Pitting oedema in the legs can be caused by venous hypertension due to varicose veins, right heart failure due to several causes, or hypoalbuminaemia and renal disease. Look for signs of heart failure, lung disease, and ascites and hepatomegaly. Test the urine for protein, and arrange blood tests for blood count and biochemistry. If other causes are excluded, venous hypertension can be treated in primary care with support stockings and diuretics, with checks of the patient's renal function.

Hypertension

FIVE

Clinical cases

1. A 40-year-old symptom-free man who is moderately overweight has a blood sugar level of 7 mmol/l and is worried about his blood pressure, which he checks himself frequently and he records as 150/100 mmHg. What do you do?
2. A 75-year-old known hypertensive man comes to see you with headache, and you record his blood pressure as 190/150 mmHg. What do you do?
3. A 34-year-old woman is 28 weeks into her second pregnancy, having been diagnosed as having borderline hypertension during her first uncomplicated pregnancy four years ago. She feels well, but the nurse in the hospital antenatal clinic found her blood pressure to be 145/95 mmHg. What do you do?
4. A fit 86-year-old woman has a blood pressure of 175/80 mmHg but, because she feels fine, can do the crossword and does a lot of voluntary work at the old-age home, is not keen to take any tablets. What do you advise her to do?
5. A 67-year-old obese woman with type 2 diabetes, hyperlipidaemia and mild claudication has a blood pressure of 165/95 mmHg, despite taking a thiazide diuretic and an angiotensin-converting-enzyme inhibitor. How do you manage her?
6. A 74-year-old man with a history of myocardial infarction and stroke has been taking a β-blocker for his hypertension for over 20 years. His blood pressure is well controlled. Should he remain on the β-blocker?

The public health implications of hypertension

The World Health Organization has ranked hypertension as the most important cause of death worldwide. The screening for hypertension and its continual monitoring, treatment and control, as part of a comprehensive or global strategy of cardiovascular prevention, constitutes a major part of the workload in primary care. Good hypertension management makes an important difference to the health of the individual, and a well-organised hypertension clinic reduces cardiovascular disease in the population.

Definitions and classification of hypertension

Hypertension is graded in three categories as shown in Table 5.1.

TABLE 5.1: Classification of blood pressure

Category	Systolic (mmHg)	Diastolic (mmHg)
Optimal	< 120 and	< 80
Normal	120–129 and/or	80–84
High normal	130–139 and/or	85–89
Grade 1 hypertension	140–159 and/or	90–99
Grade 2 hypertension	160–179 and/or	100–109
Grade 3 hypertension	> 180 and/or	> 110
Isolated systolic hypertension	> 140 and	< 90

Hypertension is defined as a systolic blood pressure of > 140 mmHg and/or a diastolic pressure of > 85 mmHg. Optimal blood pressure is defined as < 120/80 mmHg. Isolated systolic hypertension is a systolic pressure of >140 mmHg and a diastolic pressure of < 90 mmHg.

> Systolic and diastolic pressures are prognostically equally important, although some studies have shown a stronger relationship between hypertension and stroke than between hypertension and coronary events.
>
> There is a graded independent relationship between systolic and diastolic pressure with heart failure, peripheral artery disease and end-stage renal disease.

Current issues in hypertension

* The cause of hypertension is unknown in over 90% of patients.
* Hypertension remains under-diagnosed. Many patients with 'mild' hypertension are untreated, and the majority of those with 'severe' hypertension are under-treated or not taking the prescribed medication. Thus, large numbers of people who do not regularly see their GP (notably middle-aged men) are at unnecessarily high risk of coronary heart disease and stroke.
* Less than 10% of hypertensive patients are controlled at 'target' levels.
* There is a reluctance to treat elderly patients with 'mild hypertension' and isolated systolic hypertension.
* White coat hypertension is recognised by clinicians and patients, but its prognostic implications and the need for treatment remain unclear.
* The roles of ambulatory blood pressure recordings and self-monitored recordings as useful diagnostic and monitoring tools, and their use and place in diagnosis and treatment, are becoming clearer. They are recommended to provide a more comprehensive view of a patient's blood pressure. High home recordings may be due to anxiety but not 'white coat syndrome.' The readings still need careful interpretation.
* β-blockers are less effective than other classes of antihypertensive drugs in reducing major cardiovascular events (particularly stroke) and diabetes. They are no longer recommended as either first- or second-line medication unless there are good clinical reasons for using them (e.g. angina, previous infarction).
* Most patients with hypertension will require more than one type of drug to reduce their blood pressure to the target level.
* Combination treatment as initial therapy is not yet recommended, but would probably be more effective than initial treatment with a single drug.
* Consensus guidelines have recommended lower target blood pressure levels for patients with a high absolute cardiovascular risk, including diabetics, smokers and those with coronary artery disease or target organ damage, particularly left ventricular hypertrophy. It is important that these groups of high-risk patients are identified and treated effectively.
* Compliance with drug and non-pharmacological treatment can be improved by explaining to patients the nature of hypertension, its complications and potential drug side-effects, and by continual clinical monitoring and checks on tablet intake. Once-daily dosing improves compliance.

Hypertension as a primary care specialty

The vast majority of patients with hypertension are diagnosed, treated and monitored within primary care. Patients with suspected secondary hypertension and who may need further complex investigations, individuals with important postural hypotension and those whose blood pressure is not adequately controlled need referral to hospital. Pregnant women with hypertension should be referred for a specialist opinion, although these cases would be detected during antenatal checks. Accelerated or malignant hypertension is now rarely seen, and these patients should be referred to hospital for urgent assessment and treatment.

Tasks for primary care clinicians in managing hypertension

- Identify people with hypertension.
- Establish blood pressure values.
- Identify people with secondary hypertension.
- Evaluate the total cardiovascular risk.
- Look for end-organ damage and complications.
- Look for other diseases.
- Carry out at least annual monitoring of blood pressure and response to medication. Young patients may need less frequent evaluation.
- Start the most appropriate medication.
- Plan and explain long-term management.

Recording the history in a patient with hypertension

This information can be obtained by asking the patient to fill in a tick-box history sheet. The data can then be entered into their computerised records.

1. *Duration and previous level of blood pressure.* Women should be asked about hypertension during pregnancy.
2. *Clues to possible secondary hypertension*:
- family history of renal disease due to polycystic kidney disease
- renal disease, urinary tract infection, haematuria, analgesic abuse causing renal parenchymal disease
- drugs/illicit substances – oral contraceptives, liquorice, carbenoxolone, cocaine, amphetamines, steroids, non-steroidal anti-inflammatory drugs, cyclosporin
- sweating, headache, anxiety, palpitation – phaeochromocytoma
- muscle weakness and tetany – aldosteronism.

3. *Cardiovascular risk factors*:
- family history of hypertension and cardiovascular disease
- family and personal history of dyslipidaemia
- family and personal history of diabetes
- smoking
- dietary habits
- obesity
- exercise habits
- snoring and sleep apnoea
- stress.

4. *Clinical features of cardiovascular disease*:
- angina, heart failure, carotid bruits, fundal examination (haemorrhages, exudates and papilloedema are now rarely seen in modern practice)
- transient ischaemic attacks

✧ claudication (radio-femoral delay, decreased foot pulses)
✧ waist measurement and weight.

Routine investigations in hypertensive patients

Sub-clinical organ damage is a bad prognostic sign.

Tests are done to determine whether there is left ventricular hypertrophy, diastolic dysfunction, atherosclerotic vascular disease or kidney damage, all of which put the patient in a poor prognostic group, and necessitate vigorous risk factor modification. The tests listed in Table 5.2 are widely available and cost-effective.

TABLE 5.2: Routine tests in hypertensive patients

Test	Clinical indication
ECG	Left ventricular hypertrophy, ischaemia, infarction
Echocardiography	Heart murmurs or hypertension, left ventricular hypertrophy
Carotid ultrasound	Carotid bruits or a history of transient ischaemic attacks
Renal function[a]	Creatinine clearance, eGFR, urinary protein by dipstix
Spot urine[b]	Microalbuminuria, relate to urinary creatinine if dipstix is negative
Quantitative proteinuria	If dipstix is positive, measure albumin excretion
Ankle-brachial index	Claudication or reduced leg pulses
Glucose tolerance test	If fasting glucose level is > 5.6 mmol/l (100 mg/dl)
Home and 24-hour BP recording	Suspected white coat syndrome, episodic symptoms

a Hypertension-induced kidney damage is shown by reduced renal function and/or increased excretion of albumin. The estimated glomerular filtration rate (eGFR) is calculated using the patient's age, gender, race and serum creatinine concentration. There are two methods of estimating the eGFR, both of which identify patients with renal disease even if the creatinine level remains normal. Values below 60 ml/min/1.73 m^2 indicate chronic renal disease stage 3.

b Urinary protein should be measured with a dipstick. In both hypertensive and diabetic patients, micro-albuminuria is associated with increased cardiovascular disease.

Haemodynamic changes in hypertension

Hypertension occurs when excessive vasoconstriction and/or volume are not compensated by adequate pressure natriuresis or suppression of the renin–aldosterone system.

Hypertension and pulse pressure as cardiovascular risk factors: benefits of lowering blood pressure

Hypertension is the most common cause of stroke, the most common reversible cause of heart failure and an important cause of coronary heart disease (particularly in diabetics) and renal disease. The relationship between blood pressure and cardiovascular disease is continuous and graded, and there is no cut-off value that separates those patients who will and those who will not develop a cardiovascular event.

The risk of an individual developing cardiovascular disease depends on the level of the blood pressure and coexisting risk factors. Because hypertension and other risk factors are common, most hypertensive patients have other risk factors and also sub-clinical organ damage. Risk is directly proportional to systolic blood pressure and inversely proportional to diastolic blood pressure.

Isolated systolic hypertension is defined as a systolic blood pressure of ≥ 140 mmHg and a diastolic pressure of < 90 mmHg. It is the most common form of hypertension, occurring in over two-thirds of people over 65 years and three-quarters of those over 75 years of age. In patients over 50 years of age, elevation of systolic blood pressure predicts the risk of stroke better than increases in diastolic blood pressure. Lowering systolic blood pressure to less than 150 mmHg is associated with reductions of 40% in stroke, 16% in coronary events, 50% in heart failure and 15% in mortality.

In patients under 50 years of age, diastolic blood pressure is a stronger predictor of fatal and non-fatal coronary artery disease. Above the age of 60 years diastolic pressure is inversely related to coronary risk so that *pulse pressure* (systolic pressure minus diastolic pressure) is a better predictor of cardiovascular events than systolic blood pressure. The increasing systolic blood pressure increases left ventricular work and the risk of hypertrophy. The lowering of the diastolic blood pressure compromises coronary blood flow. Thus a blood pressure of 150/85 mmHg carries a higher risk than a blood pressure of 150/95 mmHg in patients over 60 years of age. A wide pulse pressure is an important risk factor, and lowering of the systolic blood pressure alone is a primary objective of treating hypertension, but difficult to achieve. Pulse pressure is also highly predictive of cardiovascular risk. This is because the higher the pulse pressure, the greater the pressure stress on arterial walls, and the more likely it is that organ damage will occur. A blood pressure recording of 150/95 mmHg has different implications for a 70-year-old man to those it would have for a 35-year-old man. The 70-year-old man has a higher absolute cardiovascular risk, but the 35-year-old man has a higher relative risk compared with normal men of his age.

Observational studies suggest that the lower the blood pressure the better, although this notion is not confirmed by individual outcome trials, except in diabetics.

New epidemiological and clinical trial data has reshaped treatment guidelines. An understanding of absolute and relative risk is essential when making treatment decisions for individual patients.

> Treatment decisions should be based on a formal estimation of 10-year coronary heart disease risk using the programme 'Cardiac Risk Assessor' or the coronary heart disease risk chart issued by the Joint British Societies. The treatment threshold is flexible, based on the level of blood pressure and the total cardiovascular risk. For example, a blood pressure of 140/85 mmHg is normal in a low-risk individual, but should be treated in a diabetic with a high overall cardiovascular risk.

Cardiovascular risk estimation according to age: the risk of under-treating the young and over-treating the elderly

All patients should have a global or total cardiovascular risk estimation based on their risk profile, organ damage and disease. The risk should be categorised as low, moderate, high or very high. The estimated risk determines the treatment strategy, whether the patient should be treated, the target blood pressure level, the use of combination therapies, and the need for a statin and other non-hypertensive drugs.

The commonly used British Societies' risk tables are based on Framingham data, which apply to only some European and US populations. The SCORE model is recommended by the European Society of Cardiology, available on their website (www.escardio.org).

An understanding of absolute and relative risk is important when deciding upon treatment for patients with hypertension. An individual's cardiovascular risk is recorded using risk charts to estimate their *absolute risk* of a cardiovascular event over the next 10 years. Risk estimation is used to make treatment decisions 'intelligent' so that limited resources are targeted to those most at risk. In the UK, the guidelines recommend treatment only if an individual's risk of a cardiovascular event over the next 10 years is greater than 20%. This is an arbitrary cut-off value and is not universally used. Risk estimates are inaccurate, and strict adherence to this treatment threshold would mean that an individual who was estimated to be at a marginally lower risk would not be treated.

Age is a heavily weighted risk factor. An elderly patient's *absolute risk* is much higher than that of a young patient, almost irrespective of their level of blood pressure and the presence of other risk factors. Most men aged over 70 years will justify treatment, although their relative risk will be similar to that of their 'normal' peers. The absolute risk in a young woman is unlikely to reach treatment thresholds even if she has a major risk factor, although she is at much higher relative risk compared with a woman of the same age without risk factors.

The consequence of basing treatment on absolute rather than relative risk is that most resources would be concentrated on older people, whose long-term mortality may not be improved, although their cardiovascular event rate may be reduced. Less attention is paid to preventing cardiovascular disease in young people who may be at significant long-term risk and who may develop irreversible cardiovascular problems when still relatively young. To reduce long-term risk in young patients, treatment decisions should be guided by their *relative risk* (their risk compared with people of the same age who have no risk factors). These problems highlight the importance of using guidelines as guidelines and not as prescriptive protocols. Clinicians need to use evidence-based guidelines as a flexible foundation for deciding on treatment for each individual patient.

> In young patients, management should be based on relative rather than absolute risk.

Risk factors that influence prognosis in hypertension

These should be assessed and used to estimate risk in order to determine whether a patient should be treated. The decision to start treatment for hypertension depends on the blood pressure level and the patient's total cardiovascular risk. Levels above those given below constitute a significant risk factor.

The following risk factors influence prognosis in hypertension:
- levels of systolic and diastolic blood pressure
- pulse pressure in the elderly
- smoking
- dyslipidaemia:
  - total cholesterol > 5.0 mmol/l or
  - LDL-cholesterol > 3.0 mmol/l or
  - HDL-cholesterol < 1.0 mmol/l or
  - triglycerides > 1.7 mmol/l
- fasting glucose 5.6–6.9 mmol/l
- abnormal glucose tolerance test
- family history of premature coronary artery disease (men aged < 55 years and women aged < 65 years)
- abdominal obesity (> 102 cm in men and > 88 cm in women)

- diabetes (fasting glucose > 7.0 mmol/l, or random measurement > 11.0 mmol/l)
- end-organ damage:
  - left ventricular hypertrophy on ECG or echocardiogram
  - carotid wall thickening or plaque
  - ankle-brachial blood pressure index < 0.9
  - renal impairment (eGFR < 60 ml/min)
  - microalbuminuria (30–300 mg/24 hours)
  - diabetes (fasting glucose > 7.0 mmol/l)
- vascular disease in the brain, heart, kidneys, legs or eyes.

Metabolic syndrome

This is defined as the presence of three or more of the following: abdominal obesity, high fasting glucose, blood pressure > 130/85 mmHg, low HDL-cholesterol levels and high triglyceride levels. It is most common in middle-aged and elderly patients, and is associated with a significantly higher cardiovascular risk. Other associated features include microalbuminuria, left ventricular hypertrophy and arterial stiffness.

Because patients are at greater risk, a more detailed investigation of sub-clinical organ damage is recommended. Twenty-four-hour ambulatory blood pressure recording and self-recorded blood pressure readings are helpful.

Angiotensin-converting-enzyme (ACE) inhibitors and/or angiotensin II receptor antagonists are recommended for treating hypertension in patients with metabolic syndrome. Calcium-channel blockers and/or thiazide diuretics can be added. β-blockers are not recommended as first-line therapy.

Statins and anti-diabetic medication are also used when necessary. The role of insulin sensitisers has not been defined.

Classification of cardiovascular risk

Classification of risk is easiest in individuals at high risk. It is most difficult and inaccurate in those who fall between high and low risk, who are classified as intermediate risk.

High-risk individuals are those who have one or more of the following:
- systolic blood pressure > 180 mmHg and/or diastolic pressure > 110 mmHg
- any form of vascular disease
- metabolic syndrome
- organ damage (microalbuminuria – low-level albuminuria), left ventricular hypertrophy
- type 1 or type 2 diabetes mellitus
- one or more severely elevated risk factors
- older patients (men aged > 55 years and women aged > 65 years).

Low-risk individuals are those who:
- are under 50 years of age
- have no risk factors.

Recording devices

Health and safety regulations have relegated the mercury sphygmomanometer to history in hospitals, which now use mainly automated, semi-automated and aneroid devices.

Measuring blood pressure

Blood pressure is a very labile haemodynamic parameter that varies with each heart beat, hour of the day, season of the year, activity and position of the individual. Therefore, a diagnosis of hypertension should be based on many recordings made over several weeks. If blood pressure is only slightly high, many recordings should be taken over a period of months before a diagnosis of hypertension is made. However, if the patient has a very high recording and evidence of end-organ damage and other cardiovascular risk factors, the diagnosis is more secure.

> Blood pressure recordings can be taken not only by a doctor or nurse, but also by other trained healthcare professionals, and assuming the recordings have been taken accurately under correct conditions, by the patient or carer at the patient's home.

Accurate recordings are inexpensive, easily obtained, non-invasive determinants of cardiovascular status and cardiovascular events.

* Blood pressure should be measured with the patient sitting at ease and as relaxed as possible, in a quiet room (or standing if elderly or diabetic, or if orthostatic hypertension is suspected). Two recordings separated by at least one minute should be taken, and more if the recordings are very different. Measure the blood pressure in both arms at the first visit, to investigate the possibility of coarctation. The patient should be relaxed.
* Current guidelines recommend that recordings should be taken in all patients at least every five years, but the frequency of recordings will be determined by the patient's clinical state. Patients with borderline readings and those with hypertension that is difficult to control will require more frequent recordings and clinical assessments.
* The recording device should be validated, calibrated and regularly maintained. The blood pressure cuff must be of an appropriate size for the patient's arm, which should be at the level of the heart, and the cuff deflated slowly enough to aim to measure the blood pressure to the nearest 2 mmHg.
* The cuff should be inflated above the systolic level by feeling the brachial artery pulsation disappear as the cuff is inflated. The stethoscope should then be applied over the brachial artery as the cuff is gradually and slowly deflated.
* The systolic pressure should be recorded as the level when the pulse sounds reappear with cuff deflation (Korotkov phase 1). The diastolic level should be recorded as the pulse sounds disappear (Korotkov phase 5). The average of at least two readings should be taken.
* Because of the weighting given to blood pressure in cardiovascular risk assessment, use the average recording from several visits when estimating the 10-year risk.

White coat syndrome

In white coat syndrome, the blood pressure in the surgery is > 140/90 mmHg, but the home recording is < 130/85 mmHg. Cardiovascular risk is less than in individuals with raised surgery and ambulatory or home recordings.

Self-measurement of blood pressure

Self-measurement of blood pressure is of clinical and prognostic value. The normal value of home, self-recorded blood pressure is < 130–135/85 mmHg. Doctors used to be reluctant to advise patients to record their own blood pressure, because they were not confident about the accuracy of the recordings, which may be taken when patients are stressed or anxious, or shortly after exercising. However, in the same way as some people like to check their weight, or measure their heart rate while exercising (both of which are sensible things to do), self-recording devices are popular with some patients who like to keep an eye on their blood pressure to check whether they are 'healthy' and their blood pressure is within normal limits. Accurate recordings assist the evaluation of treatment, and encourage patients to take their tablets.

However, some patients may become obsessed with their blood pressure measurements, and this is undesirable. If patients become obsessed and feel anxious, they should be advised to stop taking their blood pressure. Patients should be told that irrespective of their recordings, they must not alter their medication without consulting their doctor.

There are several blood pressure machines available for self-recording. In general, semi-automatic arm recorders are more accurate than wrist recorders. The patient should sit while measuring their blood pressure, and should have rested for several minutes beforehand. Recordings should not be taken shortly after exercise or if the patient feels stressed. Self-recorded home measurements are lower than clinic or surgery recordings. It is useful for patients to check their device and the accuracy of their self-recording against a simultaneous recording performed in the surgery.

Ambulatory blood pressure recording

This is a very useful and accurate method for non-invasive measurement of the blood pressure during usual daily activities over a 24-hour period. It provides blood pressure data when the patient is asleep, driving, working or engaged in activities that would be expected to have a significant effect on blood pressure, and when self-recordings or clinic recordings would be difficult to obtain. Many GP surgeries now have their own machines as well as software on their computers to analyse the data, and this greatly improves the quality of care for patients with established or suspected hypertension.

Ambulatory blood pressure recording is a much stronger predictor of cardiovascular morbidity and mortality than conventional blood pressure recordings. It should be available to all patients with known or suspected hypertension.

Ambulatory blood pressure recordings have shown the natural circadian variation in blood pressure, with an early-morning surge, which accounts for the peak incidence of cardiac and cerebrovascular events in the morning. High recordings are associated with stress, and low levels are obtained when the patient is asleep or resting. This type of recording provides a full 24-hour 'panorama' of the patient's blood pressure, rather than a 'snapshot' measurement taken when both the patient and possibly the GP or nurse are stressed in a busy clinic.

Ambulatory blood pressure recordings and white coat syndrome (hypertension only in clinic or the surgery)

Twenty-four-hour ambulatory blood pressure recording is particularly helpful for evaluating the possibility of white coat syndrome, which is present in around 15% of the general population.

> White coat hypertension is defined as high clinic readings (> 140/90 mmHg) but normal ambulatory blood pressure recordings (< 130/80 mmHg), apart from the first stressful and unfamiliar hour of the ambulatory recording.

Although patients with this common condition do not generally appear to benefit from antihypertensive treatment, the prevalence of end-organ damage is higher than in individuals without white coat syndrome, so it is not a completely benign condition. Patients with white coat syndrome should be screened for risk factors and organ damage.

> Antihypertensive medication is recommended for patients with white coat syndrome who have cardiovascular risk factors or organ damage.

Patients who have raised clinic recordings but an average 24-hour blood pressure level of < 130/80 mmHg are no more likely than normotensive people to have a cardiovascular event. They do not need medication unless they have significant risk factors or organ damage, and thus drug side-effects are avoided. Excluding hypertension has important employment and insurance benefits for the patient and reduces healthcare costs.

Ambulatory blood pressure recordings are a better predictor of cardiovascular outcomes than isolated clinic recordings in patients with treated hypertension. High ambulatory recordings (a mean blood pressure of > 135/85 mmHg), particularly at night, are also reliable in predicting cardiovascular events. Patients with raised clinic blood pressure recordings should be considered for ambulatory recordings.

Indications for 24-hour ambulatory blood pressure recording
- Diagnosis of white coat syndrome.
- Deciding the diagnosis in patients with borderline clinic readings.
- Marked variability of clinic recordings.
- Resistant hypertension (> 150/90 mmHg despite three or more drugs).
- Suspected hypotension, particularly in diabetics or the elderly.
- Patients with a blood pressure of > 160/100 mmHg with no target organ damage and an estimated 10-year cardiovascular risk of < 15%. If the average ambulatory blood pressure recording is normal, medication may not be necessary.
- Deciding treatment in elderly patients with isolated systolic hypertension.
- Patients with hypertension in pregnancy.
- When a previous ambulatory blood pressure recording is normal but the patient has borderline hypertension or significant cardiovascular risk for other reasons.
- Evaluation of the efficacy of treatment.
- Sleep apnoea.

Interpreting the results of ambulatory blood pressure recording
Patients should be asked to fill in a diary recording their activities during the day, when they rested and went to bed, and how well they slept. They should not exercise vigorously while wearing the cuff. They can take the cuff off when they have a bath or shower. At least 70% of the recordings should be 'valid' and not affected by artefact.

The decision to treat should be based on the average daytime readings, not the average 24-hour recording. The threshold for starting treatment should be 12/7 mmHg lower than clinic readings, because blood pressure recordings are systematically lower with ambulatory recordings. Thus, an average ambulatory recording of 148/83 mmHg, which equates to a clinic blood pressure of 160/90 mmHg, may require treatment.

> An average ambulatory blood pressure of 130/80 mmHg is normal in low-risk individuals, but a level of < 120/75 mmHg is optimal in diabetics.

Ambulatory 24-hour blood pressure recordings identify patients whose blood pressure does not fall normally at night – so-called 'non-dippers' – who are probably at high risk.

Exercise-induced hypertension

Blood pressure increases with both mental stress and physical exercise.

High blood pressure values in response to mental stress have been found to predict those who develop hypertension later in life.

Normally, during exercise, the systolic blood pressure increases and the diastolic pressure falls. These changes rely on an intact response of the peripheral vessels (reduced systemic vascular resistance to leg exercise), a normal heart pump and blood supply, and a normal autonomic nervous system. An exaggerated blood pressure response to exercise (peak exercise-related systolic blood pressure > 200 mmHg) may identify patients with hypertension who have not been previously diagnosed. It also predicts cardiovascular death, and therefore adds prognostic information.

Causes of hypertension

> The most common cause of hypertension is 'essential hypertension', which accounts for at least 94% of cases.

Secondary causes of hypertension
Renal parenchymal disease

Renal parenchymal disease is the most common cause of secondary hypertension. It is suggested by urinalysis that shows erythrocytes, white cells and protein. Referral and further investigations are warranted. Two normal creatinine levels and urinalyses exclude renal parenchymal disease.

> Urinalysis and creatinine levels should be measured in all patients with hypertension to investigate the presence of renal parenchymal disease.

Bilateral polycystic kidney disease may be found on clinical examination. Ultrasound is diagnostic.

Hypertension may result from acute renal failure of any cause, including acute glomerulonephritis, vasculitis, acute obstruction, or chronic renal failure due to diabetic nephropathy or chronic glomerulonephritis.

Management

The threshold for treatment in patients with renal disease is > 140/90 mmHg, and the target is < 130/85 mmHg. These patients should be referred to a specialist to plan and monitor the long-term management of the underlying renal disease and to choose the most appropriate combination of tablets. Thiazide diuretics (e.g. bendroflumethiazide, indapamide, hydrochlorothiazide) may be ineffective and high-dose loop diuretics (furosemide) may be required. Aggressive lowering of the blood pressure may slow progression of the renal disease. Salt restriction is important in patients with impaired renal function. Patients should be considered for aspirin and statins.

Renovascular hypertension

This is the second most common cause of secondary hypertension, accounting for 2% of hypertensive patients referred to specialist centres. Reduced blood flow to either or both kidneys, due to renal artery stenosis, results in activation of the renin–angiotensin system, with increased renin levels and fluid retention. There are two causes of renal artery stenosis.

✧ *Atherosclerotic disease* (70% of cases) usually affects both renal arteries (although it is often more marked in one artery), and is a progressive disease. It should be considered in patients with resistant hypertension and those who have evidence or a high probability of vascular disease, those who have smoked, those with peripheral vascular, cerebrovascular or coronary artery disease, and those who develop increasing renal impairment when treated with ACE inhibitors or angiotensin II antagonists. Bilateral renal artery stenosis may cause 'flash pulmonary oedema' with normal left ventricular failure.

✧ *Fibromuscular dysplasia* (25% of cases) occurs typically in young females who present with hypertension and no family history of hypertension.

Diagnosis and management

Patients with suspected renal artery stenosis should be referred for a specialist opinion. Features include an abdominal bruit, hypokalaemia and progressive decline in renal function. Colour flow Doppler ultrasound, computerised tomography (CT) and magnetic resonance scanning can be used to select patients for arteriography and revascularisation with angioplasty and stenting (which can be performed at the same time as arteriography), or surgical reconstruction of the affected arteries. Three-dimensional, gadolinium-enhanced, magnetic resonance angiography may prove to be the diagnostic procedure with the highest accuracy.

Fibromuscular renal artery stenosis

Angioplasty and stenting are useful in patients with fibromuscular renal artery stenosis.

Renal angioplasty may be complicated by local problems. These include proteinuria following a sudden increase in renal artery pressure after dilatation of the stenosis, radiographic contrast agent-induced renal damage, cholesterol emboli (in atherosclerotic disease) and restenosis in 50% of patients.

Atherosclerotic renal artery stenosis

Renal angioplasty is no more effective for control of blood pressure than antihypertensive drug therapy alone in atherosclerotic renal artery stenosis. It is therefore no longer necessary to screen all hypertensive patients for renal artery stenosis with a view to angioplasty. However, it should be considered for those with uncontrolled hypertension, high serum creatinine levels, bilateral renal artery stenosis (which may present as 'flash pulmonary oedema') and severe unilateral renal artery stenosis.

All classes of antihypertensive drugs may be used. ACE inhibitors may be used in unilateral renal artery stenosis, but are contraindicated in severe bilateral disease. All patients on ACE inhibitors need regular renal function tests. Increases in serum creatinine levels are usually reversed when the ACE inhibitor is stopped. In patients who are on maximal medical treatment but who have resistant severe hypertension, the risk of continuing ACE inhibitors must be weighed against the dangers of uncontrolled hypertension. These patients require specialist assessment.

Aortic coarctation

This is a narrowing of the aorta, usually distal to the left subclavian artery, and may be associated with a bicuspid aortic valve and other heart defects. It should be diagnosed in childhood. Affected patients may have a systolic heart murmur heard over the chest and back, hypertension and decreased leg pulses. The blood pressure is high in the arms but often unrecordable in the legs and feet. The resulting hypertension usually resolves if the coarctation is resected during childhood. Stenting can also be used. Hypertension usually persists if surgery is performed in a patient over 40 years of age. Affected patients are vulnerable to hypertensive complications at a younger age.

Management

These patients should be referred for investigation and consideration of surgery or angioplasty. Even after correction of the coarctation, patients require follow-up for hypertension and its complications.

Cushing's syndrome

Hypertension affects 80% of patients with Cushing's syndrome, thus accounting for less than 0.1% of the total population. The diagnosis can be made on the basis of the typical physical appearance.

Management

A 24-hour urinary cortisol level of > 110 mmol/l suggests the diagnosis. This is confirmed with a two-day low-dose dexamethasone suppression test (0.5 mg every six hours for eight doses). In the two-day test a urinary cortisone excretion rate higher than 27 mmol/l per day on day two is diagnostic of Cushing's syndrome. A normal result excludes the diagnosis. Patients should be referred for investigation and management of the underlying problem, but also require effective treatment for hypertension.

Conn's syndrome (primary hyperaldosteronism)

This condition is most commonly due to a benign, unilateral, autonomous adenoma of the adrenal gland secreting aldosterone. This results in low renin levels, increased sodium levels and low potassium levels, particularly in patients who are taking diuretics. Importantly, most patients have normal plasma electrolytes at presentation. Conn's syndrome accounts for 1% of patients with hypertension. Around 70% of cases are due to adrenal hyperplasia.

Around 30% of cases are due to adrenal adenomas, which are more common in women. The condition should be suspected in people with hypokalaemia and in those with resistant hypertension.

Management

These patients should be referred for confirmation and categorisation of the diagnosis and guidance on the most appropriate medical treatment, which is often necessary. Diagnosis is made by measuring 24-hour urinary aldosterone. The plasma aldosterone:plasma renin ratio after withdrawing antihypertensive treatment for two weeks is used, but interpretation of this test is difficult and controversial. Primary aldosteronism can be confirmed by the fludrocortisone suppression test (failure of four-day administration of the hormone to reduce plasma aldosterone and renin levels).

Aldosterone-secreting adenomata should be localised by either CT or MRI scanning. Adrenal hyperplasia may produce false-positive scan results. Adenomas should be removed because this leads to resolution of hypertension in 70% of cases.

Phaeochromocytoma

These catecholamine-secreting tumours are usually unilateral and limited to the adrenal glands. They account for 0.2% of cases of hypertension. They may present incidentally as a first hypertensive episode peri-operatively, or as episodic hypertension, headache, and palpitation with or without tachycardia, pallor and sweating. Other symptoms reflecting catecholamine excess include anxiety, tremor, nausea, chest or abdominal pain, weight loss and fatigue. There may be dramatic elevations in blood pressure.

The diagnosis should be suspected in patients with suggestive symptoms, resistant hypertension or severe hypertension during pregnancy, when the uterus may press on the adrenal gland.

Management

The diagnosis can be made by measuring the levels of catecholamines in the blood, or catecholamine breakdown products in the urine over a 24-hour collection period. The most sensitive test (98%) is the level of plasma-free metanephrines, but this is not widely available. The 24-hour urinary catecholamine level is the most commonly performed test. If the level is very high, no further diagnostic tests are required. Localisation of the tumour is then necessary. Around 95% of these tumours are located close to or in the adrenal glands. Large ones can be seen on ultrasound. CT is more sensitive (> 98%). A negative assay has a 98% predictive value for excluding the condition in a primary care population, and the test may be arranged with the local pathology department, which will be able to provide instructions on what the patient should do about food and medication before and during the collection.

Patients should be referred to a specialist who may wish to perform further tests, including localisation of the tumour by MRI or CT scanning. Surgical removal of the tumour(s) (now performed laparoscopically) usually results in normalisation of the blood pressure, but 25% of patients may have persistent hypertension.

Sleep apnoea

Patients with this condition are usually very overweight and stop breathing for periods while asleep. Sleep apnoea can be very worrying for the patient's partner. It can cause blood pressure that is resistant to treatment in obese individuals. Patients feel sleepy during the day and find it difficult to concentrate, and choke while asleep. Sleep studies using polysomnography are used to diagnose the condition. The problem usually responds to substantial weight loss and the use of positive pressure breathing equipment at night.

Drug causes of hypertension

All prescribed and non-prescribed medication should be noted. The following drugs cause hypertension:
◇ oestrogens and oral contraceptives
◇ β-agonists (bronchodilators, stimulant abuse, over-the-counter 'cold cures')
◇ steroids
◇ liquorice
◇ non-steroidal anti-inflammatory drugs
◇ amphetamines.

Contributory and correctable factors in relation to hypertension

◇ Being overweight.
◇ Excess alcohol consumption (> three units per day).
◇ Excess salt intake.
◇ Lack of exercise.

Complications and target organ damage

✧ Stroke and/or transient ischaemic attack.
✧ Multi-infarct dementia.
✧ Left ventricular hypertrophy.
✧ Heart failure.
✧ Coronary artery disease.
✧ Peripheral arterial disease.
✧ Retinal hypertensive changes.
✧ Proteinuria.
✧ Renal impairment (raised serum creatinine, microalbuminuria).

Rationale for effective treatment of hypertension

> Hypertension increases the risk of vascular diseases, particularly stroke and coronary heart disease and renal disease.

Reducing cardiovascular risk necessitates treatment of hypertension and all other risk factors. Blood pressure values in the range 130–139/85–89 mmHg are associated with a greater than two-fold increase in the relative risk of cardiovascular disease compared with people with a blood pressure of 120/80 mmHg. Reducing blood pressure by 12/6 mmHg reduces the risk of stroke by 40% and the risk of coronary disease by 20%.

Those at highest cardiovascular risk derive the most benefit from treatment of hypertension.

> Blood pressure lowering reduces fatal and non-fatal cardiovascular events. Treatment of hypertension in the elderly reduces the risk of dementia. Treatment of hypertension in people aged over 80 years reduces the risk of stroke and myocardial infarction.
> All classes of antihypertensive drugs appear to be similar in their effects.

Aims and principles of treatment

✧ The aim is to achieve maximal reduction in the long-term risk of cardiovascular disease.
✧ Treatment should start before end-organ damage and cardiovascular disease occur.
✧ The blood pressure should be reduced to target levels, and all associated reversible risk factors should be treated.
✧ Blood pressure should be reduced to below 140/90 mmHg, and to lower levels if tolerated, in all patients.
✧ In diabetics, patients with renal impairment and proteinuria, and those with vascular disease (stroke, myocardial infarction), the target level is < 130/80 mmHg.
✧ Patients aged over 80 years should be treated in a similar way to patients aged over 55 years.
✧ Isolated systolic hypertension (systolic blood pressure > 160 mmHg) should be treated in the same way as combined systolic and diastolic hypertension.

✧ Most patients will need more than one antihypertensive drug to achieve target levels.

✧ Compliance is better if once-daily dosing is used.

✧ Non-proprietary drugs reduce treatment costs.

✧ Patients should be advised about common side-effects so that they can make informed choices about their treatment.

✧ Treatment should be started if the blood pressure is > 160/100 mmHg, and if it is >140/85 mmHg in patients with vascular disease and those with an estimated 10-year cardiovascular risk of > 20%.

✧ Patients with accelerated (malignant) hypertension (papilloedema, fundal haemorrhages or exudates) should be referred and admitted to hospital for immediate treatment, but treatment should be started in the surgery if there is a delay.

✧ Treatment should be started immediately in patients with a blood pressure of > 220/120 mmHg.

✧ Drug therapy should be started in all patients with sustained (monitored over a four-week period) systolic blood pressure of > 160 mmHg or sustained diastolic blood pressure of > 100 mmHg despite non-pharmacological measures.

✧ Drug therapy should be started in patients with sustained systolic blood pressure > 140 mmHg or diastolic blood pressure > 90 mmHg *only* if:
   — target organ damage is present, *or*
   — there is evidence of cardiovascular disease and/or diabetes, *or*
   — the 10-year coronary heart disease risk is > 15%.
      Otherwise, patients with a blood pressure of < 160/100 mmHg and *no* target organ damage or cardiovascular complications, no diabetes and a 10-year coronary heart disease risk of < 15% do not need drug treatment, but should be given advice about non-pharmacological measures and be monitored monthly.

✧ Patients with a blood pressure of < 135/85 mmHg should be reassessed every five years.

> The aim of treatment is to lower blood pressure sufficiently to prevent cardiovascular complications with no drug-induced adverse effects. The choice of drug is of secondary importance.
>
> Response to treatment is mainly determined by the patient's age, assuming that there is good compliance.

Patient education

One of the major problems in treating hypertension is that most patients are symptom-free and do not like taking tablets. Treatment means total management, not just tablets. It is important that patients understand what hypertension is, what their blood pressure is and what their target level is, what the risks of uncontrolled hypertension are, what general measures they can and should instigate and maintain for themselves which reduce blood pressure and cardiovascular risk, what tablets they should take, and how frequently they should be monitored. They should understand that treatment is for life and that when their blood pressure becomes controlled they must continue to take tablets, and these may need to be increased if their blood pressure increases.

Although the prevention of cardiovascular complications is the principal aim and, hopefully, result of treatment, antihypertensive treatment also prevents dementia, which suggests that it improves the quality of life both mentally and physically in symptom-free patients.

After establishing a diagnosis of hypertension, patients need to understand that treatment and lifestyle measures are for life. Medication may need to be adjusted or changed depending on the response or the development of side-effects.

Blood pressure targets

In general, the lower the blood pressure the better, particularly in diabetics.
The target for all patients of all ages is < 140/90 mmHg.
The target for patients with diabetes and/or target organ damage or cardio-vascular disease is < 130/80 mmHg.

Targets are helpful to clinicians, but are difficult to achieve even in fully compliant patients. The blood pressure levels suggested as 'audit standards' in the current guidelines are higher than the recommended targets. These different levels cause confusion.

Because blood pressure increases with age, life events and other factors, the recommended targets become increasingly difficult to achieve. Blood pressure reduction, particularly reduction of systolic pressure in people aged over 60 years, is important in reducing cardiovascular events.

When the target blood pressure is not achieved

Patients with resistant hypertension may become anxious and feel that they have 'failed' by not achieving their blood pressure target. They should be told that resistant hypertension is not uncommon even with perfect compliance and appropriate medication. Occasionally, this anxiety and frustration may lead to a preoccupation with their blood pressure levels, making control more difficult. When starting drug therapy, it may be helpful to advise patients that it may not be possible to achieve the target blood pressure despite perfect compliance and the best medication. Further emphasis on non-pharmacological measures is often helpful to the patient's morale.

Target achievers

Some responders may feel that the diagnosis was wrong and may stop or ask to stop their tablets. If hypertensive patients stop taking their tablets, their blood pressure will inevitably increase within a few weeks, but it may occasionally be necessary to go through this exercise in order to convince doubtful patients.

TABLE 5.3: Target blood pressures during antihypertensive treatment (both the systolic and diastolic blood pressure targets should be attained)

	Clinic blood pressure (mmHg)		Mean daytime ABPM or home blood pressure (mmHg)	
	No diabetes	Diabetes	No diabetes	Diabetes
Optimal BP	< 140/85	< 130/80	< 130/80	< 130/75
Audit standard[a]	< 150/90	< 140/85	< 140/85	< 140/80

ABPM, ambulatory blood pressure monitoring.

a The audit standard is the minimum recommended level of blood pressure control, recognising that only 10% of patients have blood levels at target.

Target achievers should be congratulated on achieving their targets and reassured that the reason why their blood pressure is 'low' is because of the medication and other measures they are taking.

Non-pharmacological measures

Quite often, overweight, stressed, inactive people with high clinic blood pressure readings respond to the measures listed below, which are effective and may make drug treatment unnecessary, or at least reduce the number of different drugs needed by enhancing the antihypertensive effect of the drugs. These measures are effective, safe and, compared with drug treatment, inexpensive. Patients need enthusiastic supervision, monitoring, encouragement, and regular supervision and support. These measures are an integral part of the initial and long-term treatment of all patients with hypertension. Drug treatment may need to be started without delay in patients with severe hypertension.

There is no evidence from controlled trials that complementary therapies (e.g. foods, acupuncture, hypnosis, spinal manipulation, herbal therapies) are as effective as conventional drug therapies.

The following non-pharmacological methods are effective:

- ✧ weight loss to achieve optimal weight and body shape
- ✧ reduction of salt intake to less than 5 g (1 teaspoonful) per day
- ✧ low-fat diet
- ✧ modest alcohol consumption (< 7 units per week for men and women). There is no controlled trial evidence on what is a 'safe' level of alcohol consumption. High levels of alcohol consumption lead to obesity and hypertension. The mode of action of alcohol on blood pressure is unclear
- ✧ cardiovascular exercise (e.g. 30 minutes of fast walking per day and avoidance of heavy isometric exercise)
- ✧ a diet rich in fruit and vegetables, rather than one with a high fat, salt and sugar content (as found in processed and 'ready meals')
- ✧ stopping smoking
- ✧ optimisation of lipids with drugs if necessary.

Treatment thresholds

These are based on an estimation of coronary heart disease risk.

> Effective antihypertensive treatment results in a relative risk reduction of 38% for stroke and 16% for coronary events.

The pros and cons of drug treatment have to be explained to patients who reach the treatment thresholds. Ultimately it is the responsibility of the patient to comply with the advice given, but additional consultations are helpful in addressing concerns that they or their family may have.

Choice of antihypertensive drug

The British Hypertension Society has provided useful information on indications and contraindications for different classes of antihypertensive drugs (*see* Table 5.4).

TABLE 5.4: Indications and contraindications of antihypertensive drugs

Class of drug	Indications	Contraindications
ACE inhibitors	Heart failure	Pregnancy
	Left ventricular dysfunction	Renovascular disease
	Diabetic nephropathy	PVD[b]
	Chronic renal disease[a]	Hyperkalaemia
	Previous MI	
	Metabolic syndrome	
	Diabetes	
β-blockers[c]	Myocardial infarction	Asthma/COAD
	Angina	Heart block
	Heart failure[d]	Bradycardia
	Women of childbearing age	Severe claudication
	Intolerance to ACE/ARB	Metabolic syndrome
	Atrial fibrillation	Diabetes
	Glaucoma	Athletes and physically active
Calcium-channel blockers (dihydropyridines)	Elderly ISH	
	Angina	
	Inadequate control with β-blockers	
	Claudication	
	Black people	
Calcium-channel blockers (rate-limiting)	Angina	Heart block
	Uncontrolled atrial fibrillation	Bradycardia
		Heart failure
Thiazides	Elderly	Gout
		Glucose intolerance
		Pregnancy
Alpha-blockers	Prostatism	Postural hypotension
	Dyslipidaemias	Urinary incontinence
Antialdosterone diuretic		Renal failure
		Hyperkalaemia

ISH, isolated systolic hypertension; ACE inhibitor, angiotensin-converting-enzyme inhibitor; ARB, angiotensin-receptor blocker; MI, myocardial infarction.

a ACE inhibitors may be beneficial in chronic renal failure, but should be used with caution, with monitoring of renal function and specialist advice if the patient has severe renal impairment.

b PVD (peripheral vascular disease) is a possible contraindication to ACE inhibitors because of its association with renal artery stenosis and renovascular disease.

c β-blockers can be continued in patients with well controlled hypertension if well tolerated, and should not be stopped in patients with angina or myocardial infarction.

d Use carefully (low dose to start with, and increasing slowly) in patients with significant left ventricular impairment or a history of heart failure.

Factors that influence the choice of antihypertensive drug

Table 5.4 provides useful clinical pointers when choosing an antihypertensive drug. The AB/CD rule is helpful when choosing drug combinations in hypertension, and refers to the first letter of the four main classes of drugs used.

Renin levels and hypertension

The recognition that younger (< 55 years) white patients are more likely to have vasoconstrictor, high-renin hypertension (type 1), whereas Afro-Caribbean and older white patients tend to have volume-dependent, high-salt, low-renin hypertension (type 2), provides a pathophysiological rationale for choosing antihypertensive drugs.

⬦ The high-renin, type 1 hypertensive patient should be treated with ACE inhibitors and/or angiotensin II antagonists (A) or β-blockers (B).

⬦ Low-renin, type 2 hypertensive patients (e.g. Afro-Caribbean patients) have too much salt. They are best treated with a diuretic (D), or if they have resistant hypertension, with two different diuretics. A calcium antagonist (C) can be added, and they should have a low-salt diet. β-blockers and ACE inhibitors may be ineffective as monotherapy, although these drugs may be used when combined with a drug that activates the renin–angiotensin system (e.g. diuretics, calcium antagonists or α-blockers).

⬦ For both types of hypertension, dietary measures are important. Compared with patients who have type 2 hypertension, salt restriction in patients with type 1 hypertension may not be as effective in reducing blood pressure.

Drug combinations

Drugs from different classes have additive effects when combined. Sub-maximal doses of two drugs may avoid or reduce side-effects from maximal doses of a single drug. The A or B + C or D rule applies.

Rational drug combinations are as follows:

⬦ a diuretic (D) + either a β-blocker (B) or an ACE inhibitor or angiotensin II antagonist (A), *or*

⬦ a calcium antagonist (C) + either a β-blocker (B) or an ACE inhibitor or angiotensin II antagonist (A)

⬦ if a third antihypertensive drug is necessary, a calcium antagonist (C) can be added to a diuretic (D) and ACE inhibitor (A) and to a diuretic (D) and β-blocker (B).

Less than half of all hypertensives will be controlled on one drug, and one-third of patients will require three or more drugs.

Recommendations for treatment of hypertension

⬦ In hypertensive patients over 55 years of age, or black patients of any age, the first choice for initial therapy should be either a calcium-channel blocker or a thiazide diuretic.

✦ In hypertensive patients under 55 years of age, the first choice for initial therapy should be an ACE inhibitor or an angiotensin-II receptor antagonist if the ACE inhibitor is not tolerated.

✦ If initial therapy was with a calcium-channel blocker or a thiazide diuretic, and a second drug is required, add an ACE inhibitor. If initial therapy was with an ACE inhibitor, add a calcium-channel blocker or a thiazide-type diuretic.

✦ If treatment with three drugs is required, the combination of an ACE inhibitor, a calcium-channel blocker and a thiazide diuretic should be used.

✦ If the blood pressure is still not controlled on three drugs, add a fourth drug (another diuretic, an α-blocker or a β-blocker). Careful monitoring of renal function is necessary if two diuretics are used.

✦ When blood pressure is not controlled, consider non-compliance. A specialist opinion may be required.

✦ β-blockers are no longer recommended for *initial* treatment of hypertension. They are used in young patients who cannot tolerate ACE inhibitors or angiotensin-II receptor antagonists, and in women of childbearing age. In these circumstances, a calcium-channel blocker should be added to the β-blocker.

✦ β-blockers do *not* need to be stopped in patients whose blood pressure is well controlled (< 140/90 mmHg).

✦ β-blockers should be continued in patients for whom there are compelling reasons for β-blockade (angina or myocardial infarction), unless there are significant side-effects.

✦ β-blocker doses should be reduced gradually.

✦ An ACE inhibitor would be appropriate for patients with diabetes and/or vascular disease.

✦ For patients with cardiac failure, a combination of a diuretic and an ACE inhibitor plus a β-blocker is appropriate.

✦ Dihydropyridine calcium antagonists can be used as an alternative to a diuretic in elderly patients with isolated systolic hypertension, and have been shown to prevent strokes.

✦ Drug treatment is generally for life.

Monitoring response to treatment

Follow-up is essential to assess the patient's response to treatment. The aim of treatment is to achieve the target blood pressure without intolerable side-effects. Some patients may need to be reviewed every few weeks initially. Six-monthly review is recommended for patients with well-controlled hypertension and no organ damage or renal impairment. Home recordings allow less frequent surgery review.

Follow-up allows the clinician to review all of the cardiovascular risk factors.

It may be possible to reduce antihypertensive medication in patients who were previously overweight and taking little exercise, but who have now become slim and fit.

Inappropriate drug combinations

The following drug combinations are not recommended:

✦ β-blocker + verapamil or diltiazem (bradycardia)

✦ ACE inhibitor + angiotensin II antagonist (renal failure and hyperkalaemia)

✦ potassium-sparing diuretic + ACE inhibitor.

Compliance

Drugs don't work if they are not taken.
Is treatment failure due to the drug or to the patient?

However appropriate and rational the choice of antihypertensive drugs, there is little chance of lowering the patient's blood pressure if they do not take their medication as prescribed. It is essential that patients understand why, despite feeling well, they need to take tablets as prescribed for life, and that medications may need to be increased if their blood pressure remains high.

Non-compliance is an important cause of failure to achieve blood pressure targets. Failure to recognise this leads to the clinician prescribing a higher dose of the prescribed medication or alternative additional tablets. Most patients take approximately 75% of doses as prescribed across a variety of medical disorders. Compliance does not correlate with intelligence, personality, age, education or the number of drugs prescribed. Compliance is probably increased just before and after surgery appointments. Whether it is affected by whom the patient sees (GP or practice nurse) is unclear.

Non-compliance should be suspected and explored as the first reason for persistent hypertension.

There are several reasons for non-compliance that may be viewed as 'part of human nature.'

- ◇ Non-compliance is more likely with frequent dosing during the day, and can be improved with once-daily dosing.
- ◇ Non-compliance may develop in previously compliant patients if they feel that the medication is not necessary or they become relaxed about their condition.
- ◇ Patients, particularly the elderly or those who are very busy, may simply forget to take the tablets at the prescribed times.
- ◇ Some patients may become lax and disinterested, perhaps because they feel that the medication is unnecessary.

Potential dangers of non-compliance

Patients may not take their tablets because they may be unconvinced that they need tablets for a condition that does not cause symptoms. Careful, and if necessary, repeated education is therefore important. Patients need to understand the risks of the condition and the benefits of treatment. The treatment side-effects may be intolerable. Non-compliance is a common cause of resistant hypertension. Omission of short-acting drugs (e.g. calcium antagonists, β-blockers or vasodilators such as doxazocin) may result in blood pressure surges with the risk of vascular events.

Improving drug compliance

Patient education is fundamental to compliance. The patient and their family must understand the risks of hypertension and the benefits to them of having their blood pressure controlled.

1. Select drugs that can be given together, preferably once a day and at a time that the patient will remember and schedule as part of their daily routine. Ask the patient what time of day they would prefer and would be more likely to remember their tablets. This depends on the patient having some routine to their day. This may be with their first cup of tea, with breakfast, on arriving at work or with lunch. Competent patients have to take responsibility for taking their medication. The patient's family can be helpful. Patients who travel frequently for work or social purposes need to establish a routine for taking their tablets.
2. Provide clear written information about the treatment and all non-pharmacological treatments.
3. Advise patients that self-recorded blood pressure recordings may help them to take an interest in their condition.
4. Warn patients about possible important side-effects, and advise them what to do if these occur. This is difficult because some patients attribute symptoms to the tablets. These problems can be dealt with at further reviews or by the practice nurse over the telephone.
5. Combination tablets, prescribed once a day, improve compliance.
6. Check compliance whenever the patient comes to the surgery.

Aspirin in hypertension

Treating a hypertensive patient with aspirin reduces cardiovascular events by 15% and myocardial infarction by 36%, but the benefit depends on the individual's absolute cardiovascular risk. The number of aspirin-related bleeds is similar to the number of cardiovascular events prevented by aspirin. Mortality is not affected. Therefore, aspirin confers only a marginal benefit.

Hypertension must be controlled before starting aspirin.

Aspirin is recommended in hypertension for primary prevention to patients:

✧ aged > 50 years with target organ damage (left ventricular hypertrophy, proteinuria or renal impairment) with no contraindication *and* a blood pressure level of < 150/90 mmHg
✧ with a 10-year coronary heart disease risk of > 15% (antihypertensive treatment reduces this risk by 25%, and aspirin will reduce this risk by a further 15%)
✧ with type 2 diabetes.

The numbers needed to treat analysis for aspirin:

✧ 90 hypertensive patients will need to be treated with aspirin for five years in order to prevent one cardiovascular complication
✧ 60 hypertensive patients will need to be treated with aspirin for five years in order to prevent one myocardial infarct

Aspirin is recommended in secondary prevention for patients with hypertension who have cardiovascular disease, provided that there is no excessive risk of bleeding.

Treating hypertension in diabetics

Hypertension is present in 70% of patients with type 2 diabetes, but its prevalence is not increased in patients with type 1 diabetes without nephropathy (microalbuminuria or proteinuria).

Insulin-treated diabetes without nephropathy

The threshold for drug intervention is > 140/90 mmHg.

Insulin-treated diabetes with nephropathy

Blood pressure reduction and ACE inhibitors slow the rate of decline in renal function and delay progression to nephropathy.

> ACE inhibitors are first-line treatment in diabetic patients, and should be given and titrated up to the maximum recommended and tolerated dose, even in patients who are normotensive.
> Statins should be considered to achieve target levels of cholesterol < 4.0 mmol/l and/or LDL < 2.0 mmol/l.

Patients should be given an angiotensin II blocker if they cannot tolerate an ACE inhibitor. The blood pressure targets are 130/80 or 125/75 mmHg if there is proteinuria or albuminuria, respectively. Patients should be considered for aspirin and a statin.

Non-insulin-treated diabetes

Hypertension is common, related to obesity and predictive of cardiovascular events.
Weight loss to the patient's optimum weight and daily exercise are fundamental aspects of treatment.
Most diabetic patients will need two antihypertensive drugs.

> Hypertension control in diabetic patients is more important than glycaemic control in improving survival. It reduces the incidence of cardiovascular events by 50%.
> The recommended threshold for intervention with antihypertensive drugs in type 2 diabetes is < 140/90 mmHg, and the target is < 130/80 mmHg.

The choice of drugs, apart from using an ACE inhibitor, does not appear to matter.
Patients with type 2 diabetes and nephropathy are at high risk from cardiovascular events, and all of their risk factors need vigorous attention. They should have aspirin. The target blood pressure is 130/75 mmHg.

Treating hypertension in patients with kidney disease

Renal impairment is a major additional risk factor. Statins and aspirin are used with antihypertensive medication to reduce cardiovascular risk.

> The target blood pressure level is < 130/80 mmHg.

Combination therapy is usually required.
An ACE inhibitor, with or without an angiotensin II receptor antagonist, is used to reduce proteinuria.

Lipid lowering in hypertension

Statins (with additional lipid-lowering drugs if necessary) are recommended to achieve a cholesterol concentration of < 4.0 mmol/l and an LDL concentration of < 2.0 mmol/l in:

✧ all hypertensive patients with cardiovascular disease and/or diabetes, *or*
✧ those whose 10-year cardiovascular risk is > 20%.

Hypertension after myocardial infarction

β-blockers are recommended for all patients without contraindications after myocardial infarction, and ACE inhibitors for patients with left ventricular systolic impairment and for diabetic patients. All vascular risk factors should be treated.

Hypertension in women

Blood pressure lowering is as beneficial in women as it is in men.

Oral contraceptives

All oral contraceptives, even those with a low oestrogen content, are associated with an increased risk of hypertension, stroke and myocardial infarction. The progestogen-only pill is an alternative option for women with hypertension, but there is little information on its influence on cardiovascular outcomes.

Hormone replacement therapy

The main indication for hormone replacement therapy (HRT) is for menopausal symptoms. HRT is not contraindicated in hypertensive women with severe flushing and other menopausal symptoms. It reduces the incidence of bone fractures and colon cancer, but is associated in certain high-risk groups with an increased risk of cardiovascular events, breast cancer, thromboembolism, gall-bladder disease and dementia. HRT is *not* recommended for cardiovascular protection in post-menopausal women.

Hypertension in pregnancy

Hypertension occurs in 10% of pregnancies, and is an important cause of maternal and fetal morbidity and mortality. It is associated with abruptio placentae and with cerebral haemorrhage in the mother, as well as fetal prematurity, stillbirth and neonatal death.

Hypertension may be the first sign of pre-eclampsia, which further increases the maternal and fetal risk and is characterised by significant proteinuria; oedema is no longer a diagnostic criterion. The mechanism of eclampsia remains unclear. It may lead to intrauterine growth restriction. The mother and the baby should be monitored carefully and may need referral to hospital if the blood pressure is not optimally controlled, if the baby is not growing or if there is proteinuria.

Hypertensive patients who become pregnant and those who develop hypertension during pregnancy should be referred to a cardiologist, who should liaise with obstetric colleagues to optimise management during pregnancy, delivery and postpartum.

Treatment thresholds during pregnancy

In the absence of evidence from randomised trials, treatment guidelines are based on observational studies, experience, and a reluctance to use drugs that could result in teratogenicity.

Blood pressure levels fall during pregnancy, so it may be possible to reduce or withdraw medication in patients with mild hypertension, although frequent monitoring is essential.

Hospitalisation may be necessary, and drug treatment is essential in patients with a blood pressure of < 170/110 mmHg. Drug treatment is also justified at levels of > 140/90 mmHg. The blood pressure should be measured and the urine checked for protein every week. If either of these is unsatisfactory, the patient should be referred to hospital.

All women with hypertension during pregnancy should be monitored after delivery to ascertain whether they need long-term treatment or further investigations.

White coat hypertension occurs in 30% of pregnant women. Ambulatory blood pressure recordings are very useful, and the confirmation of a normal or only slightly raised blood pressure can avoid unnecessary anxiety, treatment and hospital admissions in this large group of individuals.

Pre-eclampsia

Patients are usually symptom-free, and 30% of pre-eclamptic fits occur in the absence of a raised blood pressure or proteinuria.

The diagnostic criteria are as follows:

✧ a rise in blood pressure of 15 mmHg diastolic or > 30 mmHg systolic from early pregnancy, *or*
✧ a diastolic pressure of > 90 mmHg on two occasions four hours apart or a diastolic pressure of > 110 mmHg on one occasion and proteinuria.

Pre-eclampsia resolves with delivery, which has to be timed carefully to optimise fetal maturation.

Risk factors for pre-eclampsia include first pregnancy, change of partner, previous pre-eclampsia, family history of pre-eclampsia, idiopathic hypertension, chronic renal disease, diabetes, multiple pregnancy and obesity. Antihypertensive treatment has not been shown to improve fetal outcome.

> Patients with pre-eclampsia need urgent referral and treatment.

Choice of antihypertensive treatment in pregnancy

Methyldopa (750 mg to 4 g per day in three or four divided doses) remains the drug of choice because of its relatively low risk of side-effects and the long experience of its use. Other acceptable drugs include calcium antagonists and labetolol. Diuretics reduce plasma volume and may theoretically increase the risk of pre-eclampsia. ACE inhibitors are contraindicated because of the risk of renal malformation.

Hypertensive women who become or plan to become pregnant should switch to a drug regime that is recommended as safe during pregnancy, and switch back to their usual medication after delivery.

Calcium supplementation, fish oil and low-dose aspirin are not recommended. Low-dose aspirin may be used prophylactically in women with a history of early-onset pre-eclampsia.

Resistant hypertension

This can be defined as a blood pressure above target levels despite treatment with three drugs in adequate dosage, after ensuring that the blood pressure has been correctly and accurately measured, and making sure that the patient is taking their tablets. This can be very difficult to confirm. Apart from white coat syndrome, it is important to consider lack of exercise, obesity, high-salt diet, excess alcohol consumption (the quantity depends on the patient, their age, gender and other unknown factors), taking of other drugs (cocaine, liquorice, glucocorticoids, non-steroidal anti-inflammatory drugs), obstructive sleep apnoea, unsuspected secondary causes of hypertension, and volume overload.

These patients should be referred for a specialist opinion and investigation.

Treatment of resistant hypertension

Compliance must first be checked, contributing factors addressed and secondary causes of hypertension, particularly phaeochromocytoma, hyperaldosteronism (Conn's syndrome) and renal artery stenosis, excluded. Patients with a high aldosterone:renin ratio may respond to spironolactone.

For patients who are already on four or five drugs, minoxidil, a powerful vasodilator, is effective. Its side-effects include hirsutism (which may be welcomed in balding men).

A combination of a diuretic (D), a calcium antagonist (C), an ACE inhibitor (A) and/or an α-blocker is usually effective.

Hypertension in the elderly

Isolated systolic hypertension is common in elderly patients but may be overestimated by clinic readings, leading to excessive treatment and possible side-effects, including drug-related hypotension and falls. Thiazide diuretics, calcium antagonists and ACE inhibitors are useful and effective, and there is no clearly superior class of drug. Current guidelines recommend that renal function should be monitored if ACE inhibitors are used.

Ambulatory blood pressure recordings are helpful when evaluating this group of patients. Management of the elderly hypertensive patient is no different to that for the younger patient. Dose increases should be gradual.

Emergency treatment of hypertension

This is indicated for:

✧ hypertensive encephalopathy (most often due to eclampsia)
✧ left ventricular failure
✧ dissecting aortic aneurysm
✧ hypertension with an acute coronary syndrome
✧ hypertension due to recreational drugs (cocaine, amphetamines, ecstasy)
✧ pre-eclampsia or eclampsia.

Intravenous nitrate alone or with labetolol is useful for lowering blood pressure in acute aortic dissection. Nitroprusside (for a maximum of a few days only, due to cyanide toxicity) can be used for the other two causes.

Advice for patients

✧ High blood pressure is common and becomes more common with age.
✧ Treatment is generally for life. If you stop taking your tablets, your blood pressure will probably increase after a few months. It is possible that your blood pressure may increase even though you take your tablets, and you may need a change in your treatment.
✧ There is a difference between feeling 'hyper' or anxious and having the medical condition of hypertension or high blood pressure. It is quite possible that people who are 'hyper' or anxious or stressed may have a high blood pressure at the time when they feel 'hyper.' However, this is normal and expected. Hypertension is a condition where the blood pressure is high all the time, and that is why we need to measure your blood pressure throughout the day.

- If the blood pressure in your arteries is high, they are subjected to strain and become stiff and liable to get furred up. This hardening of the arteries affects all of your arteries, and this is why people with a high blood pressure get complications.
- Even though you may not feel unwell, your blood pressure is too high, and this can lead to stroke, heart attack, a weakening of the heart, kidney damage, loss of sight and an unnecessarily early death. If we lower your blood pressure, your risk is lowered.
- Even though we are quite good at lowering blood pressure with tablets, we still do not know the cause of high blood pressure in nearly 95% of the people affected by it. However, we do know that high blood pressure is more common in people who are overweight, who don't exercise enough, who drink too much alcohol (more than two units per day) or who eat too much salt.
- If you smoke you should stop, because smoking increases your risk of having a serious heart problem or stroke.
- High blood pressure also runs in families, and there are some other unusual causes that account for around 5% of cases.
- If you want to check your own blood pressure, buy a good-quality machine that you put around your arm, and follow the instructions carefully. Bring it with you to the surgery and we will check its accuracy. If you feel anxious, it is possible that your pressure will be high. It may be that you do have high blood pressure, but we need to be sure that your high blood pressure recordings are high enough for long enough to justify you taking blood pressure tablets for the rest of your life.
- Your blood pressure will fall if you lose weight until you reach your 'best' weight and do regular exercise. If your blood pressure remains high despite this, then you will probably need tablets.
- The decision to give you tablets is complex, and is not based solely on your blood pressure recordings. We estimate your risk of developing heart disease on the basis of a number of factors – for example, your age, whether you have diabetes or a high cholesterol level, whether you have had a heart attack or whether you have furring up of your heart arteries.
- Because high blood pressure does not go away, if you have this condition you will need to take tablets for life, particularly as blood pressure increases in all of us as we get older. In general, the lower the blood pressure the better.
- Most people need to take at least two different types of tablets. The key point of treatment is to take enough tablets to lower the blood pressure to a safe level. If you think that you have a side-effect to a tablet, come and see us and we will try to sort this out. There are several different tablets available, and we can usually find a combination that suits you, but we may not get the combination right at the first attempt!
- People with a low blood pressure live longer than those with a high pressure. A low blood pressure is not dangerous except if you feel faint when you stand up. The pressure needs to be lower than 90/60 mmHg before it results in you feeling light-headed. If you do feel like that, lie down quickly with your legs raised in the air. Come and see us and we will check this and see whether we need to adjust your tablets.
- People with controlled high blood pressure can and should lead a full and normal life. Driving, exercise and sports are to be encouraged.
- Holders of a passenger-carrying vehicle or large goods vehicle licence should inform the DVLA.
- Some men find that their sexual function deteriorates. If this happens, come to see us so that we can help. Sometimes it may be due to the tablets, but there are several causes that need to be investigated.
- Women who are on the oral contraceptive pill should have regular blood pressure checks (at least every six months), because some formulations of the pill increase

the blood pressure. The pill may need to be changed or stopped and another form of contraception used instead.

✧ Hypertensive women who are on HRT can continue with both treatments, but need to have their blood pressure checked.

✧ Women with high blood pressure who are pregnant need frequent blood pressure checks, and may need to have their tablets changed. In some women, the blood pressure is found to be high for the first time during pregnancy, and may remain high. Some women may need to be admitted to hospital for observation and treatment, or have their delivery induced before term.

Answers to questions about clinical cases

1. If a 24-hour blood pressure recording shows an average blood pressure of 135/85 mmHg or less, then the patient can be reassured and encouraged to exercise and lose weight. His blood sugar level will need review. If the 24-hour blood pressure recording is greater than 140/90 mmHg, he should be encouraged to pay serious attention to all of his risk factors and have another 24-hour blood pressure recording after he has lost weight and addressed all of the modifiable risk factors. If his blood pressure remains over 135/85 mmHg and a formal cardiovascular risk estimation indicates that he is at greater than 15% risk, he should be treated with either a thiazide or a β-blocker. Alternatively, if he is diagnosed as diabetic or cannot tolerate a β-blocker, he should be treated with an ACE inhibitor.

2. Treatment should be started immediately and the patient referred to hospital for further investigation.

3. If there is doubt about this patient's true daily blood pressure recordings, check her 24-hour recordings. If these show a sustained rise in diastolic pressure of 15 mmHg, or a rise in systolic pressure of more than 30 mmHg, then she fulfils the criteria for pre-eclampsia and should be referred to hospital for treatment and control. Treatment should be started if the blood pressure is > 170/110 mmHg, but many physicians would start treatment at a level of > 140/90 mmHg. Even if the result of the 24-hour recording is satisfactory, this patient's blood pressure should be monitored continually during pregnancy and after delivery, because it is likely that she will require treatment at some stage.

4. Explain to the patient the potential advantages of blood pressure control in reducing stroke, cardiovascular events, heart failure and dementia, and try her on a thiazide diuretic. Reducing her blood pressure is likely to prolong her active life. The target blood pressure level is 140/90 mmHg, and she may need an additional drug – for example, an ACE inhibitor.

5. Check the patient's blood pressure with an ambulatory recording. The target blood pressure for diabetics is < 130/80 mmHg. At this level there is a 50% reduction in cardiovascular events. If her blood pressure is not controlled, check her compliance, weight, diet and salt intake. Encourage her to exercise if she is able to do so. She should be gently reminded that she has a 30% risk of a cardiovascular event within 10 years. Combinations of an ACE inhibitor, β-blockers, dihydropyridine calcium-channel blockers, thiazide diuretics and α-blockers are all suitable. It is important to address all cardiovascular risk factors. It is clearly going to be difficult for this patient to achieve her blood pressure targets, and she will need help, encouragement and regular monitoring.

6. Yes, so long as there are no side-effects.

FURTHER READING

ALLHAT Officers and Coordinators for the ALLHAT Collaborative Research Group. Major outcomes in high-risk patients randomised to angiotensin-converting-enzyme inhibitor or calcium-channel blocker vs diuretic. The Antihypertensive and Lipid-Lowering Treatment to Prevent Heart Attack Trial (ALLHAT). *JAMA*. 2002; **288**: 2981–97.

August P. Initial treatment of hypertension. *NEJM*. 2003; **348**: 610–17.

Benetos, A, Thomas F, Bean K *et al.* Prognostic value of systolic and diastolic blood pressure in treated hypertensive men. *Arch Intern Med*. 2002; **162**: 577–81.

Blood Pressure Lowering Treatment Trialists Collaboration. Effects of angiotensin-converting-enzyme inhibitors, calcium antagonists and other blood-pressure-lowering drugs on mortality and major cardiovascular morbidity. *Lancet*. 2000; **356**: 1955–64.

Brown M. Matching the right drug to the right patient in essential hypertension. *Heart*. 2001; **86**: 113–20.

Brown MJ, Palmer CR, Castaigne A *et al.* Morbidity and mortality in patients randomised to double-blind treatment with once daily calcium channel blockade or diuretic in the International Nifedipine GITS Study: Intervention as a Goal in Hypertension Treatment (INSIGHT). *Lancet*. 2000; **356**: 366–72.

Clement DL, De Buyzere ML, De Bacquer DA *et al.* Prognostic value of ambulatory blood-pressure recordings in patients with treated hypertension. *NEJM*. 2003; **348**: 2407–15.

Fourth Joint Task Force of the European Society of Cardiology and Other Societies on Cardiovascular Disease Prevention in Clinical Practice (constituted by representatives of nine societies and by invited experts). European guidelines on cardiovascular disease prevention in clinical practice: executive summary. *Eur Heart J*. 2007; **28**: 2375–414.

Franklin SS, Khan SA, Wong ND *et al.* Is pulse pressure useful in predicting risk for coronary heart disease? The Framingham heart study. *Circulation*. 1999; **100**: 354–60.

Heart Outcomes Prevention Evaluation Study Investigators. Effects of ramipril on cardiovascular and microvascular outcomes in people with diabetes mellitus: results of the HOPE study and MICRO-HOPE substudy. *Lancet*. 2000; **355**: 253–9.

National Collaborating Centre for Chronic Conditions. *Hypertension. Management of hypertension in adults in primary care: partial update*. Update of NICE Clinical Guideline 18 (published in August 2004). London: National Collaborating Centre for Chronic Conditions; 2006.

O'Brien E. Ambulatory blood pressure monitoring in the management of hypertension. *Heart*. 2003; **89**: 571–6.

Pickering T. How common is white coat hypertension? *JAMA*. 1988; **259**: 225–8.

Ramsay LE, Williams B, Johnston GD *et al.* BHS Guidelines. Guidelines for the management of hypertension: report of the Third Working Party of the British Hypertension Society. *J Hum Hypertens*. 1999; **13**: 569–92.

Van Jaarsveld BC, Krijnen P, Pieterman H *et al.* The effect of balloon angioplasty on hypertension in atherosclerotic renal-artery stenosis. *NEJM*. 2000; **342**: 1007–14.

Wing LMH, Reid CM, Ryan P *et al.* A comparison of outcomes with angiotensin-converting-enzyme inhibitors and diuretics for hypertension in the elderly. *NEJM*. 2003; **348**: 583–92.

Heart failure

six

Clinical cases

1. An 81-year-old hypertensive woman complains of exertional breathlessness and ankle swelling but has normal left ventricular function on echocardiography. What do you do?
2. A 68-year-old man develops a dry unpleasant cough six months after starting an angiotensin-converting-enzyme inhibitor? What do you do?
3. A 76-year-old man with heart failure develops dizziness and breathlessness after starting a β-blocker. What do you do?
4. The creatinine level increases to twice the normal level in a 71-year-old man with peripheral vascular disease and hypertension, shortly after increasing the dose of an angiotensin-converting-enzyme inhibitor. What do you do?
5. A 73-year-old man with a dilated cardiomyopathy requires repeated hospital treatment for deteriorating heart failure. What do you do?
6. A 69-year-old woman develops hyperkalaemia. What do you do?

Importance of heart failure in primary care

There are nearly one million people with heart failure in the UK, and most of them are treated exclusively in primary care. The incidence and prevalence of heart failure are increasing principally because heart failure increases with age. People are living longer, partly due to public health measures, success in treating infections, cancer screening and treatment, widespread public recognition of the importance of lifestyle changes combined with improved management of cardiovascular risk factors, and improved treatment and survival after myocardial infarction.

Patients are living longer with heart failure due to improved drug and non-pharmacological treatment. Nevertheless, heart failure becomes more common with increasing age due to age-related decreases in the power of the heart.

End-stage or terminal heart failure is one of the leading causes of death in the elderly. It has a one-year mortality rate of 50%, and requires special management.

Primary care clinicians are now familiar with national guidance on the management of heart failure, and some practices have well organised multi-disciplinary services.

Specialist heart failure nurses provide domiciliary care, and this improves the quality of care and reduces the rate of hospital admissions for decompensated heart failure. Patients with decompensated heart failure can be identified and their treatment adjusted.

Treatment complexities in the management of heart failure

A greater proportion of patients with heart failure will be older and more likely to have coexisting morbidity. Memory impairment, difficulty in remembering to take tablets, difficulty in opening tablet bottles and containers, and confusion about which tablets to take all result in non-compliance with medication. Management is complicated by coexisting medical conditions and their treatments, including diabetes and renal impairment, valve disease and widespread vascular disease.

Factors that improve the community management of heart failure

Most GPs will have responsibility for the management of at least 20 patients with heart failure, and this figure will probably increase.

More patients can and should be diagnosed, treated and monitored in the community by well trained, experienced and energetic multi-disciplinary teams who are familiar with all aspects of heart failure management, and aware of the potential medical and psychological problems involved. They should be alert to situations where specialist referral is advisable. The management of heart failure in the community is improved by good communication between secondary and primary care. There should be accessible and prompt echocardiography, and links to expert subspecialty cardiology services offering electrophysiology for arrhythmia management, biventricular pacing and cardiac defibrillators, cardiac surgery and specialist nurse services.

Specialist nurses can provide:

◇ medical and lifestyle advice and information regarding fluid and food intake, smoking cessation, blood pressure control, diet, weight control, exercise and cardiovascular risk factor management
◇ psychological support and identification of patients who require assessment for antidepressants or other forms of therapy and support
◇ support and education for carers about heart failure management
◇ advice about contraception and vaccination. It is recommended that patients with heart failure should be offered an annual vaccination against flu and the single vaccination against pneumococcal disease
◇ domiciliary visits to check the clinical status, heart rhythm and fluid status, to measure weight, to ensure drug compliance and to recognise clinical deterioration that necessitates a change in medication or specialist review.

What is heart failure?

Heart failure is a syndrome resulting from any structural or functional disorder that affects the heart.

Although the long-term prognosis of heart failure remains poor despite advances in medical and non-pharmacological therapy, much may be done to reduce its incidence and progression and to improve the quality of life of the growing proportion of the population who have this common condition.

The most common type is *systolic heart failure*, usually due to impaired left ventricular contraction. This affects all age groups, mainly males, and often results from myocardial infarction and hypertension. The left ventricle is usually dilated and the ejection fraction reduced.

Diastolic heart failure occurs in around 40% of patients, and is due to abnormal filling of the ventricles. The haemodynamic and clinical consequences are similar to those of systolic heart failure. Patients with diastolic heart failure are typically elderly, female, obese, hypertensive and diabetic, and in contrast to patients with systolic heart failure, have preserved or normal left ventricular size, systolic function and ejection fraction. The diagnosis is made by finding clinical features of heart failure with normal systolic function on echocardiography, but signs of abnormal ventricular filling due to diastolic impairment.

'Remodelling' of the ventricle

The increased pressure on the left ventricle ultimately distorts its shape, and this reduces its pumping efficiency and power. The left ventricle changes from an ellipse to a round sphere. This is called remodelling, and it signifies an important reduction in left ventricular performance, a worse prognosis and usually significant symptoms. Once this occurs, most patients deteriorate quickly and die, despite medication.

'Reverse remodelling' of the ventricle

A remodelled failing ventricle can occasionally 'remodel.' Medical treatments (ACE inhibitors, angiotensin II blockers, β-blockers and aldosterone blockers) and cardiac resynchronisation devices may temporarily halt, or slow and, less commonly, in some cases, reverse the pathophysiological processes in patients with remodelled hearts, with normalisation of the ventricular shape and consequent improved function. This is called reverse remodelling. It has been reported with a combination of phosphodiesterase inhibitors and β-blockers, and with an implanted left ventricular assist device that 'unloads' the left ventricle.

Diagnostic criteria for heart failure

The European Society of Cardiology criteria for the diagnosis of heart failure are as follows:
✧ appropriate symptoms and/or signs of heart failure
✧ objective evidence of cardiac dysfunction on echocardiography and electro-cardiography
✧ appropriate response to treatment.

Clinical features of heart failure

Symptoms include:
✧ shortness of breath on exercise and in severe cases, at rest
✧ fatigue
✧ fluid retention.

Signs include:
✧ tachycardia
✧ raised jugular venous pressure
✧ added heart sounds
✧ pulmonary crackles
✧ ankle, leg and sacral swelling.

Diagnosing heart failure

Heart failure should be suspected if a patient has relevant symptoms and/or signs. However, the sensitivity of clinical features in diagnosis is poor. For example, oedema and orthopnoea have a sensitivity of only 20%. Their specificity is 80%.
    Conditions causing breathlessness and leg swelling:
✧ obesity
✧ chronic airways disease should be excluded on clinical grounds, chest X-ray and spirometry
✧ venous hypertension in the leg veins due to venous valve incompetence
✧ kidney disease

✧ liver disease
✧ severe anaemia.

Heart failure suspected because of symptoms and signs

Assess presence of cardiac disease by ECG, chest X-ray or brain natriuretic peptide

Normal:
heart failure
unlikely

Abnormal: echocardiography

Normal:
heart failure
unlikely
? diastolic heart
failure

Abnormal:

• Assess aetiology, severity, precipitating and correctable factors
• Additional tests where appropriate
• Consider referral

Choose treatment

FIGURE 6.1: Algorithm for the diagnosis of heart failure based on guidelines from the European Society of Cardiology.

Classification of heart failure

Until recently, patients with heart failure were categorised according to their functional limitation using the New York Heart Association (NYHA) classification. This classification does not take into account their risk factors for heart failure. Patients in NYHA class IV may after treatment revert to class III, although their underlying pathology remains unchanged.

A new classification published by the American College of Cardiology and the American Heart Association emphasises the evolution and progression of heart failure, highlights prevention strategies and superimposes treatment strategies. Four stages have been described.

✧ Stage A: The patient is at high risk for developing heart failure but has no structural heart abnormality.
✧ Stage B: The patient has a structural heart abnormality but has never had symptoms of heart failure.
✧ Stage C: The patient has a structural heart abnormality and current or previous symptoms of heart failure.
✧ Stage D: The patient has end-stage heart failure that is refractory to standard treatment and requires special intervention.

Although patients may show an improvement in their NYHA class, they can only deteriorate in class using the new staging classification that is analogous to staging of cancer.

Investigations

The most important and useful investigation is *echocardiography*, which may show either global (e.g. in a dilated cardiomyopathy) or regional (e.g. after myocardial infarction) ventricular wall movement abnormality. Echocardiography can distinguish systolic and diastolic heart failure with assessments of systolic function and diastolic filling patterns.

✧ Left ventricular chamber size measurement is useful when evaluating severity and prognosis, and provides a baseline. The different types of cardiomyopathy can more or less be diagnosed with echocardiography. Amyloid is an uncommon cause of heart failure and has characteristic echocardiographic features.

✧ Mitral and/or aortic valve disease should be excluded. Occasionally heart failure may be caused by infective endocarditis, which may be difficult to diagnose clinically.

✧ Using Doppler, estimate the pulmonary artery pressure. In pulmonary hypertension, the Doppler echocardiography estimate of the peak tricuspid regurgitant velocity is > 2.8m/s. In severe pulmonary hypertension, the right ventricle is dilated. There are several causes of pulmonary hypertension, most commonly left heart conditions, chronic lung disease and pulmonary emboli. Pulmonary arterial hypertension is rare but should be considered in all patients with unexplained breathlessness.

✧ A 12-lead electrocardiogram is usually normal in patients with stage A heart failure, but is rarely normal in patients with stage B, C or D heart failure. It may show atrial fibrillation or ectopic beats, signs of myocardial infarction, left ventricular hypertrophy and ST- and T-wave changes, conduction abnormalities or bundle branch block. These findings are important diagnostically and prognostically. Patients who have left bundle branch block and stage C and D heart failure should be considered for cardiac resynchronisation therapy.

✧ A chest X-ray may show an enlarged heart shadow, signs of pulmonary oedema and pleural effusions. Heart failure may develop in susceptible patients as a result of a chest infection or pneumonia.

✧ Blood tests: Check the renal function, glucose, blood count, thyroid function, liver function and blood lipids.

✧ Urinalysis: Check for protein and glucose.

✧ Brain natriuretic peptide (BNP) is a hormone released from the cardiac ventricles in response to stretch and dilatation, and is increased in patients with right or left heart systolic or diastolic failure of any cause. BNP levels rise with age.

It can now be measured in primary care. This facility for 'point of care testing' would reduce the number of patients who need to be referred for a consultation or for echocardiography with suspected heart failure. It would provide rapid results, allowing rapid changes in therapy.

— A widely accepted cut-off value for BNP is 100 pg/l.

— Heart failure can be ruled out in a patient with symptoms suggestive of heart failure if the BNP level is normal.

— If the BNP concentration is raised, there is a strong possibility that the patient has heart failure, for which they should be investigated with echocardiography.

A raised BNP level in a patient with normal ventricular systolic function on echocardiography is compatible with diastolic heart failure, left ventricular hypertrophy, unstable angina or pulmonary hypertension.

BNP measurements are helpful in confirming the diagnosis of heart failure, in triaging patients with suggestive symptoms for echocardiography and screening patients at risk of having heart failure. BNP levels decrease after effective treatment of heart failure.

The severity, cause, precipitating factors, risk factors, type of cardiac dysfunction and underlying cardiac structural abnormality should be defined.

Other tests (e.g. coronary angiography) may be required. The stage of heart failure is then classified and treatment is started.

Causes of heart failure

The common causes of heart failure in the UK, accounting for over 90% of cases, are coronary heart disease (ischaemia and myocardial infarction) and hypertension. Congestive heart failure is a term used to describe combined right and left heart failure. Right heart failure due to chronic obstructive airways disease is also common.

Hypertension	
Coronary heart disease ischaemia and infarction	
Cardiomyopathy	There are several types classified according to the echocardiographic appearance: • dilated – alcohol, post partum, viral, chemotherapy • hypertrophic – familial and genetic • restrictive – amyloid, sarcoid
Valvular heart disease	Mitral valve disease Aortic valve disease Congenital heart disease Atrial septal defect Ventricular septal defect

BOX 6.1: Causes of left heart failure.

Any cause of left heart failure. The increased pulmonary venous pressure is tranmitted to the pulmonary arteries and right ventricle.

Chronic airways disease (cor pulmonale)

Pulmonary emboli

Pulmonary arterial hypertension. When suspected, patients should be referred to a specialist centre.

BOX 6.2: Causes of right heart failure due to pulmonary hypertension.

Risk factors for heart failure

Effective management of hypertension and vascular risk factors is important and effective in preventing heart failure.

Hypertension

Even moderate hypertension increases the risk of developing heart failure; lowering blood pressure reduces the risk. Effective treatment of hypertension decreases the left ventricular hypertrophy and cardiovascular mortality, and reduces the incidence of heart failure by 30–50%. Diastolic blood pressure should be reduced below 80 mmHg in people at risk, particularly in diabetics.

Left ventricular hypertrophy

This is independent of hypertension and predicts the risk of developing heart failure.

Smoking

This is an independent and strong predictor of heart failure.

Hyperlipidaemia

A raised triglyceride level, or a high ratio of total cholesterol to high-density-lipoprotein cholesterol, is associated with an increased incidence of heart failure. Lipid lowering with statins reduces the risk of developing heart failure.

Diabetes mellitus

This is an independent risk factor for heart failure, present in around 20% of patients. It predicts death in high-risk patients who have a left ventricular ejection fraction of < 35%.

Microalbuminuria

Patients with an albumin:creatinine ratio of > 2 mg/mmol have a greater risk of developing heart failure than those with a normal albumin:creatinine ratio.

Obesity

This is an independent risk factor for heart failure – weight loss reduces the risk and helps to correct lipid abnormalities and associated hypertension.

Asymptomatic left ventricular dysfunction

This is an independent risk factor for heart failure and death, and occurs in around 1–5% of the adult population, depending on their risk profile. This highlights the interest in early diagnosis with echocardiography, although there is no evidence as yet that screening and treatment are beneficial, except perhaps in high-risk individuals.

Age spectrum of patients with heart failure

The median age at presentation is 74 years. Heart failure is rare in young people, and the prevalence increases with age. The prevalence is around 1 in 35 people aged 65–74 years, 1 in 15 in people aged 75–84 years and 1 in 7 among people aged 85 years or over.

Prognosis of heart failure

The prognosis of heart failure depends on several factors, principally the age of the patient, the severity of left ventricular impairment, coronary artery disease, vascular disease and other comorbidity, including renal function and diabetes (*see* Boxes 6.3 and 6.4). The prognosis of mild heart failure in a young patient with stage A heart failure is good, whereas the one-year mortality rate in an elderly patient with stage D heart failure is 50%.

Prompt intervention and correction of treatable, mechanical causes of heart failure improve the prognosis (e.g. valve surgery in severe aortic stenosis).

Recognition and haemodynamic resuscitation of patients with the uncommon condition of heart failure due to acute viral myocarditis may be life-saving.

Patients with chronic heart failure have a worse prognosis than patients with breast, prostate or colon cancer, with percentage survival rates of 67%, 41% and 24% at one, two and three years, respectively.

Age	
Genetic background	
Gender	
Coexisting conditions	Vascular disease
	Diabetes mellitus
	Hypertension
	Renal impairment
	Coronary artery disease
	Anaemia
	Obesity
	Sleep apnoea
	Depression
	Lung disease
Lifestyle	Smoking
	Alcohol

BOX 6.3: Non-cardiac factors that affect the prognosis in patients with heart failure.

Degree of left and/or ventricular damage (ejection fraction)	
Left ventricular hypertrophy	
Extent of myocardial ischaemia	
Hibernating myocardium	
Severity of coronary artery disease	
Valvular disease	Mitral regurgitation
	Aortic stenosis

BOX 6.4: Cardiac factors that affect the prognosis in patients with heart failure.

Effects of interventions in heart failure

The prognosis and quality of life for patients with heart failure remain poor, but have improved with new pharmacological and non-pharmacological treatments.

The prognosis of patients with heart failure enrolled in trials differs from those observed in the community. Clinical trials of ACE inhibitors, angiotensin-receptor antagonists, spironolactone, biventricular pacing, coronary artery surgery and multi-disciplinary teams have been shown to reduce the rate of hospital admissions and to reduce mortality or improve functional ability. However, data from large observational epidemiological surveys, such as the Framingham study, has not shown that the death rate from heart failure has changed significantly. This difference may be explained by the way patients in clinical trials are selected and their medication, compliance and clinical state are carefully monitored.

Economic benefits of reducing hospital care for patients with heart failure

It is estimated that heart failure, with all its management and treatment components both in hospital and in the community, accounts for 2% of all health expenditure in the UK, and this figure may become much higher in future with the introduction of expensive electrophysiological assessment and interventions including pacing and cardiac surgery. Heart failure is the cause of approximately 20% of all hospital admissions, and is consequently a major drain on healthcare resources.

Improving the effectiveness of care in the community reduces healthcare costs by reducing the frequency and duration of hospital readmissions, and also improves the morale and self-confidence of patients. A number of organisational factors have been shown to be effective and allow a greater proportion of patients to be treated comfortably and safely at home. These include:

◇ education and training of GPs and nurses in cardiovascular medicine and heart failure
◇ open access hospital echocardiography and portable domiciliary echocardiography
◇ increasing confidence among primary care clinicians in diagnosing heart failure and initiating treatment when appropriate with β-blockers, ACE inhibitors and spironolactone
◇ the establishment of hospital-based and primary care nurse-led clinics and multi-disciplinary teams providing domiciliary services. Nurses are trained in examination, weighing, dietary advice and blood testing
◇ careful and detailed continuing review of patients' drug treatment and non-pharmacological treatment
◇ recognising when patients need admission to hospital and when they need domiciliary visits by trained nurses.

Treatment of heart failure patients at home

Patients should be treated at home if it is safe, clinically appropriate and there is adequate social support. Bed rest is helpful for relieving symptoms by reducing heart rate and workload, but prolonged periods of bed rest, particularly in elderly patients, increase the risk of venous thrombosis and embolism, pressure sores, chest infection, depression and weakness of the arms and legs, making rehabilitation difficult.

Patients should be given subcutaneous fractionated heparin to reduce the thrombotic risk. Warfarin is used for patients in atrial fibrillation. The other medical treatments are discussed below.

A large proportion of patients with severe, refractory heart failure with co-morbidity will need to be readmitted to hospital for intense medical treatment (*see* Box 6.5).

Haemodynamic decompensation with pulmonary oedema or leg swelling	Deterioration in cardiac function, may be precipitated by β-blockers New myocardial infarct or ischaemia drugs that suppress cardiac function (β-blockers, verapamil) Arrhythmia, most commonly atrial fibrillation and heart block New or increasing mitral regurgitation
Right heart decompensation	Chest infection Pulmonary emboli Arrhythmia
Failure to take prescribed medication, most commonly diuretics	
Renal impairment	
Physical deterioration	Falls Weakness Stroke Inadequate social support at home
Other coexisting medical problems	
Depression, fear and anxiety	

BOX 6.5: Reasons why patients with compensated heart failure may deteriorate.

Management of acute heart failure

Patients who become very breathless should be admitted to hospital urgently. They may have had an acute myocardial infarction, pulmonary embolus or deterioration in previously stable heart failure, possibly due to an arrhythmia. Other causes of acute breathlessness, including chest infection, asthma or pneumothorax, should be investigated.

In acute myocardial infarction, the prognosis depends on the severity of left ventricular damage. Over 90% of patients with cardiogenic shock – the triad of low cardiac output, hypotension (systolic blood pressure < 90 mmHg) and oliguria – die in hospital. In contrast, the mortality of patients with myocardial infarction but no signs of heart failure is around 5%. Other causes of acute heart failure include acute decompensation of chronic heart failure.

The principles of management of patients with heart failure are to:
- relieve symptoms and improve myocardial and tissue oxygenation with oxygen (nasal continuous positive airway pressure – CPAP) and sit them up
- relieve symptoms and improve haemodynamics with diamorphine and intravenous diuretics
- treat significant arrhythmias
- maintain the circulation with inotropes, or with intra-aortic balloon pumping in severe cases
- improve the cardiac output by improving myocardial blood flow and oxygenation with thrombolysis or, if possible, primary coronary angioplasty.

Short-term infusions of positive inotropes (dobutamine with or without dopamine to improve renal perfusion) may be used in severe cardiac decompensation. Prolonged use of inotropes does not improve survival. Milrinone and enoximone increase mortality.

The reasons for the patient's deterioration should be investigated together with a re-evaluation of renal and cardiac function. Expert opinions may need to be sought for patients who might benefit from angioplasty, cardiac surgery and electrophysiological evaluation with a view to biventricular pacing and implantable defibrillators. Suitable patients with stage D heart failure require evaluation at a specialised centre for cardiac transplantation. Although this procedure is restricted to only a small fraction of the heart failure population because of the limited number of donor hearts, the long-term results are good.

The patient's social circumstances will need to be reviewed with the primary care team – this is another example of the importance of good communication and co-operation between the hospital and primary care teams, in order to provide seamless, co-ordinated care with the aim of returning the patient to their home safely and with the necessary support. Patients, their families and carers should be educated about the condition, and the reason for their deterioration explained. Advice should be given about lifestyle.

Pathological processes associated with hypertension and the rationale of heart failure treatment

Rational treatment of the syndrome of heart failure demands an understanding of its complex interrelated biochemical, neuroendocrine, structural and haemodynamic consequences. Drugs and pacing are used to target several pathological processes that result from heart failure.

Loop diuretics (e.g. furosemide, bumetanide, torasemide) reduce fluid accumulation. They are an important part of the treatment of stage C and D heart failure, and in patients where there is fluid retention or a history of fluid retention.

Thiazide diuretics (e.g. bendroflumethiazide, indapamide, metolazone) are moderately potent diuretics. They inhibit sodium reabsorption at the beginning of the distal convoluted tubule. They are effective when combined with a loop diuretic for resistant oedema. They may increase the levels of glucose and uric acid (precipitating acute attacks of gout), and lower sodium levels.

The combination of a loop diuretic and a thiazide diuretic may cause severe dehydration and renal and electrolyte disturbance. Low intermittent doses are useful, particularly in elderly patients who have renal impairment. As part of self-management of their heart failure, patients can be taught to weigh themselves and to take a thiazide diuretic if their weight increases. Biochemical monitoring is important.

ACE inhibitors and *angiotensin-receptor antagonists* are powerful vasodilators. They block the renin–angiotensin–aldosterone system, reduce salt retention by decreasing aldosterone levels (in common with the aldosterone antagonist, spironolactone), prevent the deleterious vasoconstriction and myocardial hypertrophy induced by angiotensin II, and prevent the degradation of bradykinin, which is a vasodilator and increases fluid excretion.

β-blockers (e.g. carvedilol, bisoprolol, metoprolol) are used to block production by the sympathetic nervous system of the cathecholamines (adrenaline and noradrenaline) and other vasoactive substances that trigger vasoconstriction, tachycardia, and deleterious ventricular remodelling and dilatation. They are used in patients with symptomatic, stable heart failure in conjunction with ACE inhibitors and diuretics. β-blockers decrease the rate of hospitalisation and mortality, and improve symptoms and functional class. They are used in patients with stable heart failure, and are started at a low dose and increased slowly to the maximum tolerated dose. Side-effects include deterioration of symptoms due to increasing heart failure, bradycardia and hypotension.

Aldosterone antagonists (e.g. spironolactone, eplerenone) potentiate the effects of thiazides and loop diuretics by antagonising aldosterone, with consequent hyperkalaemia and hyponatraemia. They are recommended for patients with stage C and D heart failure as adjunctive treatment to ACE inhibitors, β-blockers and diuretics. Electrolytes must be monitored. The side-effects of spironolactone include gastrointestinal disturbances, impotence and gynaecomastia. The side-effects of eplerenone include diarrhoea, nausea and hypotension.

Digoxin is a weak inotrope that slows the ventricular rate in atrial fibrillation by slowing conduction through the atrioventricular node. The risk of toxicity is high in the elderly and in patients with co-morbidity and renal impairment.

Hydralazine and *isosorbide* decrease afterload and preload, reducing cardiac work.

Cardiac resynchronisation using biventricular pacing improves left ventricular function.

Exercise improves peripheral blood flow and skeletal muscle physiology.

Anaemia is common, and is associated with decreased functional activity, worsening symptoms and increased mortality. It results from renal insufficiency and plasma volume overload. Treatment with *erythropoietin* results in improved symptoms and left ventricular ejection fraction.

Warfarin is indicated for established atrial fibrillation, a previous thromboembolic event or a mobile left ventricular thrombus.

Structural and electrical consequences of heart failure
Myocardial remodelling

This is the term used to describe the dilatation and change in shape of the heart, which leads to impaired myocardial function due to fibrosis, hypertrophy and loss of myocytes. The most common condition is myocardial infarction resulting in ventricular scarring, but remodelling also occurs in cardiomyopathy, hypertension and valvular heart disease. It is important because interventions that result in reverse remodelling and a return to a more normal heart shape and size improve cardiac function, symptoms and prognosis. Examples include ACE inhibitors, β-blockers and cardiac resynchronisation with biventricular pacing .

Mitral regurgitation

Mitral regurgitation is another consequence of left ventricular dilatation, and results in further cardiac enlargement due to volume overload. Correction of primary mitral regurgitation by valve repair or replacement can be beneficial in selected patients.

Arrhythmias and bundle branch block

Myocardial ischaemia, fibrosis and atrial dilatation may result in atrial fibrillation, which can precipitate heart failure and stroke. It is important to diagnose this promptly and treat patients with warfarin to reduce the risk of stroke.

Amiodarone is useful for treating supraventricular and ventricular tachycardias and it may, if the arrhythmia has occurred recently and the heart is not dilated, restore sinus rhythm. It is also used to improve the chances of successful electrical cardioversion in patients with atrial fibrillation. It does not improve survival in chronic heart failure, and is not indicated for primary prevention of arrhythmias. Side-effects include nausea and vomiting, taste disturbance, bradycardia, hyper- and hypothyroidism, corneal deposits, photosensitivity, hepatitis, pulmonary fibrosis, and peripheral neuropathy and myopathy. Low doses reduce the risk of side effects

Cardiac resynchronisation

Left bundle branch block is caused by ischaemia and fibrosis of the conducting tissue, and is a major predictor of sudden death due to ventricular arrhythmias. It occurs in at least 30% of patients with heart failure. It results in abnormal and discoordinated cardiac contraction and relaxation, with delayed opening and closure of the mitral and aortic valves. This leads to a reduction in ejection fraction, cardiac output and blood pressure. Biventricular pacing is used to restore synchronous ventricular contraction, improve ventricular function and exercise capacity, and reduce the need for hospital readmissions (see below).

Management of patients with heart failure
Treatment of patients with stage A heart failure
The aim is to prevent ventricular remodelling. Risk factor control and the interventions and principles discussed below should be used for patients with all stages of heart failure.

Risk factor control
Active and effective management of risk factors for heart failure is very important, and should be continually emphasised to patients and their families. The following can improve prognosis and quality of life:
✧ weight loss to an optimal level
✧ individually prescribed exercise
✧ control of hypertension
✧ treatment of hyperlipidaemia
✧ smoking cessation
✧ a low-salt diet
✧ tight diabetic control.

Alcohol should be consumed only in moderation, because it increases weight and can be arrhythmogenic in patients with more advanced stages of heart failure and structural heart disease. It should be avoided in patients with alcoholic cardiomyopathy.

Angiotensin-converting-enzyme inhibitors
ACE inhibitors improve survival and reduce by 20% the incidence of myocardial infarction and stroke in asymptomatic, high-risk patients with diabetes or vascular disease and no history of heart failure.

There is probably no significant difference between the different types of ACE inhibitors. They act by decreasing the conversion of angiotensin I to angiotensin II, which has deleterious effects including vasoconstriction, salt retention and induction of cardiac hypertrophy. ACE inhibitors also potentiate the effects of bradykinin, which is a vasodilator and causes water loss via the kidneys.

ACE inhibitors have several beneficial effects both in patients with chronic heart failure and in those with heart failure complicating myocardial infarction.

They:
✧ improve survival by 20%
✧ reduce progression to heart failure
✧ reduce the frequency of readmission to hospital by 33%
✧ improve symptoms
✧ improve cardiac performance
✧ reverse remodelling.

ACE inhibitors should be given to patients with all stages of heart failure.

The most common side-effect is a dry cough, which occurs in around 20% of patients and is thought to be due to increased levels of bradykinin. Occasionally the cough may resolve if the ACE inhibitor is stopped and another one substituted for it. Switching to an angiotensin-receptor antagonist usually solves the problem. Other ACE inhibitor adverse effects include hypotension, renal failure, hyperkalaemia and angio-oedema. These adverse effects may be avoided if the ACE inhibitor is started at a low dose and gradually titrated upward. Because ACE inhibitors are very useful, it is important to be sure that the patient's symptoms are genuine side-effects of the drug.

ACE inhibitors should be started at a low dose, and the dose should then be doubled every two weeks. *The highest tolerated dose of ACE inhibitor should be used.* High-dose ACE inhibition is superior to low-dose treatment in reducing the combined end-point of death and hospital readmission, although there is no good evidence that ACE inhibitors reduce the rate of sudden death.

ACE inhibitors can usually be started safely by GPs and 'first-dose hypotension' avoided if the first dose is low, and started when the patient goes to bed, not over-diuresed and dehydrated.

Patients should be monitored by recording lying and standing blood pressure, renal function and serum electrolytes (the potassium level may increase) at regular intervals, depending on their age and baseline levels. Contraindications to the use of ACE inhibitors include anuric renal failure, very low systolic blood pressure, a significantly raised creatinine level, hyperkalaemia and bilateral renal artery stenosis.

Angiotensin II receptor blockers

These very useful drugs block the effects of angiotensin II at the receptor, and are currently recommended for patients who cannot tolerate ACE inhibitors, usually because of a cough or, less commonly, because of angioneurotic oedema. They may also be used in conjunction with ACE inhibitors in patients with more severe heart failure (stages B, C and D).

These drugs are of similar benefit to ACE inhibitors, and may act synergistically with an ACE inhibitor in reducing death and cardiovascular events. Adding angiotensin II receptor blockers to an ACE inhibitor increases the risk of hypotension, renal dysfunction and hyperkalaemia, so these patients need careful frequent monitoring. The benefit of combined treatment may not extend to patients who are taking β-blockers. Angiotensin II antagonists are recommended for patients with stage B heart failure (symptom-free patients with hypertensive heart disease), in whom they reduce cardiovascular mortality and morbidity.

Candesartan reduces cardiovascular deaths and readmissions to hospital for heart failure in patients with left ventricular impairment by 23% reduction. These benefits apply to its use either alone or with β-blockers in patients who cannot tolerate ACE inhibitors. When added to ACE inhibitors (with or without β-blockers), it results in a further 15% reduction in cardiovascular deaths and hospital readmissions for heart failure.

A total of 23 patients need to be treated with candesartan for three years in order to prevent one cardiovascular death or hospital readmission for heart failure.

Patients who cannot tolerate ACE inhibitors or angiotensin II receptor blockers

This is unusual, but elderly patients and those with renal impairment may be tried on a combination of hydralazine and isosorbide dinitrate. They should also be prescribed a diuretic and a β-blocker.

Patient education

This is of fundamental importance to patients with all stages and types of heart failure. It is a primary function of community heart failure clinics.

Most patients are frightened when told that they have heart failure. Patients and carers will need a careful, sympathetic and gentle explanation of what this means. They should be taught the basic reasons for their symptoms and what they can and should do to mitigate and control their condition. This includes careful attention to correctable risk factors. They should be educated about their medication, what the tablets are for, what they look like and when they should be taken, and what they should do if they forget to take their medication. They should be warned about the common side-effects of their treatment and advised to report any worsening of their symptoms. It is useful for patients to have the name of a clinician they can contact for advice – this may reduce the number of unnecessary clinic visits.

Some GP practices have arranged specialist outreach clinics where a consultant cardiologist visits the surgery to see patients with known or suspected heart failure, and where 'point of care' echocardiography can be performed to either confirm or exclude the diagnosis. Primary care trusts may wish to support these initiatives, which reduce hospital outpatient waiting times and improve the quality of primary care services. This model of care is supported by the National Institute for Clinical Excellence.

Advice may need to be given about the level and type of exercise that is appropriate, and about employment, sex, contraception and vaccination.

Drug compliance

Compliance with drug treatment and lifestyle advice is crucial. Some elderly patients who for whatever reason have difficulty taking their medication may need help with this from a domiciliary nurse specialist. Medication should be prescribed in such a way as to increase the likelihood of compliance. Simplification of drug administration and reducing the frequency of administration will improve compliance and so decrease the likelihood of cardiac decompensation and the need for readmission to hospital.

Diet

This is part of patient education and is a very important component of the management of patients with all stages of heart failure.

Patients who are overweight should lose weight and aim to achieve their optimal body mass index.

A low-salt diet of around 2 g of sodium per day is desirable. 'Lo Salt' or potassium may be preferable. A minimal amount of salt should be used for cooking, and patients should be advised not to add salt to their food. 'Ready meals' and convenience meals generally contain a large amount of salt, which increases the tendency to fluid accumulation and the need to increase the dose of diuretic. Foods that have a high salt content include crisps, salted nuts, sausages, meat pies, Chinese and Indian meals, cheese, bacon, ham and tinned meats, smoked fish, chocolate and most tinned foods, including soups and vegetables. Patients should be advised that these foods contain a lot of salt and that they should be mindful of this and read the contents of any processed or packaged food.

A diet rich in fresh fruit, vegetables, fish and eggs (in moderation) is low in salt and recommended.

Fluid

Strict fluid restriction is very unpleasant for patients, who should be advised to try to avoid salty and sweet food in order to reduce their thirst.

Daily weight measurement

A reliable set of scales is essential. Patients should be advised to be vigilant about foot swelling, and diuretic dosage or route of administration may need to be changed if their weight increases by more than 1 kg over two days. The usual reason is congestion of the gut mucosa and impaired absorption of the medication.

Patients with severe heart failure may need additional nutrition, vitamins and a formal nutritional assessment because they may have a poor appetite and an increased metabolic rate.

Treatment of patients with stage B, C or D heart failure

The aims of treatment for patients with a low ejection fraction are to improve survival, slow the progression of disease, alleviate symptoms and minimise risk factors.

Non-steroidal anti-inflammatory drugs may result in cardiac decompensation and new heart failure so should be avoided.

Diuretics

These are the mainstay of treatment for patients with symptoms of pulmonary oedema or peripheral oedema, in whom they should be combined with an ACE inhibitor and/or β-blocker.

The synergistic effect of combining a loop diuretic (e.g. furosemide or bumetanide) with a thiazide diuretic (e.g. bendrofluazide, hydrochlorthiazide or metolazone) is very effective in severe, resistant cases of heart failure, particularly when the patient has peripheral oedema and right heart failure. The loop diuretic should be given intravenously if the patient is likely to have decreased and unpredictable absorption through a congested oedematous gut. The diuretic dose should be gradually increased until the oedema resolves. The most appropriate maintenance dose of loop diuretic is then prescribed, if necessary together with an intermittent dose (e.g. once or twice a week) of a thiazide diuretic.

It is very important to monitor the patient carefully both clinically, including daily weighing at the same time of day and at the same interval after drug administration, and by checking renal function and electrolytes. Sodium levels may decrease and the potassium level may increase if an ACE inhibitor is used in conjunction with a potassium-sparing diuretic (e.g. spironolactone or amiloride).

β-blockers

β-blockers blunt the effects of the sympathetic nervous system and reduce heart rate, force of cardiac contraction and blood pressure. They have been used for many years to treat patients with hypertension, angina and arrhythmias, but only recently to treat heart failure.

β-blockers improve survival, morbidity, left ventricular ejection fraction, exercise capacity, remodelling, quality of life, need for hospitalisation and the incidence of sudden death. There is no comparative trial data showing clear superiority of one β-blocker. The selective β_1-adrenergic blockers, metoprolol and bisoprolol, and the inexpensive and commonly used atenolol, appear to be as effective as the more expensive, non-selective carvedilol.

β-blockers should be used in carefully selected patients, and can be started in primary care, but only in patients with stable heart failure who do not have pulmonary oedema or significant fluid retention. Patients may deteriorate initially, but the drug can be continued unless the patient is unwell.

> β-blockers should not be started in patients with pulmonary oedema or signs of congestive heart failure.

β-blockers should be started only after fluid overload is corrected. The lowest doses should be used (bisoprolol 1.25 mg every morning, metoprolol 6.25 mg twice a day, carvedilol 3.125 mg every morning and atenolol 12.5 mg every morning). The dose should be increased gradually every two to three weeks, and the patient should be carefully monitored for signs of decompensation and hypotension. The target dose should be the dose employed in clinical trials of the β-blocker that is being used. If it results in haemodynamic decompensation, the patient should stop the drug and may need to be referred to hospital, but this is unusual if patients are carefully selected and monitored.

The dose may need to be reduced if the patient develops side-effects (bradycardia < 50 bpm, deterioration in heart failure symptoms), but not for asymptomatic hypotension.

Contraindications include asthma and chronic airways disease, bradyarrhythmias and heart block, patients who do not have a pacemaker and diabetic patients with frequent attacks of hypoglycaemia. Left bundle branch block is a relative contraindication.

Digoxin

This drug has weak positive inotropic actions and slows the heart rate through vagal stimulation. Its main indication is for lowering the ventricular rate in patients with atrial fibrillation. It is also indicated for worsening systolic heart failure in patients who are already on other treatments. It can be added to β-blockers in patients with uncontrolled atrial fibrillation, but the heart rate must be carefully monitored.

Digoxin does not reduce mortality. It has only marginal benefits in patients who are in sinus rhythm. When added to standard treatment in patients who are in sinus rhythm with reduced left ventricular systolic function, it improves symptoms and reduces hospitalisations, but does not reduce mortality. It is reasonable to continue its use in patients with persistent symptoms despite other medication.

The usual dose of digoxin, 0.25 mg every morning, should be reduced in the elderly, patients with renal impairment and those taking amiodarone. Digoxin 0.125 mg om or 0.0625 mg om is usually appropriate for small elderly patients. Side-effects or toxic symptoms including nausea, anorexia and arrhythmias may occur with 'normal' drug levels (which are rarely needed diagnostically or to control the dose), and are more likely to occur in elderly patients with renal impairment and hypokalaemia. A low drug level is as effective as a higher dose in reducing cardiovascular events, and is less likely to result in side-effects. The heart rate, atrioventricular conduction (with an ECG), and potassium and renal function should be monitored.

Additional treatment for patients with stage C or D heart failure

All potentially reversible factors should be identified and corrected. These include:

❖ poor compliance with medication

- ❖ myocardial ischaemia
- ❖ tachycardias or bradycardias
- ❖ valvular disease
- ❖ pulmonary embolism
- ❖ infection
- ❖ renal dysfunction.

Spironolactone

In severe heart failure, aldosterone levels are raised as a result of high angiotensin II levels and decreased clearance by the liver. Aldosterone stimulates the retention of salt, myocardial hypertrophy and potassium excretion. Spironolactone, an aldosterone antagonist, has been shown to reduce mortality in patients with severe systolic heart failure and may, by the same mechanisms, confer similar benefits in patients with other types and stages of heart failure, although there is currently no data available to support this.

The addition of spironolactone (25–50 mg per day) to standard treatment (ACE inhibitors, β-blockers and diuretics) reduces morbidity and mortality in patients with severe congestive heart failure.

Spironolactone should not be given to patients with hyperkalaemia (potassium > 5.0 mmol/l) or renal failure (creatinine > 220 μmol/l), because the combination of spironolactone and either an ACE inhibitor or an angiotensin II receptor antagonist blocks the renal excretion of potassium. Severe hyperkalaemia (potassium > 6.0 mmol/l) may occasionally occur in patients who are elderly or have diabetes even without renal impairment. Serum electrolytes and creatinine should be checked as part of the clinical assessment soon after starting treatment and regularly thereafter. Men who develop gynaecomastia may refuse to continue to take spironolactone.

Atrial fibrillation in patients with heart failure

Atrial fibrillation is an important precipitant of heart failure, and results in worsening symptoms and left ventricular function. Rate control and anticoagulation are important, although rhythm control may obviate the need for negatively inotropic anti-arrhythmic drugs and the practical difficulties of anticoagulation control.

Cardiac resynchronisation therapy (CRT) using biventricular pacemakers

This is a new and technically difficult treatment for patients with severe heart failure symptoms despite optimal medical treatment, and left bundle branch block. Left bundle branch block occurs in 30% of patients, and results in asynchronous and unco-ordinated cardiac depolarisation, and further impairment of cardiac contraction and function. The pacemaker is implanted to correct specific electrical abnormalities resulting from abnormal activation of the heart. Cardiac resynchronisation therapy reduces mortality in patients with severe heart failure.

Cardiac resynchronisation therapy (CRT) can be given on its own with pacing support (CRT-P), or in combination with an implantable cardioverter defibrillator (ICD) (CRT-D). The devices have similar effects in reducing mortality. Cardiac resynchronisation therapy with or without a defibrillation facility reduces mortality by around 40% compared with medical treatment.

Cardiac resynchronisation therapy does not improve the force of myocardial contraction, so patients must be carefully selected, and this evolving therapy should not at present be applied to all patients with stage C or D heart failure. Not all patients with severe symptomatic heart failure improve as a result of biventricular pacing, but the following criteria help to select those patients who should be referred to a centre with the necessary expertise.

Patients who should be referred for biventricular pacing

Patients with any of the following should be referred for biventricular pacing:

❖ systolic heart failure and an ejection fraction of < 30%
❖ sinus rhythm
❖ severe symptoms despite optimal medical treatment
❖ left bundle branch block (QRS width > 120 ms)
❖ significant mitral regurgitation
❖ patients with prior myocardial infarction who present with haemodynamically unstable sustained ventricular tachycardia
❖ those with an expectation of survival with a good functional status for more than one year.

The method involves the use of three, rather than the usual one or two, pacing electrodes, which are inserted into the right heart via the cephalic and subclavian veins. Two electrodes are positioned in the right atrium and the right ventricle, respectively, and the third electrode is positioned via the right atrium and coronary sinus into a left ventricular cardiac vein in order to pace the left ventricle and restore cardiac synchrony.

> Biventricular pacing improves exercise capacity, quality of life and, importantly, reduces the rate of hospital readmission. As yet there is no evidence that it reduces mortality.

Implantable cardioverter defibrillators

Serious ventricular arrhythmias (i.e. ventricular tachycardia or fibrillation) are common in patients with left ventricular impairment, and are the cause of death in most patients. Heart failure patients are the largest single population of patients who could benefit from prevention of sudden death. Implantable cardiac defibrillators are implanted like a pacemaker. They have been shown to reduce mortality by 30% in survivors of sudden cardiac death and in patients with ventricular arrhythmias and severe left ventricular impairment. Implantable cardioverter defibrillators are superior to amiodarone in preventing sudden death in patients with severe heart failure. The use of these devices will probably increase, and they are currently indicated for survivors of sudden death or significant ventricular arrhythmias. Biventricular pacemakers now have a defibrillator facility. They reduce all-cause mortality and readmission to hospital. Although these devices are expensive, the indications for them are becoming clearer and expanding, and patients with severe heart failure and dizzy turns or loss of consciousness should be investigated for ventricular arrhythmias and heart block, and referred to a specialist centre.

Indications for implantable cardioverter defibrillators

❖ cardiac arrest due to ventricular tachycardia (VT) or ventricular fibrillation (VF) with no reversible cause
❖ ventricular tachycardia in a patient with structural heart disease
❖ non-sustained VT or VF in a patient with coronary artery disease, myocardial infarction

❖ syncope due to VT or VF during an electrophysiological study
❖ patients with left ventricular ejection fraction of <30% at least one month after myocardial infarction or three months after coronary artery surgery.

There are other less firm indications.

Cardiac surgery

Severe left ventricular impairment increases the risks of both coronary angioplasty and cardiac surgery. Patients with heart failure and important angina should be referred for investigation, including coronary angiography, which may show suitable lesions for coronary angioplasty or bypass surgery.

Theoretically, myocardial revascularisation using either or both (hybrid) coronary angioplasty and coronary artery surgery should improve function in 'hibernating' (ischaemic but potentially recoverable) heart muscle, but there is currently no evidence that myocardial revascularisation improves survival. Hibernating myocardium is a presumed diagnosis made in patients in whom the heart muscle, when visualised by echocardiography, shows increased contractility to intravenous dobutamine. Therefore, patients with severe heart failure that is probably due to coronary artery disease should be referred for assessment of underlying myocardial ischaemia and hibernating myocardium. If these are present, coronary angiography should be performed with a view to revascularisation.

Mitral valve repair or replacement may be helpful in the 10% of patients whose heart failure results from severe mitral regurgitation or aortic stenosis disease. Surgery is not indicated when mitral regurgitation is a consequence of cardiac dilatation, as in dilated cardiomyopathy.

Resection of localised left ventricular aneurysms resulting in or contributing significantly to heart failure may be appropriate, and has been combined in a few centres with mitral valve repair (the Batista procedure). However, except in experienced centres the results to date have been poor, although this might reflect the high-risk patients (transplant candidates) studied.

Intra-aortic balloon pumps are inserted percutaneously into the aorta via a femoral artery. They augment diastolic blood pressure and myocardial blood supply and are used as a short-term haemodynamic support measure in patients with severe acute heart failure after infarction or haemodynamic impairment following heart surgery.

Left ventricular assist devices are mechanical, electrically powered pumps that may be either implanted into the left ventricle, or connected to the heart but carried outside the body. The increasing incidence of end-stage heart failure and the shortage of donor hearts for transplantation have fuelled considerable interest in developing these devices. An implanted device enables the patient to go home and lead a fairly active life. The aim of the device is to support or 'unload' the heart while it is recovering. It is implanted with the aim of explanting it when possible. It is not implanted in order to act as a replacement for the patient's heart.

The device reduces the work of the weak heart and allows drugs to be used, which might not otherwise be tolerated due to their negative inotropic (blood-pressure-lowering) effects. Conventional drugs that are used to treat heart failure are given with the aim of reversing remodelling. Other new drugs – β_2-adrenergic-receptor agonists – are given to prevent myocardial cell death.

Left ventricular assist devices improve one-year survival in patients with end-stage heart failure who are awaiting cardiac surgery or transplantation. The one- and two-year survival rates for patients with a left ventricular assist device compared with medical treatment are 50% vs 25% and 23% vs 8%, respectively. More recently, 90% of patients treated for non-ischaemic cardiomyopathy and without features of active myocarditis were found to be free from heart failure four years after device explantation.

Where some recovery of left ventricular function is expected (e.g. in dilated cardiomyopathy), left ventricular assist devices combined with medical treatments (β-blockers, ACE inhibitors, spironolactone and angiotensin II antagonists, and a new β_2-adrenergic-receptor agonist, clenbuterol, to prevent myocardial atrophy) enable the heart muscle to recover sufficiently to allow explantation of the device. Explantation is performed with a minimally invasive technique. Careful patient selection and the use of medical treatments allow the device to be explanted in most patients. However, some patients, particularly those with peripartum cardiomyopathy, may improve spontaneously, so without a control group it is not possible to show that these devices combined with medical treatment are solely responsible for cardiac reverse remodelling.

The device sucks blood out of the left ventricle and pumps it into the aorta, allowing the left ventricle to rest. They were used initially as a bridge to heart transplantation. New data suggests that they can be used to rest an 'end-stage heart', which may recover. Although the complications of bleeding, thromboembolism, malfunction of the device and infection are serious, these devices can improve survival and quality of life in patients with end-stage heart failure who are unable to have or who are not candidates for a heart transplant.

Cardiac transplantation

This is an effective operation, but the availability of donor hearts is insufficient to meet demand. The operative mortality is 10% and the survival rates at one, five and 10 years are 92%, 75% and 60%, respectively. This compares with a one-year survival rate of less than 50% for patients with stage C and D heart failure treated with optimal medical treatment. There are a few national transplant centres, and patients are usually referred by their cardiologist.

The main indication for cardiac transplantation is stage D heart failure in patients with NYHA class IV symptoms. Contraindications include active and significant malignancy (which would in itself shorten life expectancy), active infection or systemic disease (which would significantly increase the risk of the transplant or shorten life expectancy), and pulmonary hypertension or other causes of increased pulmonary vascular resistance (which would result in failure of the transplanted right heart). Transplants should not be performed if the patient is psychologically unsuitable or socially unsupported. Most transplant centres offer donor hearts preferentially to younger patients.

Accelerated small-vessel coronary artery disease is a major problem for patients after transplantation. Although the mechanism is unclear, it appears to be related to the anti-rejection immunotherapy.

Palliative care

Modern treatment has resulted in an increasingly large number of elderly patients who survive for longer, but who eventually develop symptoms that are refractory to medical treatment, and who are not candidates for specialised treatments. Palliative care similar to that provided for patients with cancer, either at home or in a hospice, should be offered to these patients, who may have severe breathlessness at rest, mental disturbances and pain.

Palliative care should take into account the wishes of the patient and their family with regard to clinical management decisions, including turning off an implantable cardioverter defibrillator, resuscitation, and supportive measures. The aim is to enable the patient to have a painless, peaceful and dignified death. Patients find visits to hospices and visits from palliative care nurses very helpful and supportive.

Opioids are used to relieve anxiety and dyspnoea. The dose of the opioid should be increased depending on the patient's symptoms.

Experimental approaches

Patients and their families may have read about experimental approaches to the treatment of heart failure.

Stem cell and progenitor cell transfer to the heart were initially claimed to be feasible and to offer benefits. However, there is not enough data from randomised controlled trials to recommend this approach.

Who should be referred to a specialist?

Indications for referral to a specialist include the following:

❖ patients for whom the diagnosis is in doubt
❖ those who remain symptomatic despite conventional medical treatment
❖ those with suspected severe valvular disease (murmurs, echocardiographic features)
❖ patients with angina and those in whom revascularisation may be indicated (e.g. triple-vessel coronary artery disease and hibernating myocardium)
❖ conditions that make pharmacological vasodilatation (ACE inhibition) risky, such as severe hypotension and left ventricular impairment, and possible renal artery stenosis
❖ arrhythmia (e.g. atrial fibrillation that is difficult to control)
❖ bradycardia and heart block that will require pacing
❖ important renal impairment or other difficult coexisting medical problems
❖ patients who wish to see a specialist.

Advice for patients

❖ Heart failure means that your heart is not working as it should be, but there are varying degrees of the condition. Some people with heart failure feel well and can do almost everything they want. Others are more breathless, feel weak and tired, and develop swelling of the feet and legs. Do not think too much about the term 'heart failure.' If you feel generally OK, then you probably are! Your symptoms are the best guide to how you are. If you can walk comfortably without getting breathless, this means that your heart is working well. If you get breathless at night and when you wake up, this is due to fluid accumulating in your lungs when you lie flat, and this means that you need to go to hospital for special treatment and tests.
❖ If you feel depressed at any time, this is to be expected and we would want you to come and see us so that we can help you. If your partner or spouse would like to come, too, that would be fine.
❖ The more you do, the better. Work if you can, and exercise as much and as often as you can. It is not dangerous, and only you can tell if you are overdoing things.
❖ If you are tired or you become breathless, listen to your body and slow down. If work or travelling gets too much for you, slow down and come to see us if you need advice about how to manage this.
❖ Heart failure is diagnosed with a clinical examination, an ECG and an ultrasound test of the heart and, in some patients, a chest X-ray and a blood test.
❖ There are several causes of heart failure. The most common causes are high blood pressure, and scarring and damage to the heart muscle due to heart attack. This is why

it is important for you to do everything you can to reduce the chances of furring up of the heart arteries, by stopping smoking (if you do smoke), getting down to your best weight, lowering your cholesterol level by switching to a healthy diet (and tablets if necessary), taking regular exercise and pushing yourself to a comfortable level every day, drinking and eating in moderation and taking the tablets that have been recommended for you. If you have diabetes, this needs to be carefully controlled.

✧ Other causes of heart failure include leaky or narrowed heart valves, which make the heart pump inefficient and weak, and a rather unusual heart muscle condition called cardiomyopathy, the cause of which is unknown.

✧ Sometimes, valve surgery or replacement may help. In extreme cases, patients may need a transplant, but there is a shortage of suitable donor hearts.

✧ In certain situations, a pacemaker is implanted to resynchronise the heart so that it contracts in a more efficient manner.

✧ There are several types of tablets, which work in different ways. Water tablets (diuretics) encourage you to pass more water and thus keep the lungs and legs free of fluid, which is a cause of breathlessness. Others tablets, called angiotensin-converting-enzyme inhibitors and angiotensin II blockers, make it easier for the heart to pump by widening the arteries. β-blockers are used and may make you feel sluggish or 'low', but they do help. It may be possible to reduce the dose of tablets if you experience side-effects.

✧ People with furring up of the arteries (those who have experienced heart attack, bypass surgery or angioplasty or leg circulation problems) should be taking aspirin.

✧ People with a weak heart are more breathless if the heart rhythm is 'out of sync', and they may need tablets or, in certain situations, an electrical shock to convert the rhythm back to normal. Patients with an irregular heart rhythm may need anticoagulants to reduce the risk of clots from the heart (emboli) circulating around the body.

✧ Try to keep to your best weight. You should try to be slim and as fit as possible. There are a number of exercises that you can do safely to keep your muscles toned.

✧ Avoid salty and fatty food. We can arrange for you to see a dietitian to give you advice. 'Ready meals', fast food and restaurant food often contain too much salt, so you should be careful about what and how you eat.

Answers to questions about clinical cases

1. This patient may have diastolic heart failure, but other causes, including mitral and aortic valve disease, chronic obstructive airways disease, anaemia and hypothyroidism, should be excluded. The principles of managing diastolic heart failure in the absence of evidence from clinical trials are control of blood pressure, heart rate, myocardial ischaemia and other risk factors.

2. Exclude pulmonary oedema with a chest X-ray and review the patient to ensure that there has not been a significant clinical deterioration. Stop the ACE inhibitor, and if the cough resolves quickly (within a few days) then either re-challenge the patient with another ACE inhibitor after explaining that this might also result in similar side-effects, or simply change the treatment to an angiotensin II blocker and ask the patient to let you know how he gets on. Take the opportunity to review all of his medication, ask about compliance, and check blood tests if they have not been checked recently.

3. This patient may be hypotensive or he may have developed heart failure or bradycardia due to the β-blocker. Ask the patient and any available witnesses about loss of consciousness and symptoms of pulmonary oedema. Examine the patient and check the lying and standing blood pressure, state of hydration, heart rate and rhythm, and also look for signs of cardiac decompensation. Perform an ECG to check the heart rate and rhythm, signs of conduction abnormality and heart block, and signs of new

myocardial infarction. The β-blocker may need to be stopped if there is heart block or profound bradycardia (< 40 bpm). Otherwise the dose can be reduced and the patient monitored, the situation explained, and the potential benefits of β-blockade reiterated. It may be possible to gradually increase the dose again. If the patient is difficult to control, discuss the case with or refer the patient to the cardiologist.

4. This patient may have important bilateral renal artery stenosis, which will need to be excluded by magnetic resonance imaging or Duplex ultrasound and referral to hospital. ACE inhibitors and angiotensin-receptor antagonists are contraindicated in patients with bilateral renal artery stenosis. The diuretic dosage may need to be reduced.

5. Causes of repeated hospitalisations are listed above and need careful review with a multi-disciplinary perspective and solution, and close collaboration with the hospital team.

6. Check the patient's diet and medication. Potassium-sparing diuretics (amiloride, spironolactone) may need to be reduced or stopped, and the doses of ACE inhibitors and angiotensin II blockers may need to be reduced. Avoid hypovolaemia. Use low doses of spironolactone, ACE inhibitors and angiotensin II blockers in patients with renal impairment, and monitor the renal function.

FURTHER READING

Reviews

Friedrich EB, Böhm M. Management of end-stage heart failure. *Heart.* 2007; **93:** 626–31.

Gomberg-Maitland M, Baran DA, Fuster V. Treatment of congestive heart failure: guidelines for the primary care physician and the heart failure specialist. *Arch Intern Med.* 2001; **161:** 342–52.

Jessup M, Brozena S. Heart failure. *NEJM.* 2003; **348:** 2007–18.

McMurray J, Pfeffer MA. New therapeutic options in congestive heart failure. *Circulation.* 2002; **105:** 2099–106, 2223–8.

Remme WJ, Swedberg K. Guidelines for the diagnosis and treatment of chronic heart failure. *Eur Heart J.* 2001; **22:** 1527–60.

Medical treatment

Brater DC. Diuretic therapy. *NEJM.* 1998; **339:** 387–95.

Brenner BM, Cooper ME, de Zeeuw D *et al.* Effects of Losartan on renal and cardiovascular outcomes in patients with type II diabetes and nephropathy. *NEJM.* 2001; **345:** 861–9.

Digitalis Investigation Group. The effect of digoxin on mortality and morbidity in patients with heart failure. *NEJM.* 1997; **336:** 525–33.

Foody JM, Farrell MH, Krumholz HM. Beta-blocker therapy in heart failure: scientific review. *JAMA.* 2002; **287:** 883–9.

Garg R, Yusuf S. Overview of randomised trials of angiotensin-converting-enzyme inhibitors on mortality and morbidity in patients with heart failure. *JAMA.* 1995; **273:** 1450–56 (erratum published in *JAMA*: 1995; **274:** 462).

Heart Outcomes Prevention Evaluation Study Investigators. Effects of an angiotensin-converting-enzyme inhibitor, ramipril, on cardiovascular events in high-risk patients. *NEJM.* 2000; **342:** 145–53 (errata published in *NEJM.* 2000; **342:** 748, 1376).

McMurray JJ, Ostergren J, Swedberg K *et al.* Effects of candesartan in patients with chronic heart failure and reduced left-ventricular systolic function taking angiotensin converting-enzyme inhibitors: the CHARM-Added trial. *Lancet.* 2003; **362:** 767–71.

Pitt B, Zannad F, Remme WJ *et al.* The effect of spironolactone on morbidity and mortality in patients with severe heart failure. *NEJM.* 1999; **341:** 709–17.

Biventricular pacing

Chow AWC, Lane RE, Cowie MR. New pacing technologies for heart failure. *BMJ*. 2003; **326:** 1073–7.

Cleland JG, Daubert JC, Erdman E *et al.* The effect of cardiac resynchronization on morbidity and mortality in heart failure. *NEJM*. 2005; **352:** 1539–49.

Exercise training

Hambrecht R, Gielen S, Linke A *et al.* Effects of exercise training on left ventricular function and peripheral resistance in patients with chronic heart failure: a randomized trial. *JAMA*. 2000; **283:** 3095–101.

Surgery

Bitran D, Merin O, Klutstein MW *et al.* Mitral valve repair in severe ischaemic cardiomyopathy. *J Cardiothorac Surg*. 2001; **16:** 79–82.

Left ventricular assist device for end-stage heart failure

Birks EJ, Tansley PD, Hardy J *et al.* Left ventricular assist device and drug therapy for the reversal of heart failure. *NEJM*. 2006; **355:** 1873–84.

Guidelines

Department of Health. *National Framework for Coronary Heart Disease*. London: The Stationery Office; 2000.

Hunt SA. ACC/AHA 2005 guideline update for the diagnosis and management of chronic heart failure in the adult: a report of the American College of Cardiology/American Heart Association Task Force on Practice Guidelines (Writing Committee to update the 2001 guidelines for the evaluation and management of heart failure). *J Am Coll Cardiol*. 2005; **46:** e1–82.

National Institute for Clinical Excellence. *Chronic Heart Failure: management of chronic heart failure in adults in primary and secondary care. A clinical guideline for the NHS in England and Wales*. London: National Institute for Clinical Excellence; 2003.

Swedberg K, Cleland J, Dargie H *et al.* Guidelines for the diagnosis and treatment of chronic heart failure: executive summary (update 2005): the Task Force for the Diagnosis and Treatment of Chronic Heart Failure of the European Society of Cardiology. *Eur Heart J*. 2005; **26:** 1115–40.

Angina

SEVEN

Clinical cases

1. A 70-year-old man presents with typical angina four months after coronary angioplasty performed for single-vessel left anterior descending coronary artery disease. What do you do?
2. A 30-year-old woman who exercises regularly and has no risk factors for coronary artery disease complains of localised left infra-mammary chest pain and wants reassurance that the pain is not related to her heart. What do you do?
3. A 68-year-old man with a history of cancer of the prostate comes to see you because of breathlessness and chest pain. What do you do?
4. A 65-year-old obese hypertensive woman with disabling arthritis of the knees and a long history of typical angina notices an increase in the frequency of her symptoms. What do you do?
5. A 55-year-old diabetic man with treated hyperlipidaemia develops mild chest discomfort, which is not consistently related to exercise. What do you do?
6. A 58-year-old man with type 2 diabetes and angina asks you for advice about impotence. What do you do?
7. A 73-year-old woman has mild stable angina. Her sister, who lives abroad, has had an angioplasty. Your patient wants to know whether she should have one, too. What advice do you give her?

The role of primary care physicians in the management of angina and coronary heart disease

GPs and primary care clinicians shoulder the main responsibility for the management of patients with coronary heart disease and angina. Cardiovascular prevention underpins the management of patients with angina and all other forms of vascular disease. The identification and treatment of patients with angina, and recognising which patients should be referred for specialist evaluation and when they should be referred, are an important part of the work in primary care. Provision of effective screening programmes, patient education and close collaboration between primary and secondary care are essential.

Primary care clinicians should understand:

- the significance of cardiovascular risk factors
- that effective secondary prevention and drugs are as effective as coronary angioplasty in reducing the risk of death, myocardial infarction and other cardiovascular events in stable angina
- the principles of cardiovascular risk estimation, and how to apply these methods to individual patients
- that angina is a clinical diagnosis, and management is guided largely by symptom severity
- the value and limitations of cardiac investigations for ischaemia and assessments for coronary artery disease in patients at different levels of risk
- the various principles of and indications for medical treatments and myocardial revascularisation.

Relationship between primary and secondary care in angina management

The GP surgery is the focal point for the long-term management of angina. Patients attend hospital for specialist evaluation and investigations that cannot be performed in primary care. After specialist cardiological review and investigation, and when the diagnosis of coronary heart disease has been confirmed or excluded in hospital, patients are referred back to primary care for long-term management, usually after only one or two hospital outpatient appointments. Patients without coronary heart disease are reassured about their heart, and they may require assessment for other conditions. After myocardial revascularisation, patients are referred back to primary care for long-term care. Patients with recurrent symptoms should be referred back to hospital for review.

Management guidelines

GPs and local cardiologists may have local guidelines for the management of angina and cardiovascular risk. These, and those published by international cardiovascular societies, are helpful for standardising management and for audit.

Primary care as a vascular disease surveillance centre

Coronary heart disease and angina are chronic conditions. Patients require lifelong follow-up to determine whether their management needs to be changed. A patient with stable angina may develop unstable symptoms and require specialist review.

Primary care clinicians should be aware of advances in treatment for angina in order to be able to offer and explain to patients the most appropriate treatment as their condition changes. As in other fields of medicine and cardiology, skill and judgement are required to tailor treatment to individual patients. Patients often consult GPs about claims in the media and on the Internet about certain heart disease treatments.

Coronary heart disease prevention, diagnosis and management curriculum for GPs and primary care clinicians

This includes:

- global risk factor management and secondary prevention
- blood pressure targets and how to achieve these
- exercise recommendations for patients with coronary heart disease with and without heart failure
- management of obesity and diet
- aspirin and/or other antiplatelet drugs, including practice after revascularisation
- lowering of treatment thresholds for statins and new target levels for total cholesterol and LDL-cholesterol
- optimising glucose control in diabetes
- ACE inhibitors and angiotensin II antagonists for both primary and secondary prevention
- indications for established and new anti-anginal drugs
- value and limitations of tests for ischaemia in different patient subgroups

✧ indications for and management after angioplasty and stenting
✧ new techniques of coronary artery surgery, including 'off-pump' (beating heart) coronary artery surgery.

In-house prevention clinics

Some practices provide risk factor clinics. These include the following:
✧ smoking cessation
✧ hypertension
✧ weight and diet
✧ exercise and rehabilitation
✧ stress management
✧ lipid management.

Prevention clinics can be run by suitably trained nurses. Some clinics (e.g. those that deal with diet and weight, smoking cessation, stress management and exercise) could be led by patients as a 'self-help' group.

These clinics offer patients advice and support, and have been shown to be both popular and helpful. It is not known whether they are cost-effective or reduce cardiac morbidity or mortality compared with traditional consultation practice.

Patients who want to help themselves are usually able to control their risk factors without attending these clinics. Equally, patients who are not interested in prevention would probably not attend these clinics. Prevention clinics are no substitute for patients effectively managing their own risk factors. GPs have to decide whether specialty prevention clinics are practical and worthwhile for their patients.

Open-access chest pain clinics

Chest pain clinics were set up several years ago to reduce waiting times for specialist assessment and stress testing, with the aim of reducing morbidity and mortality from coronary heart disease.

The Coronary Heart Disease National Service Framework target is for all patients with suspected angina to be referred by their GP to a chest pain clinic and seen within two weeks of referral. Most GPs in the UK have access to chest pain clinics at their local hospital. These clinics are generally run by cardiac-trained nurses with cardiologist support. Patients have a comprehensive clinical and cardiovascular risk assessment and, where indicated, an exercise stress test. Patients with angina and significant ischaemia are treated and advised to have coronary angiography. Those with a low probability of coronary heart disease can be reassured and referred back to their GP, and are then referred for further investigation if necessary. Cardiovascular prevention should be offered to all patients.

Chest pain clinics have led to increased rates of coronary angiography and revascularisation. There is no evidence that mortality rates have decreased. Not all patients want to be referred to a chest pain clinic, and some may want to be managed by their GP.

Pathology
Atherosclerosis

Atherosclerosis is the process of hardening, caused by lipid and calcium deposition, of the walls of medium-sized and large arteries. This process affects the brain, carotid, heart, kidney and peripheral arteries, as well as the aorta. Fatty plaques of cholesterol are deposited in the intima and subintima of the artery.

Plaque deposition

The pathological processes of atherosclerosis are unclear. It is believed to be an inflammatory condition that is triggered by arterial injury. It occurs prematurely in vulnerable people, particularly those with diabetes or hypertension.

Plaque deposition is more likely to occur in patients with certain risk factors. Arterial injury results in endothelial dysfunction and inflammation. The causes of injury are unclear, but chemical toxins (e.g. tobacco smoke and other smoking constituents, and oxidised LDL-cholesterol) are believed to play a part. A complex interaction of chemical mediators acting on smooth muscle cells, white cells, other inflammatory cells and platelets increases intimal and subintimal susceptibility to cholesterol deposition. The increased levels and activity of endothelin-1 and angiotensin II, which are proliferative and vasoconstrictor agents, lead to thickening and remodelling of the arterial wall. There is reduced production of nitric oxide, a vasodilator and antiproliferative agent, from the endothelium.

Fatty streaks

Circulating cholesterol is taken up by white cells in the endothelium, which migrate to the subendothelial layer to form plaques of atheroma. The earliest stages are called *fatty streaks*. They have been shown to be present in young people who die from a condition called *homozygous* familial hypercholesterolaemia (not to be confused with the much less dangerous and more common *heterozygous* familial hypercholesterolaemia).

Fibrous plaques

The fatty streaks swell, due to increased cholesterol deposition, to form fibrous plaques. Initially the fibrous plaques lead to expansion or remodelling of the artery (ectasia). Blood flow is not laminar, and is slower in ectatic arteries than in normal arteries. This may cause angina.

As more cholesterol is deposited in the subendothelial layer, the cholesterol plaque swells and protrudes into the vessel lumen, obstructing blood flow. Depending on the characteristics of the plaque and the state of the endothelium and various triggers, plaques of cholesterol may rupture, causing acute coronary syndromes and myocardial infarction.

Plaque rupture and acute coronary syndromes

Myocardial infarction and acute coronary syndromes are due to rupture (cracking) of the surface of the fibrous cap that covers a coronary plaque. There are no simple imaging or diagnostic tests to predict which plaques will rupture and which are stable. Those that have ruptured are referred to as *unstable plaques*. Those that have not ruptured are referred to as *stable plaques*.

Stable and unstable plaques

Histologically, unstable plaques differ from stable plaques.

- *Unstable* plaques are susceptible to rupture and thrombosis. They have a thin fibrous cap, a large necrotic lipid core and a high proportion of inflammatory cells and mediators, which are associated with endothelial dysfunction.
- *Stable* plaques have a thicker fibrous cap, a smaller lipid core and less inflammatory cells and mediators. They are less susceptible to rupture.

Causes of angina

> Angina is a clinical diagnosis made solely from the history and the probability of coronary artery disease based on the patient's age and risk factor profile.

Angina occurs when there is an imbalance between oxygen demand by the heart, and supply of blood and oxygen through the coronary arteries. Virtually all patients with angina have atherosclerotic obstructive coronary artery disease.

Angina may also occur in patients with normal epicardial coronary arteries, but where there is impaired uptake of oxygen or increased demand for oxygen by the heart muscle – for example, where there is severe left ventricular hypertrophy due to hypertension or aortic stenosis. *Calcific aortic stenosis* (most common in the elderly) and coronary artery disease share cardiovascular risk factors, and this is one of the reasons why the two conditions often coexist.

Severe anaemia results in a reduced oxygen supply to the heart muscle, although the blood flow is normal.

Tachycardia may cause angina due to reduced coronary filling time. Patients may complain of both palpitation and chest pain, or only chest pain, during an episode of tachycardia.

Other unusual causes of angina include *microvascular angina* and *vasculitis*.

Syndrome X is a combination of angina, normal coronary arteries on angiography, and exercise-induced ST depression. Mortality is low but morbidity is high. The condition is treated medically.

Rarely, *pulmonary hypertension* (which has several causes, including chronic obstructive airways disease, pulmonary emboli, any cause of left heart disease and pulmonary venous hypertension, and the less common pulmonary arterial hypertension) may cause angina because of right ventricular failure, hypoxia and low cardiac output.

Relationship between anginal symptoms and coronary heart disease

Symptoms do not predict the severity of coronary artery disease. A patient may have severe triple-vessel coronary artery disease but no symptoms. The first ischaemic symptom may be infarction and sudden death. Conversely, patients with apparently mild coronary artery disease on angiography may have severe angina. The reason why symptoms are not consistently or predictably related to coronary anatomy is not known.

Atypical anginal symptoms

Women, the elderly and diabetics may have exertional breathlessness as their main or only anginal symptom, rather than chest discomfort. Angina in women may be experienced as unusual chest, arm, neck and back discomfort.

Differential diagnosis of chest pain

- ✧ Oesophageal pain
- ✧ Gastritis, peptic ulcer
- ✧ Chest wall pain
- ✧ Pericarditis
- ✧ Chest infection, pneumonia

- ◇ Aortic dissection
- ◇ Referred pain from the neck and spine
- ◇ Anxiety

These possibilities should be considered and investigated if necessary.

Principles of management of angina

The main objectives of treatment of angina are to improve the symptoms and prognosis.

Patients with exertional chest pain and/or breathlessness usually present initially to their GP. If the diagnosis of angina is clear, the GP should:
- ◇ start treatment
- ◇ assess and treat all cardiovascular risk factors
- ◇ perform laboratory investigations
- ◇ decide whether stress testing is necessary
- ◇ review the patient to assess their response to treatment
- ◇ refer any patient with unstable angina directly to hospital for specialist assessment
- ◇ medically manage patients with stable angina who are at low or intermediate risk, and who become symptom free in primary care
- ◇ refer high-risk patients for specialist review. Most of these patients will have coronary angiography and assessment for revascularisation
- ◇ refer patients who remain symptomatic for specialist review for coronary angiography and revascularisation.

Many GPs now refer all patients with suspected angina to chest pain clinics, where stress testing is usually done and then, depending on the result, a decision is made to proceed to coronary angiography.

Prognostic risk stratification and referral

The prognosis depends on the age of the patient, the extent of coronary artery disease and left ventricular function, previous myocardial infarction, and coexisting vascular and other medical conditions, including hypertension, dyslipidaemia, renal disease, lung disease and diabetes.

Risk stratification is important and should be undertaken at the first consultation. The aim is to identify patients who are at high risk from infarction or other vascular events, and who may benefit from myocardial revascularisation.

Patients who present with possible ischaemic symptoms should have a complete vascular risk examination and assessment.

High-risk patients should be referred to a cardiologist. Those at low risk, with mild stable angina, can be managed in primary care. Those at intermediate risk can also be managed in primary care, but require careful assessment and monitoring, and specialist referral, if their symptoms become unstable. Those who show important signs of ischaemia on stress testing should be referred.

Coronary heart disease, angina and ischaemia

These terms are often confused.

❖ *Coronary heart disease* (or coronary artery disease) is an anatomical term. It is the visible presence of atherosclerotic disease in a coronary artery. It is inferred from a history of angina (although a small minority of patients with angina may have normal coronary arteries), myocardial infarction or myocardial revascularisation. It is diagnosed with coronary angiography, magnetic resonance or computerised tomographic imaging, or at post-mortem.
❖ *Angina* is a clinical diagnosis made from the history.
❖ *Ischaemia* (lack of oxygen) is a pathophysiological term. It is most commonly diagnosed with an ECG recording the hallmark sign of ST depression induced during stress (exercise or dobutamine) testing. It may be suggested by a reversible perfusion defect with nuclear myocardial perfusion imaging.

Types of angina

Management of angina depends on whether the patient has stable or unstable angina.

Stable angina

Symptoms have to be assessed taking account of the patient's age and risk factor profile. Exertional chest pain in a very young person is very unlikely to be angina. Angina has to be considered even if the symptoms are atypical, if the patient is at high risk of having coronary heart disease.

Angina is typically central chest discomfort, fullness or tightness, or difficulty in breathing, on exertion or with stress. The symptoms may be in the throat and/or the chest, and radiate to the arms. Some patients experience angina only in the face or jaw, or the arms. The symptoms are consistent.

Symptoms occur predictably and often, reproducibly, only when patients exert themselves to a certain level (e.g. climbing up more than two or three flights of stairs, or running fast for a bus). The symptoms disappear quickly when they stop or slow down, or take a glyceryl trinitrate (GTN) spray or tablet.

Patients with stable angina are at low risk from a heart attack. Their 10-year risk of infarction or death is less than 20%. This equates to an annual event rate of less than 2%, and patients should be told that this condition is generally associated with a good prognosis. Morbidity and mortality may be reduced significantly by aggressive risk factor reduction. Patients with stable angina can be managed conservatively with risk factor modification and medical treatment, although they may need to adjust their exercise activities (e.g. not go skiing).

Unstable angina

This is new-onset angina, or when patients with stable angina notice that their symptoms occur at a lower level or intensity of exertion. For example, they may previously have been able to walk a long distance quite fast on the flat, but now find that they experience angina after walking a short distance or even when they are at rest. The management of unstable angina demands urgent specialist assessment and further investigations at hospital.

Symptoms inconsistent with angina

Localised, pin-pricking or needle-like chest pain is rarely due to angina. Chest wall tenderness excludes angina.

Grading the severity of angina

The Canadian Cardiovascular Society grading of the severity of angina is often used by cardiologists in their correspondence, so it is helpful for primary care clinicians to understand this classification.

⬧ Class I: Minimal limitation of ordinary activity. Angina occurs only with strenuous, rapid or prolonged exertion.

⬧ Class II: Slight limitation of ordinary activity. Angina occurs on walking or climbing stairs quickly, walking in cold weather or when under emotional stress.

⬧ Class III: Marked limitation of ordinary physical activity. Angina occurs on walking 50–100 metres at level ground or climbing one flight of stairs at a normal pace in normal conditions.

⬧ Class IV: Inability to perform any physical activity without discomfort; angina may also occur at rest.

Examination

There are no specific signs of coronary heart disease, and examination is usually unremarkable. The main purpose is to measure the blood pressure, and to look for signs of risk factors, thyrotoxicosis, heart failure, mitral regurgitation or aortic stenosis.

Measure the pulse rate and assess the rhythm. Feel for foot pulses and if they are not present, feel for all the leg pulses. Feel for dilatation or abnormal pulsation of the abdominal aorta, which would prompt investigation (ultrasound or CT) for an aneurysm. Feel the carotid artery upstroke. If it is slow, aortic stenosis should be suspected. If it is hyperdynamic, this may be due to severe anxiety, thyrotoxicosis or another cause of high cardiac output, or to aortic regurgitation. Patients with a heart rate of < 50 bpm or > 100 bpm should have an ECG. If the heart rate is < 50 bpm, β-blockers, diltiazem and ivabradine as antianginal treatments are contraindicated.

Vascular disease checklist

⬧ Measure blood pressure.

⬧ Feel both radial arteries. They should be equal.

⬧ Auscultation of the heart (heart sounds, added sounds, valve disease – aortic stenosis or mitral regurgitation).

⬧ Listen for carotid bruits.

⬧ Feel for foot and leg pulses and measure the pulse wave with Doppler if a leg pulse is reduced or absent.

⬧ Listen for femoral artery bruits.

⬧ Feel for a dilated aortic aneurysm.

⬧ Look for the presence of varicose veins. The absence of suitable leg veins reduces the choice of bypass conduit for coronary artery surgery.

⬧ Look for signs of high cholesterol (xanthelasma, premature corneal arcus, tendon xanthomata).

⬧ Measure the fasting lipid profile.

Assessing ischaemia and prognosis with stress testing

Stress testing, using either a treadmill or a cycle, is used to assess reversible ischaemia. The results provide both prognostic and diagnostic information. The results are evaluated in conjunction with the patient's cardiovascular risk profile, history and examination findings in order to estimate the probability of coronary heart disease, and the consequent risk of cardiovascular events.

Patients who develop ischaemia (chest discomfort and/or ST depression or breath-lessness) at a low heart rate and workload, and who have an inadequate blood pressure response to exercise, are likely to have significant coronary heart disease and a worse prognosis. These patients are likely to gain prognostic benefit from myocardial revascu-larisation.

Patients who can exercise for more than 10 minutes on either the Bruce treadmill protocol or the WHO cycle protocol, without angina or signs of ischaemia, and who have a normal haemodynamic response to exercise, are at low risk from cardiac events.

> The result of exercise testing should not be simply 'positive' or 'negative' based solely on the presence or absence of ST depression. It should report on all relevant aspects of the test, together with a clinical assessment of the probability of coronary heart disease.

Principles of management of angina

Management is determined mainly by the severity of symptoms, and by an assessment of the patient's cardiovascular risk based on a number of factors, including age, the threshold for inducible ischaemia during stress testing, coronary anatomy and left ventricular function.

> The patient's views on how they want to be treated are important, particularly when symptoms are mild or intermittent and when there is no clear advantage to be gained from revascularisation.

◇ Patients with non-cardiac chest pain should be reassured. They may need further investigation and referral.
◇ Cardiovascular risk should be assessed and treated.
◇ Patients with chronic stable angina may be managed in primary care.
◇ In patients with stable angina, effective control of risk factors and serum lipids, combined with antiplatelet treatment, β-blockers and ACE inhibitors, is as effective as coronary angioplasty and stenting in reducing the risk of death, myocardial infarction and other major cardiovascular events.
◇ Patients with acute coronary syndromes and suspected myocardial infarction need urgent referral to hospital.
◇ Evaluation of the probability of coronary heart disease using global cardiovascular risk analysis, investigation of the presence of reversible ischaemia and, when necessary, exclusion of coronary heart disease simplifies future management. Identifying patients at high and low risk is important for the patient and the primary care team.

> In patients at intermediate or higher cardiovascular risk, coronary heart disease should be investigated before other potential causes of chest pain.

Likelihood of angina according to age and gender

The patient's age, risk factor profile and, most importantly, the character of their symptoms determine the probability of coronary heart disease (*see* Table 7.1).

In a 30-year-old woman with no cardiovascular risk factors, it is very unlikely (12% risk) that coronary artery disease accounts for symptoms of even severe chest pain. The severity of symptoms has a low predictive value in diagnosing angina.

However, typical anginal symptoms in a 70-year-old man are highly likely (94% risk) to represent angina. If he complained only of atypical symptoms, the probability of coronary heart disease would still be 72%. If his symptoms were not consistent with either typical or atypical angina, the probability of at least single-vessel coronary artery disease would be 27%.

Patients aged less than 50 years, with non-anginal chest pain, are very unlikely to have coronary heart disease.

TABLE 7.1: Probability (%) of at least single-vessel coronary artery disease (taken from the American College of Cardiology/American Heart Association guidelines on management of stable angina) in patients with non-anginal chest pain, atypical angina and typical angina

Age (years)	Non-anginal chest pain (%)		Atypical angina (%)		Typical angina (%)	
	Men	Women	Men	Women	Men	Women
30–39	4	2	34	12	76	26
40–49	13	3	51	22	87	55
50–59	20	7	65	31	93	73
60–69	27	14	72	51	94	86

Principles of management of patients with suspected angina

The aim of treatment is to relieve symptoms and to reduce mortality and cardio-vascular events, so that the patient may have a full and active life.

1. Patients with acute coronary syndromes and myocardial infarction need to be referred urgently to hospital for specialist evaluation and exclusion of myocardial infarction.
2. If the probability of angina and coronary artery disease is low, other non-cardiac diagnoses should be investigated and the patient referred to the appropriate specialist.
3. The prognosis of patients with angina depends on the presenting symptoms, the patient's age, clinical characteristics and risk profile, left ventricular function and extent of coronary artery disease, previous infarction, and their functional capacity and extent of inducible ischaemia on exercise. Diabetes, peripheral vascular disease, hypertension, obesity and renal function are all important adverse prognostic risk factors.
4. Exclude and assess associated conditions:
   ⬦ severe anaemia
   ⬦ dyslipidaemia
   ⬦ hyperthyroidism
   ⬦ uncontrolled hypertension

❖   tachyarrhythmia and bradyarrhythmias

❖   valvular conditions (aortic stenosis)

❖   left ventricular hypertrophy and hypertrophic cardiomyopathy, which may cause and exacerbate angina.

5. The patient and their family should be informed about all aspects of the condition and its long-term management. This includes simple advice about what to do in order to reduce the frequency of their symptoms (e.g. if they are stress or exertion related), and what to do if their symptoms become unstable.

6. All cardiovascular risk factors should be investigated and treated.

7. GTN should be taken prophylactically as well as to abort attacks of angina.

8. Alcohol should be taken only in moderation (less than seven units per week as a guide, although there is no satisfactory data on quantity).

9. A diet low in fat and salt but rich in oily fish is recommended.

10. Daily exercise is recommended and has several benefits.

11. Although sexual intercourse may trigger angina and often precipitate presentation, it is generally safe. Prophylactic nitroglycerin may prevent angina. Phosphodiesterase-5 inhibitors (sildenafil, tadalafil or vardenafil) can be prescribed safely for men with angina and coronary heart disease, but should not be used by patients who are taking long-acting nitrates.

12. Evaluate the patient's cardiovascular risk both clinically and with stress testing. Mild stable angina has a good prognosis and can be managed medically. Patients with unacceptable or unstable symptoms should be referred promptly for coronary angiography and myocardial revascularisation.

The **ABCDE** mnemonic is useful for remembering the 10 most important aspects of treatment for patients with stable angina, which together reduce the risk of cardiovascular events:

Aspirin and **A**nti-anginal treatment
Beta-blockers and **B**lood pressure control
Cholesterol reduction and **C**igarette cessation
Diet and weight advice and **D**iabetes control
Education and **E**xercise

Unstable angina or myocardial infarction

Patients should be treated with aspirin 300 mg and, if in severe pain, diamorphine 5 mg IV, Maxolon 10 mg IV and oxygen. They should be sent urgently by ambulance to the nearest hospital emergency department that can deal with this problem. Patients with acute ST elevation myocardial infarction should be sent to a hospital with the facilities and staff to perform emergency (primary) coronary angioplasty.

Stable angina not requiring urgent hospital admission

These patients can be treated in primary care and referred, if necessary, for specialist review and investigation. They may be referred to a chest pain clinic.

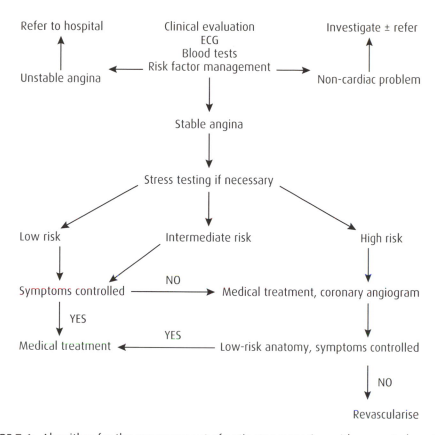

FIGURE 7.1: Algorithm for the management of patients presenting with suspected angina.

Investigations

◇ Blood tests: full blood count, creatinine. Estimated glomerular filtration rate (eGFR) is now commonly measured in UK hospitals. Fasting lipid profile, particularly LDL-cholesterol and glucose.

◇ Exercise testing gives prognostic and diagnostic information. Stress echocardiography is helpful in patients who cannot exercise or when the exercise test is inconclusive.

◇ Radionuclide imaging is sometimes helpful in patients whose ECG is uninterpretable or when the exercise ECG is inconclusive.

◇ ECG: the sensitivity and specificity are increased if this is recorded during an episode of chest pain. T-wave inversion or Q-waves suggest myocardial injury or infarction. ST depression and T-wave changes suggest ischaemia. ST elevation (convex upwards) is a sign of myocardial infarction. In pericarditis, ST elevaton is characteristically concave up.

◇ Chest X-ray in patients with suspected heart failure or murmurs, and those with chest symptoms and who have smoked. Occasionally, clinically silent lung cancer or other lung pathology is diagnosed.

◇ Echocardiogram in patients with suspected heart failure, heart murmurs, previous myocardial infarction or hypertension, and for assessment of left ventricular function.

Medical treatment of angina
Antithrombotic drugs
These are given for primary and secondary prevention of thrombotic cardiovascular and cerebrovascular disease. Aspirin 75 mg every morning or, in the rare aspirin-allergic patient, clopidogrel 75 mg every morning, is given as maintenance. Aspirin and a proton pump inhibitor are used in patients with a history of gastrointestinal bleeding. Clopidogrel, a thienopyridine, has a similar risk profile to aspirin. It is used in combination with aspirin for one year following coronary stent implantation. There is no evidence that dipyridamole reduces cardiovascular mortality; it is not indicated in angina.

Lipid-lowering drugs
Statins have a major impact in reducing cardiovascular risk in patients of all ages with vascular disease (secondary prevention). This benefit is independent of lipid lowering. They are the most effective drugs for lowering cholesterol. They have other beneficial effects on vascular inflammation, blood clotting and renal function.

Statins are also indicated for primary prevention in patients with a 10-year cardiovascular risk of more than 20%. All cardiovascular risk factors should be considered in this decision.

There are five different statins (atorvastatin, fluvastatin, pravastatin, rosuvastatin and simvastatin), which all competitively inhibit 3-hydroxy-3-methylglutaryl coenzyme A (HMG CoA) reductase, an enzyme that regulates cholesterol synthesis in the liver. Simvastatin is currently the statin preferred by the NHS funding authority, and can now be bought 'over the counter' as 10 mg tablets.

Statins reduce the risk of stroke and heart attack by 30%. They have greater impact in patients at higher risk – that is, those with vascular disease (secondary prevention), diabetes and diabetes coexisting with vascular disease, the elderly (> 70 years of age), and all patients with at least one cardiovascular risk factor.

Adverse side-effects of statins are more likely in patients with liver disease and high alcohol consumption. Liver function tests should be checked before and one to three months after starting treatment, and thereafter at least once a year. These drugs should be stopped if the liver transaminase levels are persistently raised to three times the upper limit of normal. Muscle problems (myopathy and myositis) are rare. Statins should also be stopped if the symptoms are intolerable or if the creatine kinase level is raised by fivefold.

Patients with angina and vascular disease, and others at high risk, should be treated with the optimum statin dosage – that is, simvastatin 40 mg, atorvastatin 10 mg or pravastatin 40 mg every morning. Older patients can be started at a lower dose. The target levels for patients with vascular disease are cholesterol < 4.0 mmol/l and, more importantly, LDL-cholesterol < 2.0 mmol/l. If these targets are not met, higher doses should be used. However, there is not a proportional decrease in lipid levels as the statin dose is increased. Doubling the dose of statin achieves only a relatively small (6%) further decrease in LDL-cholesterol levels. High dose atorvastatin (80 mg daily) reduces cardiovascular risk but not mortality. Side-effects are more common, the costs are greater, and very-high-dose atorvastatin (80 mg) is recommended only for high-risk patients.

Additional drugs to lower a persistently high cholesterol level
Combination therapy using a statin and another lipid-lowering drug, most commonly ezetimibe, together with a low-fat diet, weight loss and exercise, is usually effective in achieving target lipid levels. This is particularly important in patients with vascular disease and a high global cardiovascular risk.

Ezetimibe (a selective cholesterol-transport inhibitor) may be used alone in patients who cannot tolerate a statin. It is well tolerated.

Nicotinic acid in doses of 1.5–3 g daily lowers total cholesterol and triglyceride levels and increases HDL-cholesterol levels. It may be added to a statin in order to achieve target lipid levels, or used alone in patients who cannot tolerate statins. Adverse effects, including flushing, diarrhoea, nausea, rash, palpitation, shortness of breath, peripheral oedema and headache, are common.

Omega-3 fatty acids are used in combination with statins. Gastrointestinal side-effects may occur. There is no evidence that foods purported to be 'rich in omega-3 fatty acids' are beneficial.

Principles of lipid lowering in high-risk patients

- All patients with angina or other forms of vascular disease, and those at high risk, should be on a statin.

- The decision to prescribe a statin is based not solely on cholesterol level, but on the patient's overall cardiovascular risk.

- The lower the cholesterol level, the better.

- It is essential to educate patients about cardiovascular risk reduction and compliance with therapy.

Angiotensin-converting enzyme inhibitors

ACE inhibitors inhibit the conversion of angiotensin I to angiotensin II. They are beneficial in treating hypertension and heart failure, they reduce left ventricular remodelling after myocardial infarction, and they are recommended for patients with asymptomatic left ventricular dysfunction and diabetes.

ACE inhibitors are started early and continued long term in patients after myocardial infarction. Ramipril and perindopril have been shown to reduce cardiovascular mortality and morbidity in patients with stable coronary heart disease without heart failure. Trandalopril did not have these benefits.

ACE inhibitors should be prescribed to patients with angina who also have at least one of the following: hypertension, diabetes, heart failure, asymptomatic heart failure or previous myocardial infarction.

Ramipril and perindopril may be prescribed to patients with angina without these conditions.

β-blockers

β-blockers reduce cardiac work, relieve symptoms of angina and increase exercise tolerance. They improve the prognosis in patients with angina who have had a heart attack or who have heart failure. They are recommended as first-line treatment for patients with angina who have no contraindications (e.g. second- and third-degree heart block, worsening unstable heart failure, asthma, Raynaud's disease). There is no convincing evidence of the superiority of one β-blocker over the others. However, some patients tolerate one of these drugs but not the others.

Nitrates

Nitrates are useful in angina because they are potent coronary vasodilators. Their main action is through venodilatation and reducing ventricular stretch and work. Unwanted side-effects include flushing, headache and postural hypotension (which with large doses of GTN spray may cause a nitrate faint).

Sublingual GTN tablets (which are inactivated by stomach acid and should therefore be sucked or chewed) are very effective. GTN sublingual spray avoids the problems of gastric acid inactivation.

Isosorbide dinitrate and mononitrate

Isosorbide dinitrate can be used sublingually, orally and transdermally (as a patch stuck on to the skin). It is metabolised to isosorbide mononitrate, which is also useful in angina prophylaxis.

Tolerance to all long-acting nitrates occurs in a significant proportion of patients within six months of treatment. This is the diminution or disappearance of a clinical effect of the drug, and it should be expected in all patients. It is difficult to diagnose and may be confused with a deterioration of the condition. Tolerance can be at least partly avoided by reducing blood levels of nitrate. This is achieved by removing nitrate patches for a few hours per day and, in the case of nitrate tablets, taking the second dose of nitrate several hours earlier, to allow the nitrate blood level to fall before it increases following the next dose.

Calcium-channel blockers

There are three different types of calcium-channel blockers, each with different effects on cardiac conduction, cardiac contractility and vascular smooth muscle. In general, they are as effective in reducing symptoms as β-blockers, particularly in the rare condition of vasospastic angina due to coronary artery spasm.

Diltiazem is a useful anti-anginal drug. The long-acting preparation is used for hypertension. It works mainly by reducing heart rate and myocardial oxygen demands, so it should be used with caution when used with β-blockers. Diltiazem has less negative inotropic activity than verapamil. It can be given once or twice a day.

Verapamil is useful for angina and hypertension, and due to its effect on the atrioventricular node, it slows the ventricular rate in atrial fibrillation. It has a significant negative inotropic action, and therefore may precipitate left ventricular failure in patients with impaired left ventricular function. It should not be used with β-blockers. Constipation is quite a common side-effect.

Nifedipine, amlodipine, nicardipine and *felodipine* are also licensed for the treatment of angina. They relax smooth muscle and peripheral arteries, and exert little negative inotropic action. They have no anti-arrhythmic effects. Side-effects include flushing, ankle swelling and, initially, headache.

Sudden withdrawal of calcium-channel blockers may precipitate angina.

The following treatments reduce the risk of death and cardiac events or reduce symptoms in patients with angina:

✧ aspirin 75 mg every morning, or clopidogrel 75 mg if aspirin is contraindicated
✧ liberal *prophylactic* glyceryl trinitrate, and its use to abort attacks
✧ β-blockers (they are all equally effective) *or* slow-release diltiazem if the patient cannot tolerate β-blockers. The combination of a β-blocker with diltiazem may result in bradycardia, and is not recommended
✧ ACE inhibitors for patients with vascular disease and/or diabetes and/or left ventricular impairment

✧ add in, or substitute, slow-release and long-acting dihydropyridine calcium antagonists for patients who cannot tolerate β-blockers

✧ statins (with additional ezetimibe if necessary) to lower total and LDL-cholesterol levels to recommended targets

✧ patients should be encouraged to lose weight, exercise as much as they can without getting angina, and stopping smoking. Any cause of serious stress should be indentified and managed.

If anginal symptoms persist despite treatment, add in or substitute long-acting nitrates. Review the patient's treatment and compliance and their cardiovascular risk factors. Further stress testing may be helpful, but specialist referral and coronary angiography, with a view to myocardial revascularisation, represent the next step.

Newer drugs for angina

Ivabradine (5 mg twice a day or 7.5 mg twice a day) is licensed for the treatment of angina in patients with normal sinus function when β-blockers are contraindicated or not tolerated. This drug lowers the heart rate (negative chronotropic effect) by inhibiting the intrinsic pacemaker (sinus node) rate. This results in reduced myocardial oxygen consumption. It has no effect on intracardiac conduction or contractile function (i.e. no negative inotropic activity). This property, compared with β-blockers, is useful in patients with impaired left ventricular function.

Ivabradine is contraindicated in patients with a resting heart rate of < 60 bpm, cardiogenic shock, acute myocardial infarction, sinus node disease or unstable angina. It should be used with caution in patients with atrial fibrillation or atrioventricular block, and when combined with verapamil or diltiazem. There is a theoretical risk in patients with retinal disease. Long-term comparative trials are awaited.

Nicorandil 10 mg twice a day is licensed for treatment of angina. It is a potassium-channel activator with a nitrate component, and has both arterial and vasodilating properties. It is a coronary artery vasodilator. It has similar efficacy to other anti-anginal drugs, and is most commonly used as an additional treatment. Nicorandil has not been shown to reduce the number of deaths. It reduces the incidence of acute coronary syndromes and hospitalisation for angina.

It may precipitate pulmonary oedema in patients with myocardial infarction and hypotension in patients with hypovolaemia. Side-effects include headache, flushing, nausea and dizziness.

Inhibitors of fatty acid oxidation

These are not yet licensed in the UK, but have been given limited approval in the USA. They are reserved for patients with refractory angina.

Ranolazine improves exercise performance, but it prolongs the QT interval and there is a theoretical risk of torsade de pointes (ventricular tachycardia).

Trimetazidine improves exercise performance and reduces attacks of angina, but further large studies are required.

- The aims of treatment are to abolish symptoms and prevent myocardial infarction and death.

- It is appropriate to treat patients medically if they do not have high-risk coronary anatomy and left ventricular impairment.

- Short-acting nitrates, aspirin and β-blockers together with aggressive, comprehensive risk factor treatment are the foundations of medical treatment of angina.
- Optimise the anti-anginal drug dosage before adding in a different drug.
- Coronary angiography with myocardial revascularisation is usually required for patients whose symptoms remain unacceptable despite two anti-anginal drugs.

Revascularisation for chronic stable angina

The two indications for myocardial revascularisation in angina are to improve or abolish symptoms, and to improve prognosis.

In patients without angina or with only mild symptoms, revascularisation is only necessary if there are clear prognostic advantages.

The method of myocardial revascularisation should be tailored to the patient. Drug-eluting stents and other complementary interventional devices, including atherectomy, cutting balloons and rotablation, and antiplatelet treatments, have resulted in lower peri-operative complications and lower restenosis rates. They have stimulated and supported an expanding role for angioplasty. Patients with acute ST elevation myocardial infarction, multi-vessel disease, distal disease, left main stem disease or bypass graft disease are treated with angioplasty and stenting.

Revascularisation options for angina

There are a number of possible treatment options:
- coronary artery surgery
  - open chest approach (conventional coronary bypass)
  - 'beating heart' ('off-pump') technique
  - minimally invasive approach
  - robotic approach for isolated left anterior descending coronary artery disease
- coronary angioplasty and other interventional techniques
- combined angioplasty and coronary artery surgery.

Aggressive secondary prevention is crucial for all patients, whether treated medically or with myocardial revascularisation.

Making the choice

The method of revascularisation is usually chosen by the cardiologist who performed the coronary angiogram, in consultation with colleagues. Interventional cardiologists usually favour coronary angioplasty unless they consider that coronary artery surgery will provide the patient with a better long-term result, or the risks of angioplasty are too high.

Most large cardiac and cardiothoracic centres hold regular angiogram review meetings at which cardiologists and cardiac surgeons debate the benefits and risks of each method. There are a number of situations where there is an advantage of one form of myocardial revascularisation over another. In other situations, although there is no evidence of the superiority of one approach, technical, convenience and cost considerations influence the decision. Coronary artery surgery would be preferred if patients were to have valve surgery. However, a combined or hybrid approach using coronary artery surgery, valve surgery and coronary angioplasty is occasionally used.

Ultimately, the cardiologist responsible for the care of the patient makes the decision. This is straightforward when one strategy has clear advantages over the others.

In situations where either coronary artery surgery or coronary angioplasty would be appropriate, the merits and potential drawbacks of each approach should be discussed with the patient. It is the responsibility of the cardiologist to explain the pros and cons of each possible approach to the patient and allow them to make their own judgement. Some patients may wish to have a second opinion.

Coronary artery surgery

> Coronary artery surgery effectively reduces the symptoms of angina and ischaemia. In certain subsets of patients, it also improves the prognosis.

Coronary artery surgery should be performed in symptom-free patients only when there is evidence that revascularisation would result in prognostic benefit. Compared with medical treatment, coronary artery surgery confers prognostic benefits in the following situations:

- ⬦ left main stem coronary disease
- ⬦ proximal three-vessel coronary artery disease
- ⬦ significant stenosis of two major coronary arteries, including high-grade stenosis of the proximal left anterior descending coronary artery
- ⬦ three-vessel coronary artery disease and severe left ventricular impairment.

Risks of coronary artery surgery

The peri-operative risks depend on the patient's age, the presence of co-morbidity, particularly diabetes, renal disease, liver disease, vascular disease in any territory (aorta, brain, kidneys, carotids, peripheral arteries) and left ventricular impairment, recent infarction, previous stroke, immune state and lung function. Overall, the operative mortality is in the range 1–4%. The risk of stroke is lower using the 'off-pump' approach compared with traditional cardiopulmonary bypass with clamping of the aorta.

The now widespread use of the left internal mammary artery to graft the left anterior descending artery improves survival and reduces the incidence of late myocardial infarction and recurrent angina and the need for further cardiac interventions.

Patients who undergo 'off-pump' coronary artery surgery may be discharged after only four days and generally within one week of surgery.

Coronary artery surgery is generally preferred to coronary angioplasty for diabetic patients, because the peri-operative mortality is lower. However, coronary angioplasty is often a reasonable approach in selected patients who have good diabetic control.

Coronary angioplasty (percutaneous coronary intervention, PCI)

Coronary angioplasty and stenting play a key role in the treatment of unstable angina and myocardial infarction. Their place in the treatment of stable angina has recently been examined and reassessed.

Coronary angioplasty is considered an alternative to coronary artery surgery for relief of symptoms.

> Coronary angioplasty improves symptoms but does not improve survival in patients with stable angina.

Compared with coronary artery surgery, the initial costs are lower, the peri-operative risks are lower, there is less discomfort, and patients can return to work and drive one week after the procedure. Coronary angioplasty is performed as a day case. After primary angioplasty for acute ST elevation myocardial infarction, patients are discharged from hospital the following day. When offered the choice, most patients opt for coronary angioplasty.

Unless a patient has characteristics that would make coronary artery surgery the unequivocal, preferred method of revascularisation, either PCI or coronary artery surgery would be appropriate treatments. Coronary artery surgery does not offer survival benefits over coronary angioplasty except in high-risk cases.

Coronary angioplasty is usually offered to patients with single- or two-vessel coronary artery disease, assuming that the lesions are suitable.

Recurrent angina after coronary artery surgery

Coronary angioplasty is the preferred treatment for patients with recurrent angina after previous coronary artery surgery, because of the risks of redoing surgery, the risks of repeat anaesthesia, damage to the left internal mammary artery graft, post-operative sternotomy problems, and there may not be sufficient good-quality vein to use as a bypass conduit.

Restenosis after coronary angioplasty

This is due to fibromuscular hypertrophy following inevitable trauma to the vessel wall at the site of balloon dilatation. Drug-eluting stents were developed in order to try to reduce this problem. The risks of restenosis, and therefore the need for further revascularisation, are significantly lower with a drug-eluting stent compared with a bare metal stent. However, there is no evidence that restenosis is of prognostic importance. Unexpected atheromatous plaque rupture, rather than restenosis, is the cause of infarction and death.

In large coronary arteries (> 3 mm in diameter), bare metal stents (i.e. with no drug-eluting coating) are used because there is no evidence that drug-eluting stents offer any advantage.

> In stable angina, coronary angioplasty does not provide survival benefit compared to medical treatment.
>
> With regard to symptoms, coronary angioplasty is superior to medical treatment, reducing attacks of angina and breathlessness, and need for hospitalisation.
>
> Compared to bare metal stents, restenosis is less likely with a drug-eluting stent.
>
> Drug-eluting stents may increase late deaths, possibly due to cancer and stent thrombosis. Not all patients should have a drug-eluting stent.

Indications for coronary angioplasty

✧   Patients with angina refractory to medical treatments.
✧   Symptomatic one-, two- or three-vessel proximal coronary artery disease suitable for angioplasty and satisfactory left ventricular function and no diabetes.
✧   Symptomatic coronary artery disease in patients with previous angioplasty or coronary artery surgery to the previously treated artery or a different artery.
✧   Symptomatic patients with coronary artery lesions suitable for angioplasty but not suitable for coronary artery surgery.
✧   Symptomatic patients in whom coronary artery surgery is too risky.

Risks of coronary angioplasty

The risk of stroke, myocardial infarction or death is 1% in each case. The risk of vessel occlusion or damage requiring emergency coronary artery surgery is less than 2%.

Late thrombosis after the use of drug-eluting stents

There is an increased risk of in-stent thrombosis occurring several months after implantation of drug-eluting stents (6%)compared with bare metal stents (4%). The risk of thrombosis increases over time from 1% at 30 days to 3% at three years after implantation. In-stent thrombosis may lead to myocardial infarction and death. These concerns do not outweigh the benefits of drug-eluting stents in appropriately selected patients. It is important that antiplatelet drugs are prescribed and that patients take the prescribed medication. These include aspirin 75 mg every morning indefinitely, and clopidogrel 75 mg every morning for one year unless the patient is at high risk of bleeding. It is not yet clear whether clopidogrel should be taken for a longer period of time, particularly in diabetic patients.

Indications for either coronary artery surgery or coronary angioplasty

Patients with two-vessel coronary artery disease involving the proximal left anterior descending coronary artery with either abnormal left ventricular function or ischaemia shown on non-invasive stress testing.

Treatments for which there is no evidence of benefit, or where harm may result

There is interest among members of the public in alternative medical treatment for angina and coronary heart disease. However, there is no evidence that any of the following have any beneficial effect:

✧   chelation
✧   homeopathic and other treatments, including aromatherapy, reflexology, massage, hypnosis, acupuncture or other non-conventional treatments
✧   hormone replacement treatment
✧   vitamin C or E supplements
✧   garlic
✧   stress reduction
✧   folic acid
✧   special foods or fruits.

New invasive treatments for refractory angina

There is an increasing problem of managing older patients with a long history of coronary heart disease who have angina that is refractory to medical treatments but where both angioplasty and coronary artery surgery are no technically practical. The prevalence of refractory angina is not known, but is estimated to be around 5% of the total population of patients with angina. The problem is best dealt with in a multi-disciplinary team consisting of cardiologists, cardiac surgeons, pain specialists, psychologists, exercise physiologists, dietitians and the GP. Continuous and frequent support is required.

Treatments for this difficult problem are available in only a few centres in the UK. The management principles are:

◇ confirm that the symptoms are due to angina and not another condition that is mimicking chest pain
◇ investigate the location and extent of reversible ischaemia with imaging
◇ ensure effective and aggressive secondary prevention
◇ optimise the patient's weight, diet and medical regime
◇ reassess the possibility of revascularisation
◇ treat anxiety, fear and depression, and educate and reassure the patient as much as possible
◇ encourage the patient to take up daily physical rehabilitation and exercise that is tailored to their ability.

Specific treatments

These have been generally disappointing. There is no consistent evidence from randomised placebo-controlled trials that laser revascularisation, neurostimulation using spinal cord stimulation or angiogenesis improve symptoms or prognosis in this increasingly large group of patients who continue to experience significant angina despite medical treatment, and in whom revascularisation is not an option. It is not understood why some patients with chronic angina develop a collateral circulation. Various explanations, including exercise, have been proposed.

Stellate ganglion block (temporary sympathectomy)

This may reduce angina and allow patients to exercise. It is a safe and simple procedure. The effects last for one month, so patients need repeat procedures.

Neuromodulation

Transcutaneous electrical nerve stimulation (TENS)

This is quite effective, but there are practical problems. Patients have to wear electrodes, pads and the device and use it several times per day, prophylactically as well as during attacks of angina.

Spinal cord stimulation

The spinal cord between C7–T2 is stimulated using an electrocatheter introduced into the epidural space. The catheter is connected to a pacemaker-like device implanted in a subcutaneous abdominal pouch. The proposed mechanism is to suppress cardiac neuronal activity during myocardial ischaemia.

Only small numbers of patients have been studied. It is a safe procedure but as yet an unproven one because no placebo-controlled studies have been performed. There was initial enthusiasm and optimism about the technique, which in small numbers of patients was shown to relieve symptoms, reduce hospital admissions and increase quality of life. Spinal cord stimulation had a similar anti-anginal effect to coronary artery surgery but a lower six-month mortality. Spinal cord stimulation has been shown to be beneficial in patients with microvascular angina (angina where the visible epicardial coronary arteries appear normal, but patients have angina and signs of reversible ischaemia).

Enhanced external counterpulsation

Although there is some evidence of benefit, there is insufficient data to support this approach, which is similar in principle to invasive aortic balloon counterpulsation. Cuffs are wrapped around the patient's legs and arms and inflated using compressed air, and high pressures (300 mmHg) are applied sequentially in the lower legs to lower and upper thighs in early diastole to propel blood back to the heart. The cuffs are deflated at the beginning of systole. During inflation, there is an increase in blood pressure and venous return to the heart, increasing diastolic pressure and coronary filling. During deflation, there is a decrease in peripheral vascular resistance and cardiac workload, reducing left ventricular work and oxygen consumption.

The risks and contraindications include arrhythmias, bleeding, active thrombophlebitis, aortic aneurysm and pacemaker, aortic regurgitation, uncontrolled hypertension, severe left ventricular impairment and peripheral vascular disease. Local side-effects include pain during cuff inflation, oedema and skin lesions. This treatment is not available within the NHS.

Stem cell therapy

This is an experimental and unproven technique. Autologous bone marrow cells are injected into the coronary sinus of the heart to stimulate the formation of new coronary vessels. Only small numbers of patients have been treated using this approach, but there have been no deaths at one year of follow-up. There is no evidence that this approach improves symptoms of myocardial ischaemia. Complications may occur because this is an invasive treatment. Proliferative diseases in other organs and immunonological reactions may occur.

Percutaneous transmyocardial laser revascularisation

Small channels through the myocardium between the epicardium and endocardium are produced by a laser in order to bring oxygen to ischaemic areas. The channels block off quite soon after they have been created. Complications of open surgical laser revascularisation include death (3% in low-risk and 20% in high-risk patients due to stroke, infarction, heart failure or cardiac perforation). These risks are reduced with percutaneous revascularisation. There is no evidence that this technique is beneficial.

Considerations when requesting exercise tests

Before requesting an exercise test, it is important to appreciate the value and limitations of an exercise test result based on an understanding of Bayes' theorem and how the test result will influence management.

Patient's ability to exercise

Patients have to be willing and able to exercise. The test procedure should be explained to the patient before requesting the test, and patients with musculoskeletal, neurological or psychological conditions that would make the test impossible or unhelpful should not be referred.

Cycle or treadmill?

Most hospitals in the UK and the USA use treadmills, although European centres favour cycles. Many patients find it easier and less worrying to cycle.

Analysis of test results

Bayes' theorem helps to explain the fairly common occurrence of a false-positive exercise test result (exercise-induced ST depression but normal coronary arteries) in low-risk individuals, and this has implications for screening 'healthy' individuals.

Bayes' theorem

Test results cannot be interpreted adequately without knowing the prevalence of disease in the population under study.

The *pre-test likelihood* is the probability of disease in a patient to be tested

$$= \frac{\text{number of patients with disease in the test population}}{\text{total number of patients in the test population}}$$

The *post-test likelihood* is the probability of disease in a patient showing an abnormal test result

$$= \frac{\text{number of patients with disease showing an abnormal test result}}{\text{total number of patients with an abnormal test result}}$$

The *sensitivity* of a test (expressed as a percentage) is the probability that a patient with disease will be correctly identified by an abnormal test result

$$= \frac{\text{number of patients with disease with an abnormal test result}}{\text{total number of patients with disease tested}}$$

$$= \frac{\text{TP}}{\text{TP} + \text{FN}}$$

The *specificity* of a test (expressed as a percentage) is the probability that an individual without disease will be correctly identified by having a normal test result

$$= \frac{\text{number of individuals with a normal test result}}{\text{number of normal individuals tested}}$$

$$= \frac{\text{TN}}{\text{TN} + \text{FP}}$$

The *predictive value of a positive (abnormal) test result* is the probability that a positive (abnormal) test result correctly indicates that the patient has disease

$$= \frac{\text{number of patients with disease}}{\text{total number of patients with a positive test result}}$$

$$= \frac{TP}{TP + FP}$$

The *predictive value of a negative (normal) test result* is the probability that a normal test result correctly indicates that the individual does not have disease

$$= \frac{\text{number of individuals without disease}}{\text{total number of individuals with a negative test result}}$$

$$= \frac{TN}{TN + FN}$$

✧ If the prevalence of coronary heart disease in a population of patients similar to the patient tested is high, as in the case of a population of patients with typical angina, then both the pre-test and post-test probabilities of disease will be high.
✧ Conversely, if the prevalence of disease in a population of patients similar to the patient tested is low, as in young patients without angina and with no cardiovascular risk factors, then the pre-test and post-test probabilities of coronary heart disease will be low.

Sensitivity, specificity and false-positive and false-negative test results

Patients are generally aware that exercise testing is not a perfect test. It has a sensitivity of around 75% and a specificity of around 85%.

Consider the case of a 30-year-old woman with non-anginal chest pain. It can be seen from Table 7.1 that her pre-test probability of coronary heart disease is 2%. If she is referred for an exercise test, what is the probability that a 'positive' test result, showing ST depression, truly indicates coronary heart disease?

The exercise test will detect only 75% of the true positives = 1.5.

The total number of patients with a positive test result will be 75% of the true positives (1.5) + 15% of the true negatives (14.7)

$$= \frac{2.25}{16.2}$$

$$= 14\%$$

Therefore, the predictive accuracy of a positive test in an individual with a low pre-test probability of having coronary artery disease is low. However, the predictive accuracy of a negative test result in this individual is high

$$= \frac{85\% \times 98}{25\% \times 2 + 85\% \times 98}$$

$$= 99\%$$

In the case of a 70-year-old man with typical angina, the predictive value of a positive test result is 99%, while the predictive value of a negative test result is 18%.

Exercise testing in both high- and low-risk patients adds very little diagnostic information. The approach is of greatest diagnostic value in patients with an *intermediate risk* of having coronary artery disease.

Indications for exercise testing

◈ To diagnose obstructive coronary artery disease in patients with an intermediate pre-test probability of coronary artery disease, including those with right bundle branch block.

◈ For risk assessment and prognosis in patients undergoing initial evaluation.

◈ To guide prognosis and exercise capacity in patients with an abnormal resting ECG and those with known coronary artery disease.

◈ To assess new symptoms in patients with significant cardiovascular risk factors.

◈ To evaluate the response to treatment (stress imaging may be performed in patients after coronary artery surgery).

◈ Evaluation of the blood pressure response in patients with suspected hypertension.

◈ Evaluation of functional capacity in patients with impaired cardiac function.

Non-invasive stress tests assess the effects of obstructive coronary artery disease on myocardial blood flow, which, if impaired, may be revealed by an abnormal test result. In the most commonly used test – exercise testing – the hallmark of exercise-induced myocardial ischaemia is ST depression, but there are other markers of ischaemia (*see* Table 7.2).

Exercise testing will add very little diagnostic information in a patient with typical symptoms of angina, although certain features of the exercise test will help in prognostic risk stratification – identifying patients at high and low risk from cardiovascular events – and these features are used to identify patients for coronary angiography and revascularisation.

TABLE 7.2: Exercise test variables used in risk stratification assessed using either the Bruce treadmill or WHO cycle protocols

Exercise test variable	High risk	Low risk
Exercise time (min)	< 3	> 12
Time to angina (min)	< 3	No angina
Time to 1 mm ST depression (min)	< 3	No ST depression
Extent of ST depression (mm)	> 2.5	< 1
Duration of ST depression[a] (min)	> 5	Immediate resolution
Blood pressure response[b]	Abnormal	Normal
Heart rate response[c]	> 70% APMHR	< 70% APMHR
Ventricular ectopics and tachycardia	Present	No arrhythmias
ST elevation[d]	Present	Not present

a Adverse prognosis and multi-vessel coronary artery disease are associated with widespread, pronounced ST depression lasting for more than five minutes after the end of exercise.

b During maximal, symptom-limited exercise the systolic blood pressure should increase by at least 20 mmHg, reflecting normal left ventricular systolic function, myocardial blood supply and cardiovascular reflexes. If it does not rise, or if it falls at any stage during exercise, particularly below the resting level, this suggests impaired left ventricular function and/or blood supply, and a poor prognosis.

c The age-predicted maximal heart rate (APMHR) is estimated by subtracting the patient's age from 220. Thus, the age-predicted maximal heart rate of a 70-year-old man is 150 bpm. Some exercise ECG centres use 70% of the age-predicted heart rate as an exercise end point, but patients on β-blockers would have a blunted heart rate and blood pressure response. However, it is potentially dangerous to stop β-blockers suddenly. It is neither practical nor necessary to stop them prior to an exercise test, even though the sensitivity of the test may be reduced.

d ST elevation occurring in Q-wave-bearing leads in patients after myocardial infarction is associated with a poor prognosis, and is related to left ventricular impairment.

Exercise test scoring systems to assess prognosis

All of the exercise test variables listed in Table 7.2 are useful for predicting prognosis.

Various scoring systems have been devised, but these are not commonly used in routine clinical practice. One of the strongest prognostic markers is maximum exercise capacity, so it is important to request a symptom-limited exercise test.

The Duke University score combines exercise time on the treadmill, the extent of ST depression and the severity of angina to produce a score that identifies young patients at risk of cardiovascular death ranging from low (0.25%) to high (5.25%). It is not commonly used in hospitals in the UK. The score was derived from data obtained in patients with a mean age of 49 years, and is unreliable in predicting events in patients over the age of 75 years. It is not applicable to cycle exercise tests.

Other tests that are used to assess myocardial ischaemia and angina
Stress echocardiography

This is used to evaluate ischaemia in patients who cannot exercise or who have resting ECG abnormalities, and after myocardial revascularisation. Interpretation of the results is very subjective. It has a high specificity (excluding disease in low risk individuals) and provides information about cardiac anatomy. It is used to differentiate between infarcted (dead) heart muscle and hibernating and ischaemic heart muscle, which might improve after revascularisation.

Stress perfusion imaging

This involves the injection of radioactive material and imaging the left ventricle both at rest and after stress (either exercise or dobutamine). It is expensive and available in only a few centres in the UK. Some patients may feel disinclined to have a radioactive injection.

Coronary angiography

This is the 'gold standard' that provides the most accurate information about coronary anatomy and left ventricular function. It shows the location, severity and extent of atherosclerotic disease – the most powerful predictors of prognosis – and identifies patients with normal arteries. In patients with angina, coronary angioplasty is now commonly performed immediately after the coronary angiogram, and this avoids the need for the patient to return to the cardiac catheter laboratory.

Indications for coronary angiography

✧ Chronic stable angina despite medical treatment.
✧ Patients identified as being at high risk on clinical criteria or non-invasive tests.
✧ Survivors of sudden death.
✧ Angina and signs of heart failure.
✧ Suspected coronary artery disease but indeterminate non-invasive test results.
✧ When non-invasive tests are not practical.

GPs are now familiar with the limitations of non-invasive testing for ischaemia, and many of them refer patients directly for coronary angiography. Suitable patients include those with a high risk of coronary artery disease, those who cannot exercise, those with recurrent symptoms after revascularisation or infarction, and occasionally those in whom coronary artery disease needs to be excluded for occupational or insurance reasons.

Coronary angiography provides essential information about revascularisation. At present no other investigation can provide this information with sufficient accuracy.

Advice for patients

✧ Angina is a feeling of tightness, breathlessness or discomfort. It is occasionally described as pain felt in the chest, arms, gums or throat. It is associated with exertion, stress or cold weather, and is promptly relieved by rest. If you have these symptoms, come to see us straight away. If you have angina but you think it is getting more frequent and lasting longer, or if you are getting it at rest, you should see us straight away because the artery or arteries may be blocking off.
✧ Angina is caused by a lack of blood and oxygen supply to the heart muscle because one or more of the arteries that supply the heart with blood are narrowed with fat (cholesterol) and other material.
✧ Cholesterol is deposited in the wall of the arteries of the heart and elsewhere for reasons that are unclear.
✧ The risk of cholesterol formation on the inside of the arterial wall is higher in people who have a high cholesterol level, and in those who smoke, have a high blood pressure, are diabetic, are overweight, take little exercise or have a family history of heart attacks and angina. Heart disease is also more common in Asian people for reasons we do not understand.
✧ Angina is not diagnosed by tests but by your description of your symptoms. If your symptoms don't fit with a diagnosis of angina, you are unlikely to have it, particularly if it is unlikely that you have arterial disease. However, this does not mean that you don't have furring up or blockages in the heart arteries. The only way to find this out is by doing certain tests.
✧ The most commonly performed test is a stress test or exercise ECG. The aim is to increase your heart rate and blood pressure to see whether there is enough blood and oxygen getting to your heart muscle through the heart arteries. It does not tell us if the heart arteries are blocked or, if they are, by how much. The exercise test tells us the probability of you having narrowed heart arteries. The test involves you either walking on a treadmill at increasing speed and inclination, or cycling against increasing resistance. Your heart rate, blood pressure and ECG are monitored during the test. If you do well, and do not experience any chest discomfort or breathlessness, and there are no ECG changes, it is unlikely that you have any serious heart problem, although the test does not exclude this.
✧ If you have definite angina or the exercise test is abnormal, the specialist (cardiologist) may suggest that you have a special X-ray of the heart arteries called a coronary

angiogram. This is done as a day case in hospital. You will be told what to do by the hospital team. You are not allowed to eat or drink (but you should take your tablets with a little water) for four hours before the angiogram. The test is done with a local anaesthetic in the skin of the right groin (or occasionally the left groin or right arm or wrist). Very thin tubes are inserted into the heart and the heart arteries through the groin artery. You will not feel this, but you might feel a flushing sensation when the contrast fluid is injected into the pumping chamber of the heart, and possibly some chest pain when the heart arteries are injected. Pictures are taken of the arteries and if you wish you will be able to stay awake and watch the movie. Most patients find it interesting, and it should not be unpleasant. The test takes about 15 minutes, and you have to lie flat and fairly still for a few hours after the test so that you do not bleed from the small puncture site in the groin. A small collagen plug is now often inserted into the artery to seal the puncture in the artery wall. The doctor will usually explain the result to you after the test. You should not walk home after the test, nor should you drive or cycle or do any heavy lifting until the following day. If your groin bleeds or you notice a lump, come to see us immediately. Most patients have some bruising in the groin. The angiogram is generally safe and the test is done in patients of all ages and even those with recent heart attacks. Rarely, elderly patients and those with bad arteries and very weak hearts may have a heart attack. The risk of a serious complication is one in 1000 cases.

* Angina only occurs very rarely in patients with normal arteries.
* Not all patients with furred-up heart arteries experience angina. They may have no warning system. This is why, for quite a lot of people who do have furring up of the heart arteries, the first they know about it is when they have a heart attack, or worse!
* If you know that you have heart disease and you get an attack of angina, come to see us and we will give you treatment. You may also need some tests.
* We will give you aspirin and a nitroglycerin spray to use both before you do anything which might bring on the symptoms, and also when you get the symptoms. The nitroglycerin may give you a headache, and if you take more than one spray or tablet, it may make you feel faint because it lowers your blood pressure.
* Angina is unlikely to be the cause of prickly chest pain lasting for only one or two seconds.
* Angina-like chest pain associated with sweating and breathlessness lasting for more than 20 minutes in a person with a high chance of having arterial problems may be due to a heart attack. The best advice is to phone for an emergency ambulance and go straight to hospital.
* If you have furring up of any artery, you should come to see us at least once a year for an assessment of your blood pressure, and blood tests for cholesterol, kidney function, liver function and blood sugar (diabetes).
* Treatment for angina depends on the severity and frequency of the symptoms, the severity of the arterial disease and the heart function.
* It is very important for all patients with angina to do everything they can to help themselves. They should stop smoking, get down to their best weight, exercise every day, have a low-fat, low-salt and low-sugar diet, and take statins to lower their cholesterol. There are other drugs that may be helpful.
* Patients with mild symptoms who only occasionally get angina can be treated with aspirin and a GTN spray or tablets.
* Patients with bad angina are usually referred to a cardiologist for further tests, including an angiogram, which is the only way to see if the arteries are furred up, narrowed or blocked, or whether they are normal. No other test provides similarly accurate information.

Answers to questions about clinical cases

1. The most likely diagnosis is restenosis in the left anterior descending coronary artery, which may occur in up to 30% of cases after angioplasty, usually within six months of the procedure. It is less frequent after stenting (20%), and even less frequent if a drug-eluting stent was implanted (10%). Restenosis is due to fibromuscular hypertrophy occurring as a result of trauma to the vessel wall during dilatation. This is more likely than new atheroma occurring in the two other apparently normal arteries. Exercise testing or other non-invasive tests for reversible ischaemia will add little to management, and are unnecessary in view of the symptoms, which are the same as the patient experienced before angioplasty. Review all of his cardiovascular risk factors, his treatment (he should be on aspirin 75 mg every morning, a β-blocker and prophylactic GTN) and other anti-anginal medication. Because the artery may have an important stenosis and an anatomical diagnosis is required, this patient should be seen quickly, ideally by the cardiologist who performed the angioplasty. A repeat angiogram should be performed and followed, if appropriate, by repeat intervention or coronary artery surgery.

2. It is highly unlikely that this patient has coronary heart disease (pre-test probability < 3%), so exercise testing would not offer any useful diagnostic information. If she is very anxious, an exercise test showing a good exercise tolerance and no ST depression, together with (if she wished) a cardiology opinion, might reassure her.

3. The question is whether this patient's chest pain and breathlessness are due to prostatic secondaries, other possible causes, or due to cardiac problems including angina and/or heart failure. Before embarking on cardiac tests, investigations are needed for his prostate and chest, and it might be easier for him and his family if he were admitted to hospital under the care of his urologist, who should liaise with the cardiologist. If he would prefer to avoid going into hospital, some of the preliminary tests could be done as an outpatient in consultation with both specialists. These should include a chest X-ray, haematology and biochemical screening, and a bone scan.

4. This patient's arthritis would probably preclude her from exercise testing. Left ventricular hypertrophy and obesity complicate the interpretation of both nuclear perfusion scanning and stress echocardiography. If her symptoms are disabling, coronary angiography would be the most accurate and useful investigation. It would allow coronary angioplasty to be performed at the same time. As in all patients with vascular disease, check her cardiovascular risk factors and treat them. Cardiac revascularisation may be necessary before orthopaedic surgery.

5. This patient is at intermediate cardiac risk on the basis of risk factors and the questionable history. If exercise testing shows a good exercise tolerance (more than 10 minutes on the Bruce treadmill protocol or WHO cycle protocol), he could be reassured and followed up with careful cardiovascular risk management. He should be referred for coronary angiography if the exercise test shows reversible ischaemia or if the test result is equivocal.

6. Erectile dysfunction is particularly common for a number of reasons in men of this age who have diabetes and vascular disease, and should be identified by direct questioning in primary care because of its psychosocial effects on the patient and his partner, and because it is often a marker for vascular disease. This patient's cardiovascular risk factors should be reviewed and treated, and if he is on a β-blocker, this should be discussed with him and withdrawn slowly and an alternative anti-anginal medication prescribed. Drug treatment with sildenafil (Viagra) or a similar drug would probably improve his symptoms, but he should be told not to take either long- or short-acting nitrates because of hypotension, and he should be warned about the possible side-effects of headache and facial flushing.

7. Patients with mild stable angina generally have a good prognosis. Myocardial revascularisation is undertaken in order to control symptoms or improve the prognosis in certain subsets of patients (those with left main stem disease, or triple-vessel coronary artery disease and impaired left ventricular function). If this patient's symptoms are well controlled on medical treatment and you have assessed and treated all of her cardiovascular risk factors, she could be treated medically. Angiography should be considered if her symptoms become unstable.

FURTHER READING

British Cardiac Society, British Hypertension Society, Diabetes UK, HEART UK, Primary Care Cardiovascular Society and Stroke Association. Joint British Societies' guidelines on prevention of cardiovascular disease in clinical practice. *Heart.* 2005; **91 (Suppl. 5):** v1–2.

Department of Health. *National Service Framework for Coronary Heart Disease.* London: Department of Health; 2000.

Fox K, Garcia MA, Ardissino D *et al.* Guidelines for the management of stable angina pectoris: executive summary. *Eur Heart J.* 2006; **27:** 1341–81.

Gibbons RJ, Abrams J, Chatterjee K *et al.* ACC/AHA 2002 guideline update for the management of patients with chronic stable angina – summary article: a report of the American College of Cardiology/American Heart Association Task Force on Practice Guidelines (Committee on the Management of Patients with Chronic Stable Angina). *J Am Coll Cardiol.* 2003; **41:** 159–68.

Gruentzig AR, Senning A, Siegenthaler WE. Nonoperative dilatation of coronary artery stenosis: percutaneous transluminal coronary angioplasty. *NEJM.* 1979; **301:** 61–8.

Handler C, Coghlan G. *Living with Coronary Disease.* London: Springer; 2007. ISBN-10:1-84628-550-X.

Libby P, Ridker PM. Inflammation and atherothrombosis: from population biology and bench research to clinical practice. *J Am Coll Cardiol.* 2006; **48:** A33–46.

Mannheimer C, Camici P, Chester MR *et al.* The problem of chronic refractory angina. Report from the ESC Joint Study Group on the treatment of refractory angina. *Eur Heart J.* 2002; **23:** 355–70.

Patil CV, Nikolsky E, Boulos M *et al.* Multivessel coronary artery disease: current revascularisation strategies. *Eur Heart J.* 2001; **22:** 1183–97.

Pocock SJ, Henderson RA, Seed P *et al.* Quality of life, employment status and anginal symptoms after coronary angioplasty or bypass surgery: 3-year follow-up in the Randomized Intervention Treatment of Angina (RITA) Trial. *Circulation.* 1996; **94:** 135–42.

Schofield PM. Indications for percutaneous and surgical intervention: how far does the evidence base guide us? *Heart.* 2003; **89:** 565–70.

EIGHT

Myocardial infarction and other acute coronary syndromes

Clinical cases

1. The daughter of an 82-year-old woman who has never smoked and whose blood pressure is normal telephones you because her mother has suddenly become breathless and sweaty. She thinks her mother has caught a cold. What advice do you give her?
2. A 58-year-old man who had an angioplasty and drug-eluting stent implanted three months ago complains of indigestion. He asks you whether he can stop his aspirin and the clopidogrel. What do you advise?
3. A 60-year-old man is discharged from the accident and emergency department on the same day as he went in for chest pain. He brings a discharge note from the hospital stating that the troponin and ECG were normal. He is still experiencing chest pain. What do you do?
4. A 57-year-old man comes to see you complaining of a cough. You discover that he had been admitted to hospital in another town while visiting a family member three months ago. He had not volunteered this information and does not really understand what he was told in hospital. What do you do?
5. A 79-year-old woman with a long history of hypertension complains of sudden onset of back pain and breathlessness. What do you do?

Changes in management and improved prognosis for patients with acute coronary syndromes

The diagnosis and management of acute coronary syndromes have changed beyond recognition in the past 30 years. Prolonged bed rest (six weeks until the 1950s), cocktails of questionable potions and the instilling of a lifelong fear of stressful situations have been replaced by standardised, proven therapies administered within a strict timeline, and an early return to full activities. In certain circumstances a patient who is admitted with a 'full blown' ST elevation MI (STEMI) can have the event essentially aborted, be discharged the following day, and be back to work within a week. Not only has the in-hospital mortality fallen from 25% to less than 10% over the last 20 years, but also the frequency of subsequent heart failure and recurrent heart attacks has been reduced dramatically.

Of all patients who have a myocardial infarction, 25–35% will die before they receive medical attention, usually because of ventricular fibrillation. In-hospital mortality in the high-risk group of patients with ST elevation myocardial infarction has fallen. Improved survival is due to prompt medical attention and improvements in initial treatment, including thrombolysis (clot-busting drugs) and primary angioplasty (angioplasty with or without stenting), as soon as patients arrive at hospital.

> Primary coronary angioplasty restores blood flow to the heart muscle through a previously blocked artery in more than 90% of cases, compared with 50% by thrombolysis (fibrinolysis).

Vigorous and effective primary cardiovascular prevention has reduced the incidence of myocardial infarction, and secondary prevention has reduced the incidence of further infarction, associated heart failure and other complications.

Definition of acute coronary syndrome

The diagnosis of acute coronary syndrome (ACS) refers to one of the following acute ischaemic states:

- ✧ unstable angina (defined as angina at rest lasting > 20 minutes, new-onset severe angina, or angina occurring more frequently and lasting longer, without ECG changes or enzyme rise)
- ✧ non-ST-elevation myocardial infarction (non-STEMI)
- ✧ ST-elevation myocardial infarction (STEMI).

Patients with unstable angina and non-ST-elevation myocardial infarction (non-STEMI) present in a similar manner. It may not be possible to distinguish them until several hours after presentation, when ECG changes develop, or when levels of bio-chemical markers of myocardial necrosis (troponins T and I) become raised. Both conditions may progress to STEMI with new Q-wave formation (Q-wave myocardial infarction), which is associated with more extensive myocardial damage and a worse prognosis. This highlights the necessity for early diagnosis of the condition and prompt referral.

Role of primary care clinicians in the management of acute coronary syndromes

GPs play a major role in diagnosing acute coronary syndromes, educating patients about 'danger signals' and managing the return to normal life after the event.

However, the immediate management of acute coronary syndromes requires a dedicated team, access to equipment (e.g. cardiac monitors) and the provision of 24-hour access to the same level of care, and is thus beyond the remit of general practice. All patients with suspected acute coronary syndromes should be referred to the emergency department or rapid-access chest pain clinic, where the diagnosis can be confirmed or excluded within a few hours.

Occasionally patients with acute coronary syndromes, having been reassured by the hospital staff, visit the GP for further evaluation. Especially in cases where the presentation is atypical (breathlessness, autonomic symptoms, confusion and/or loss of consciousness), the greater experience of the GP (compared with an accident and emergency SHO) can be pivotal. In such situations, requesting immediate review by a cardiologist can be life-saving.

GPs need to understand the indications and contraindications for drugs used after patients have left hospital, and how long they should be prescribed for. Patients will expect guidance from their primary care team with regard to diet, alcohol, sex, work, exercise, and managing and coping with stress.

Differential diagnosis of acute coronary syndromes

The differential diagnosis of acute coronary syndromes includes:

- ✧ pericarditis (pain worse when lying down)
- ✧ dissection of the aorta (sudden-onset tearing pain in the back)
- ✧ pulmonary embolism (sudden-onset pleuritic pain and breathlessness)
- ✧ peptic ulcer and gastro-oesophageal pain (food-related burning pain)

✧ biliary tract disease (cholangitis) (fatty-food-related, severe pain, fever and rigors, and symptoms of biliary obstruction)
✧ pancreatitis (severe abdominal pain with little tenderness, amylase).

All of these conditions are important, and some of them are life-threatening. It is not possible to exclude or diagnose these conditions without investigations.

> All patients who have severe symptoms, or in whom any of these conditions is suspected, should be sent to hospital as an emergency for assessment and treatment.
> Without an ECG recording or blood tests, it is not possible to confirm or exclude an acute coronary syndrome.
> Patients who have symptoms consistent with an acute coronary syndrome should be assessed in hospital, preferably where there are facilities for primary coronary angioplasty, as an emergency.

Pathology of acute coronary syndromes (identifying patients at high risk)

Coronary artery endothelial injury and dysfunction result in adhesion and migration of leukocytes from the circulation into the arterial intima. There is migration of smooth muscle cells from the media into the intima. These two events lead to formation of an atherosclerotic plaque in the artery.

Thrombosis occurring in a coronary artery due to rupture of an atheromatous plaque is the pivotal event that leads to an acute coronary syndrome. Plaques containing a lot of fat are more likely to rupture than stable plaques, which characteristically contain very little fat and have a firm fibrous cap. Platelets and inflammatory cells, together with thrombin and fibrin, are deposited at the ruptured plaque and form a thrombus.

Stable coronary plaques

Patients with angina may have significant narrowing of their coronary arteries to at least 75%. Large plaques containing a lot of calcium, covered with a thick, fibrous cap, are generally stable and, compared with an unstable plaque, much less likely to rupture. Patients with stable plaques are at low risk of heart attacks and acute coronary syndromes. The annual mortality rate in patients with stable angina is 2%. The main aim of treatment is symptom control. Myocardial revascularisation is usually not necessary if the patient's symptoms are well controlled on tablets.

The vulnerable or unstable plaque

Most heart attacks, particularly in young people, are due to rupture of a thin layer of fat, which is not big enough to obstruct blood flow down the coronary artery or cause angina. The plaque becomes inflamed, and the thin cap covering the layer of soft fat then cracks, attracting platelets and other cells. The clot or thrombus obstructs the artery and the blood flow down the artery, causing a heart attack. This is manifested as an acute coronary syndrome or a myocardial infarction, with or without ST segment elevation on the ECG.

Some plaques of atheroma are more likely to rupture ('vulnerable' plaques) than others. However, no non-invasive tests are reliable in identifying 'vulnerable' plaques. Plaques with a thin fibrous cap and many soft, lipid, inflammatory cells and mediators are more likely to rupture than stable plaques, which have a firm fibrous cap and a comparatively small lipid core.

At present the best evidence that a patient has a vulnerable plaque is a history of an acute coronary syndrome within the past six months. The likelihood of a further event is around 20% in the first six months after hospital discharge (without modern management strategies). Patients who have had stenting of their coronary arteries for stable angina are also at increased risk of an acute coronary syndrome for around six months after the procedure (longer for drug-eluting stents), because a stable situation has been rendered relatively less stable. The pay-off for this increased risk is the improved overall perfusion of the heart and, hopefully, improved symptoms.

Intracoronary thrombosis and myocardial infarction

All of the myocardium supplied by the blocked coronary artery becomes ischaemic. This causes chest pain and ST elevation on the ECG, usually with Q-waves. The changes can be delayed. As soon as the heart becomes ischaemic, the myocardial cells die and there is a wave front of cell death and destruction, starting in the endocardium (inner wall) and spreading to the epicardium (outer wall). Within a few hours, the full thickness of the heart muscle dies. This is called transmural infarction, and it is reflected in the ECG as Q-waves overlying the area of infarcted muscle. Q-waves in the inferior leads (II, II and aVF) are diagnostic of inferior wall infarction. Q-waves in the anterior (V1–V3) or lateral (I, aVL and V4–6) ECG leads are diagnostic of anterior and lateral infarction, respectively.

Rationale for reperfusing ischaemic heart muscle

The aim of reperfusing the myocardium, using thrombolysis or angioplasty, is to delete quickly stop the spreading 'wave front' of cell death, thereby reducing myocardial damage.

This is referred to as *salvage of jeopardised myocardium* – that is, saving heart muscle that is in danger of death. Reducing the amount of heart muscle damage improves the prognosis. The more quickly the ischaemic heart muscle is re-supplied with blood, nutrients and oxygen, the less damage occurs.

Methods of reperfusion

Reperfusion therapy (angioplasty or thrombolysis) is indicated for patients whose infarction occurred within the last 12 hours and who also have ST elevation of more than 1.0 mV in two contiguous ECG leads, or left bundle branch block (for the purposes of thrombolysis or primary angioplasty, left bundle branch block is presumed to be 'new').

Angioplasty and stenting

Angioplasty for acute myocardial infarction is termed primary angioplasty. Angioplasty is preferred if the procedure can be performed within *90 minutes of the chest symptoms* appearing. Patients who present to a hospital without primary angioplasty facilities, and within this time frame, should ideally be moved to a hospital that does have appropriate staff and facilities.

Even if primary angioplasty cannot be performed within 90 minutes, it is preferred to thrombolysis:

✧   when thrombolysis is contraindicated (recent surgery, or stroke)
✧   for patients with a high risk of bleeding with thrombolysis (age > 75 years)
✧   for complicated infarcts or cardiogenic shock.

Restenosis after primary angioplasty

Restenosis in a treated artery is less likely to occur after stenting than after angioplasty without stenting. Therefore, so long as the infarct-related artery is wide enough to take a stent, and there are no reasons why the platelet inhibitor clopidogrel cannot be used for one year, stenting is generally utilised. In order to reduce the risk of thrombosis, aspirin is also administered.

Fibrinolytic (thrombolytic) therapy

Fibrinolytic therapy is preferred:
✧   when primary angioplasty is not available within 90 minutes
✧   in patients who present almost immediately after the symptoms occur (fibrinolytic therapy may abort the infarct)
✧   when angiography and angioplasty are too risky (e.g. in patients with renal impairment or serious allergy to contrast materials).

In a fairly high proportion of cases, spontaneous thrombolysis occurs. This is due to the body's own thrombolytic system dissolving clots in arteries. Some ruptured plaques heal leaving little or no visible trace of an arterial problem when imaged with angiography. However, inflamed plaques remain potentially unstable, high-risk lesions.

Cooling off hot lesions

If there is removal of damaging stimuli (e.g. smoking, stress, hypertension), together with aggressive medical management (statins, β-blockers, aspirin and other antiplatelet drugs), these high-risk, 'hot' lesions may 'cool down.' The inflammatory process in the arterial wall resolves and the vulnerable plaque may become stable.

Problems of atheroma imaging in identifying high-risk patients

It is important to identify unstable, vulnerable plaques, which often contain little or no calcium. High-risk, soft, non-calcified lesions highlight the deficiency of certain forms of atheroma imaging. Electron beam computed tomography (EBCT) is claimed to identify patients with coronary artery disease on the basis of their 'calcium score', and thus to identify patients at risk. However, this form of imaging, which is not available on the NHS, detects calcium in the wall of arteries but may fail to identify non-calcified but nevertheless vulnerable plaques. The results of EBCT scanning may therefore be misleading. Patients with a high calcium score, and who are often symptom-free, may be advised to have coronary angiography and coronary angioplasty. Patients with large amounts of calcium in their arteries, who are often the elderly, may have a high calcium score but a benign prognosis because their plaques are stable. Young people, who may have vulnerable high-risk plaques with little or no calcium in the walls of their arteries, would have a low calcium score and be misclassified as being at low risk.

What happens in hospital?

Whenever an ACS is strongly suspected, the patient should immediately be given aspirin 300 mg and a 999 call made for an emergency ambulance with trained paramedics.

Assessment by paramedics

Patients are assessed by a trained paramedic team. The ECG, pulse, blood pressure and oxygen saturation are recorded and monitored. Patients are treated with oxygen, pain relief (morphine), aspirin, and in some cases thrombolysis.

ST elevation myocardial infarction (STEMI)

Patients with ST elevation or left bundle branch block (ST elevation myocardial infarction) are taken directly to a cardiac catheter laboratory for coronary angiography and coronary angioplasty and stenting, without the delay of going to an accident and emergency unit. If there is no angioplasty centre nearby, patients are taken to an accident and emergency department for assessment. Thrombolysis is given if this has not already been done by the ambulance staff.

There is no additional benefit of treating patients with myocardial infarction with thrombolysis before prompt primary coronary angioplasty.

Patients with ST elevation usually develop a rise in activity of their cardiac enzymes. However, these enzyme activities increase approximately six hours after the onset of infarction and therefore play no role in immediate management, because patients would already have been treated with either primary angioplasty or thrombolysis.

Biochemical markers of heart muscle damage

Troponins T and I are sensitive and specific markers of myocardial damage. A normal level in a patient with chest pain identifies that patient as being at low risk.

After infarction, levels are raised for at least 12 hours and may persist for over one week. False-positive increases in troponin levels are caused by myocarditis, cardiomyopathy and pericarditis.

Levels of creatine kinase (CK) and the more specific enzyme released from heart muscle, CK-MB, are raised 4–8 hours after STEMI and return to normal within a few days. A high false-positive CK level is found after an alcohol binge, skeletal muscle injury, vigorous exercise and intramuscular injections.

Treatment of ACS in hospital

On arrival at hospital, all patients with suspected ACS have an immediate ECG (unless this has already been done by the ambulance staff), and are given aspirin 300 mg and clopidogrel 300 mg (unless these have already been given). They are assessed, given pain relief and oxygen, and heart failure is treated. Other potential complications are also evaluated.

Risk stratification of patients with non-ST elevation myocardial infarction (NSTEMI)

Patients with ischaemic chest pain, a raised troponin or CK-MB level but no ST elevation are classified as having NSTEMI. They are given thrombolysis and admitted to the cardiac care unit. Patients who have no ST elevation on their ECG are divided into low-risk and high-risk groups. Low-risk patients have no ST depression on their ECG, are young (< 65 years), have not had previous infarction or heart failure, and do not have diabetes or haemodynamic upset. If the troponin level is not raised 12 hours after the onset of chest pain, they are discharged from hospital with a view to non-invasive testing within one month.

High-risk patients are admitted and treated for threatened infarction, usually including antiplatelet agents (aspirin, clopidogrel and glycoprotein IIb/IIIa antagonists) and low-molecular-weight heparin.

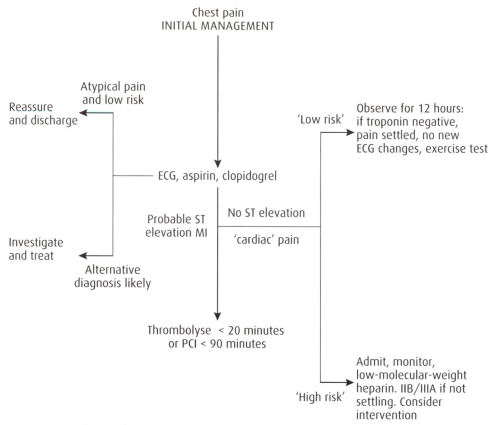

FIGURE 8.1: Risk stratification and mangement of acute chest pain.

Hospital management
Day 1
Clinical management on the first day after admission is fundamental to ensuring an optimal long-term result. Not only is this the period associated with the highest risk of arrhythmia, development of heart failure and death, but it is also a time of great uncertainty, as the precise diagnosis may not be known. The need of the patient and their family for information frequently cannot be met adequately, and trust can be eroded, leading to stress and frustration.

The patient and their family should be educated about their condition and all aspects of cardiac prevention during the patient's hospital admission.

During this period it is important to establish whether the initial working diagnosis is correct ('Is this an ACS?'), and if so, whether myocardial necrosis has occurred, and if so, how much. One must establish what immediate complications are present, and obtain sufficient information to adequately estimate the likelihood of future complications. The patient's cardiovascular risk factor profile must be assessed. It is important for the medical and nursing staff to get to know the patient and to try to understand how this event is likely to impact on their future. Finally, it is important to gain the trust of the patient and their family in order to ensure that the programme of treatment necessary is likely to be followed.

Day 1
ACS admission

Diagnosis confirmed?
- Typical ECG evolution
- Enzyme rise (yes or no) and magnitude

Complications identified and managed?
- Hypotension
- Tachycardia
- Pulmonary oedema
- Intracardiac thrombus

Likely course clear?
- Recurrent pain
- Amount of myocardium lost
- Co-morbidities identified

Thrombotic risk managed?
- Aspirin long term
- Clopidogrel for one year

Risk factor strategy?
- Statin: aim for LDL < 2 mmol/l
- Smoking cessation advice
- Blood pressure < 140/85 mmHg long term
- HbA_{1c} < 6.5 long term
- Family history: screening required?
- ACE inhibitor titration programme

Social context addressed?
- Driving issues
- Home support
- Date of return to work
- Long-term exercise programme
- Sex

FIGURE 8.2: Management of acute coronary syndromes.

Management according to risk

During the first day the situation is evolving at a variable rate from the initial 'emergency' management to long-term planning. One may be facing a patient who needs reassurance that nothing is wrong, or still dealing with a patient who requires mechanical support for blood pressure and ventilation. In general, however, most patients feel well and are beginning to wonder whether they need to be in hospital at all.

Patients who have had a successful angioplasty on admission are very unlikely to have a further coronary event, so in the absence of any other complications one should plan for discharge the following day. Most patients can be discharged within three days.

For the remainder, those in the 'high-risk' group should be reassessed and generally proceed to intervention before discharge. Those now regarded as 'low risk' should undergo non-invasive testing, ideally before discharge. All patients should have an assessment of their long-term coronary risk profile, and their risk factors should be treated. Major social problems must be evaluated.

Discharging patients after an ACS admission

One of the least well managed aspects of care is hospital discharge. As this has been a traditional area of failure, many GPs expect discharge planning and communication to be poor, and therefore rarely complain or try to improve matters. Hospitals do not audit the impact of poor discharge planning, so may be unaware of the size of these problems. Thus unless one develops a minimum standard of discharge that the general practice community expects, it is difficult to make progress.

The patient's GP should be informed in writing of their discharge within 24 hours. The summary should state whether or not a firm diagnosis of an ACS has been made, whether or not a myocardial infarction occurred, whether or not the ejection fraction is likely to be below 40%, what medicines the patient has been discharged on, whether the GP is being asked to titrate these or to check for adverse effects (e.g. electrolytes and renal function testing two weeks after discharge for patients on ACE inhibitors), what procedures have been performed, whether there are medicines that are essential to continue (e.g. clopidogrel after stenting), and what arrangements for hospital follow-up are in place.

All patients who have had an ACS remain at increased risk for around six months. They should be followed up frequently in primary care and assessed for angina, breathlessness, compliance with medication, lifestyle advice, diet and exercise, and their blood pressure and pulse should be checked. Patients who present with recurrent ischaemic symptoms need prompt and comprehensive assessment and, if necessary, referral to a cardiologist. GPs may find it convenient to have a post-discharge checklist.

Post-discharge checklist for patients with ACS
1 Has the patient had an ACS?

A transient rise in cardiac enzymes or dynamic ST or T-wave changes in association with chest discomfort consistent with an ACS is sufficient to be certain of the diagnosis. Angiography showing thrombus in the coronaries is also confirmatory. Otherwise one may be assuming that an ACS occurred on the basis of a compatible history, with or without some evidence of ischaemia on stress testing.

It is important to establish whether the patient had an ACS, as only those who have had an ACS are at very increased risk over the subsequent months.

2 Has the patient had a substantial infarct?

Increases in CK levels above 2000 IU and troponin T levels above 5 μg/l indicate substantial myocardial necrosis and a poor prognosis. Even small heart attacks in patients with previously impaired hearts can have a substantial impact.

Larger myocardial infarctions tend to be associated with more complications, such as heart failure, pericarditis and arrhythmias. This is the group that needs extra input in terms of ensuring compliance with medicines, and support in returning to work.

3 Is the patient at risk of heart failure?

An ejection fraction of ≤ 40% mentioned in the discharge summary is important. Cardiac function may improve over time after the infarct, but this group should receive heart failure therapy even if they are asymptomatic. Patients who had symptomatic heart failure during the admission are more likely to have ongoing heart failure. Crackles in the lung bases, a heart rate of more than 100 bpm and hypotension are all suggestive of significantly impaired cardiac function at discharge. Pulmonary oedema on chest radiography indicates important left ventricular impairment. These patients require long-term diuretics and ACE inhibition.

Patients who are at risk of heart failure will particularly benefit from ACE inhibitors, which should be prescribed at the maximum tolerated dose. β-blockers are important in patients who have had myocardial infarction. Metoprolol or bisoprolol rather than atenolol is given, and an appropriate dose prescribed to achieve a lowering of the pulse rate.

4 Is the patient on appropriate medicines?

All post-ACS patients should be discharged on aspirin 75 mg daily, clopidogrel 75 mg daily, simvastatin 40 mg daily, an ACE inhibitor (e.g. ramipril 10 mg daily) and a β-blocker (e.g. atenolol 25–50 mg daily) (unless the patient has heart failure). If they are not on one of these, the reason should be clear. β-blockers are contraindicated in patients with asthma.

The dose of ACE inhibitors should be optimised. Discharging a patient on ramipril 1.25 mg daily with no plans to increase the dose is suboptimal, except in persistently hypotensive patients or those with significant renal impairment (creatinine levels > 200 μmol/l). Clopidogrel should be continued for one year, after which the GP can stop it if the hospital staff do not do so. β-blockers are important only in cases where myocardial necrosis has been confirmed.

5 Are the medicines tolerated and effective?

Unless a patient has had their renal function monitored while on ACE inhibitors (usually because they have been in hospital too ill to be discharged) or they have been on ACE inhibitors for several months, it cannot be assumed that ACE inhibitors are safe and have not resulted in renal dysfunction. Primary care clinicians should check electrolytes and renal function two weeks after the patient leaves hospital.

Liver function tests and creatine kinase levels should be checked within six weeks of starting a statin. Gastrointestinal symptoms might be an indication to consider proton pump inhibition in patients who are taking aspirin and clopidogrel, rather than stopping these important antithrombotic drugs, which could lead to serious coronary thrombosis and myocardial infarction. These drugs should be stopped and the patient referred to hospital as an emergency if there is a gastrointestinal bleed.

6 Has appropriate follow-up been arranged?

Many patients are discharged over the weekend, and systems for ensuring outpatient follow-up out of hours are patchy. If by the time the patient sees you they do not have a follow-up date, one is unlikely to materialise spontaneously. Unless an ACS has been excluded, follow-up at least once within three months is appropriate. Patients should also have had contact from the rehabilitation department, to ensure that lifestyle issues are addressed after discharge. Long-term regular hospital follow-up is now rarely necessary, since recurrent symptoms are a better guide to the need for further evaluation than periodic testing (e.g. exercise testing), being better predictors of future events.

7 When can the patient get back to normal?

Patients cannot drive for one week after an ACS and for one month after a myocardial infarction. If the patient holds a PCV or LGV licence, an exercise test should be arranged for six weeks to three months after the event if they are otherwise well. Most patients nowadays should be considering getting back to work within a couple of weeks of discharge, unless the infarct is large and their work is physically demanding, in which case a more individualised approach is required.

Stress: exercise and work

An ingrained belief is that after a heart attack, patients must 'mind' themselves because they have become like china dolls that may crumble under the slightest strain. Health professionals reinforce this belief as they are fearful of the 'health and safety' implications of giving advice that may be perceived as leading to adverse events.

There is of course no smoke without fire. It is known that stressful events such as the loss of a partner or indeed airline flights are associated with an increased rate of acute coronary events. Furthermore, there is the so-called 'snow shovellers' infarct', where a patient who has done no exercise for three months goes out into the cold to remove snow from the path and is found dead.

Equally it is known that individuals who return to work have a better prognosis than those who do not, and that exercise improves coronary perfusion and myocardial function over time.

The problem therefore is that the precise response to stress and exercise is an unknown quantity for each individual in their particular situation. At the same time, the risk of another event occurring is increased for six to 12 months after an event, and if one advises exercise, one increases the risk that the patient might happen to be doing something one has advised at the time when nature takes its natural course.

There is general agreement on the following:

✧ Stress is only harmful if it is associated with frustration. People who enjoy stress do not 'suffer' from engaging in these stressful activities.

✧ Graded exercise programmes are not associated with an increased cardiac event rate, whereas inconsistent exercise may well be.

✧ Work improves self-esteem and improves psychological adjustment to major life-changing events.

It is therefore apparent that getting the patient back to work, taking regular exercise and engaged in stressful situations with which they feel comfortable is the optimal outcome after an acute coronary event. At present we have only commonsense to guide us in terms of determining the rate at which this should be achieved. It is clear that the longer one is away from normal activities, the less likely one is to return to full engagement. We therefore advise that from hospital discharge a patient should walk for 20 minutes per day at a pace at which they could not comfortably talk at the same time, stopping if they have chest discomfort or significant breathlessness. When they can walk a mile comfortably (or the equivalent if they have musculoskeletal limitations), they are fit to return to most occupations and to resume sex. If they are involved in heavy manual labour, an early return to work with support for activities that might require straining until they can do these tasks without undue 'isometric' effort is the sensible approach. Obviously for airline pilots and LGV drivers different rules apply.

The primary assumption underlying this advice is that the patient has been rendered essentially symptom free at rest and with normal levels of effort. If not, further efforts at revascularisation or medication are required.

Medications used and rationale
Aspirin
Aspirin blocks platelet cyclo-oxygenase and platelet aggregation. It reduces the risk of death from cardiac causes and fatal and non-fatal myocardial infarction by around 60% in patients presenting with unstable angina. The initial dose for newly diagnosed acute coronary syndromes is 300 mg, and 75 mg per day thereafter indefinitely.

Clopidogrel
This is a thienopyridine that affects the ADP-dependent activation of the glycoprotein IIb/IIIa complex and thereby inhibits platelet aggregation. The initial dose is 300 mg, and thereafter the dose is 75 mg per day for patients with acute coronary syndromes. Clopidogrel is also used in conjunction with aspirin long term to reduce the risk of thrombosis occurring within coronary artery stents. In addition, it has been shown to reduce the likelihood of recurrent acute coronary syndromes when given for nine months after an index event in patients who do not receive stents. Finally, it improves the efficacy of thrombolytic agents if administered during ST elevation myocardial infarction.

Glycoprotein IIb/IIIa inhibitors
GPs may not initiate treatment with these new powerful drugs, but should be aware of their use in hospital. They inhibit the final common pathway involved in platelet inhibition, activation and aggregation. There are three classes:

✧ an antibody form – abciximab – that is used intravenously with aspirin and heparin

during coronary angioplasty in patients with or at high risk of developing intra-coronary thrombus
- ⬦ a synthetic peptide form (e.g. eptifibatide)
- ⬦ a non-synthetic form (e.g. tirofiban).

Warfarin

Before the use of antiplatelet drugs, warfarin was given to patients for secondary prevention with myocardial infarction. Warfarin has been shown to reduce the incidence of death, stroke and reinfarctions, and is at least as effective as aspirin, but the logistics and costs of controlling the INR and the three times greater risk of bleeding make it less attractive. It is not used in the UK except in a few situations, including patients with extensive intravascular or left ventricular thrombus, those with atrial fibrillation, patients who are already taking warfarin and those with aspirin resistance.

Heparin

Most hospitals now use subcutaneous, low-molecular-weight heparin rather than unfractionated heparin because the former has a lower side-effect profile, a longer half-life and a more predictable dose–response curve, so clotting does not need to be monitored. The dose is determined by the patient's weight. Enoxaparin, a low-molecular-weight heparin, is superior to unfractionated heparin in reducing the incidence of myocardial infarction and the need for emergency revascularisation in patients with unstable angina. It is not yet clear whether heparin should be given with glycoprotein IIb/IIIa inhibitors in acute coronary syndromes.

Thrombolysis

Thrombolytic drugs are given as soon as possible and preferably within six hours to patients with ST elevation myocardial infarction, and those with left bundle branch block and symptoms consistent with infarction. They are not suitable for patients with unstable angina or non-Q-wave myocardial infarction because they increase the incidence of death and myocardial infarction. Thrombolytic drugs are contraindicated in patients with a recent history of bleeding, stroke, recent surgery, prolonged resuscitation or possible aortic dissection.

Streptokinase was the first thrombolytic agent used for acute myocardial infarction. It is given as an infusion, followed by an infusion of heparin. Recombinant-DNA-manufactured tissue plasminogen activators given as a single bolus offer the advantages of simplicity and speed of administration, greater efficacy in arterial recannalisation and myocardial perfusion, and do not stimulate antibody production that allowed streptokinase to be given to the same patient only once. Hospitals vary in their choice of thrombolytic drug.

β-blockers

These are well-established and effective agents for the treatment of hypertension, angina and heart failure. They reduce mortality in acute myocardial infarction and are used (with a smaller evidence base) in acute coronary syndromes. Small doses of short-acting β-blockers are used initially. Patients are often discharged from hospital on β-blockers.

Nitrates

These are used in acute coronary syndromes, although there is little evidence that they reduce mortality or the rate of new myocardial infarction. Intravenous nitroglycerin is used rather than oral long-acting nitrates because of its ease of administration, titration and rapid resolution of side-effects when the infusion is discontinued. Patients may be discharged on oral long-acting or short-acting (sublingual) nitrates. Nitrate tolerance developing after 24 hours of administration is a disadvantage of continuous nitrates. It may be avoided by switching to an oral or transdermal form and allowing an eight-hour nitrate-free period.

Calcium-channel blockers

Both dihydropyridines (e.g. nifedipine, amlodipine) and non-dihydropyridines (e.g. diltiazem, verapamil) dilate coronary arteries and reduce blood pressure, and are useful for the symptomatic treatment of angina. Neither group of drugs reduces mortality or the incidence of myocardial infarction. Diltiazem is the preferred calcium antagonist because it slows the heart rate and, unlike verapamil, is not contraindicated with β-blockers. It is recommended for patients who cannot tolerate β-blockers or for patients with refractory symptoms despite treatment with nitrates and β-blockers.

Advice for patients

✧ Heart attacks are due to blockage of a heart artery with a clot. The clot forms on fatty material in the wall of the artery. Patients with certain lifestyle factors or habits are more likely to have deposition of this fatty material. Stopping smoking, controlling high blood pressure, controlling diabetes, reducing high cholesterol levels, losing weight and taking daily exercise are helpful in preventing heart attacks and important in reducing the likelihood of a second heart attack.

✧ If you experience chest discomfort or breathlessness, arm pain or symptoms occurring with exercise or stress, come and see us. If you have had a heart attack, heart bypass surgery or angioplasty and develop similar symptoms again, come to see us as soon as possible. Do not ignore worrying symptoms. Sometimes it may be safest to dial 999 and go directly to the accident and emergency department to have an ECG and blood tests. GPs usually advise patients with prolonged angina (more than 15 minutes) to go directly to hospital in case they are having a heart attack.

✧ You will be given tablets to take after the heart attack, and you may need to continue on some of these tablets longterm. Please come to see us so that we can monitor your progress and decide which tablets need to be taken and at what dose.

✧ Some patients benefit from attending the hospital rehabilitation course. You may have already enrolled on this while you were in hospital.

✧ After the heart attack you will have tests to see how much, if any, heart muscle has been damaged and what further tests you need. Some patients have an X-ray of the heart arteries called an angiogram, and may have ballooning or opening of the arteries (angioplasty). Occasionally, coronary artery bypass is necessary.

✧ Most patients understandably feel anxious, depressed and lacking in self-confidence after a heart attack. Your confidence will improve as you do more exercise, and the doctors and nurses may have given you advice about how much to do. Fears of dying or of having another heart attack are common. If you are worried, please come to see us and we can help by arranging an exercise test or, if necessary, arranging for you to enrol on a rehabilitation course or see the cardiologist.

✧ The tablets that you have been given together with the lifestyle changes that have been suggested to you will reduce the chances of you having another heart attack. Try to remain optimistic and confident.

✧ You should not drive or do any heavy lifting for a month. Inform your insurance company about your heart attack.

✧ Inform the DVLA if you have a LGV or PCV licence. You will need tests before they let you know whether you can keep your licence.

✧ If you have done well during an exercise test after the heart attack, this is good news and means that you are at low risk and can start to exercise without fear. Regular fast walking is good for you. If you feel tired, rest. If you feel in the mood to exercise, walk progressively further and faster each day. Only you know how much you can do. If you can exercise without chest pain or breathlessness, keep going, but be sensible! Stairs are good exercise, as is gentle treadmill, cycling, swimming, housework and gentle gardening.

✧ Most people can return to work within six weeks of a heart attack. If you have a physically demanding job, start slowly with reduced duties and hours. Talk to your employers, and we can help too by writing a letter, with your permission.

✧ Sex is good exercise unless it results in chest pain or undue breathlessness. If you can walk upstairs quickly or fairly long distances easily, it is safe to have sex. Men may be impotent after a recent heart attack, and this may be due to fear, depression or some of the tablets that you have been prescribed. Speak to us about this problem. It usually improves.

✧ Avoid drinking too much alcohol, but a small amount (a glass or two of wine, or a glass of spirits) may make you feel better and more relaxed. Everything in moderation!

✧ You can fly 10 days after a heart attack. Make sure that you have travel insurance, take enough tablets with you and avoid going to places where there are few hospital facilities. Avoid stressful journeys.

Answers to questions about clinical cases

1. Her mother may have a chest infection, but the possibility of an acute coronary syndrome must be considered. Myocardial infarction and acute coronary syndromes may present as breathlessness in the older patient. The daughter should phone for an emergency ambulance for assessment and transport to hospital for investigation. The patient needs a prompt clinical assessment with blood tests and troponins, an ECG and a chest X-ray. The ambulance team will record an ECG. If this shows an acute ST elevation myocardial infarction or left bundle branch block, they may take her directly to a cardiac catheter laboratory for coronary angiography and primary angioplasty, if she presented within 90 minutes of symptoms appearing. If the ECG is normal, she should go to the nearest accident and emergency unit for evaluation.

2. Stopping either drug, and particularly stopping both drugs, will increase this patient's risk of thrombosis in the drug-eluting stent. He should take his tablets on a full stomach, and you should prescribe a proton pump inhibitor and review him. Tell him that the risks of stopping the tablets could lead to the stent blocking off, and that he could then have another heart attack. Ask him about angina and other symptoms, examine him and check his blood pressure, and ensure that he is taking all relevant secondary prevention treatment.

3. This patient may have been given a date for a chest pain clinic appointment for an exercise test or an appointment for upper gastrointestinal endoscopy. Check this with the letter. If such appointments have not been made, arrange for these tests, with the exercise test first. There are other causes of chest pain (e.g. biliary pain, pericarditis, pleurisy, aortic dissection, musculoskeletal pain) and all of these have to be evaluated. Retake the history and examine the patient with these possibilities in mind. Depending on what you find, you may wish to request some further tests.

4. You need to find out why this patient was admitted, which hospital it was, and the diagnosis and treatment that he was given. You discover that he had a myocardial infarction, but he presented a day too late for either thrombolysis or angioplasty. He was given an ACE inhibitor, aspirin, a β-blocker and a statin. He is only taking the ACE inhibitor. He needs a full review. The cough could be due to the ACE inhibitor, pulmonary oedema or a chest infection. A full history and examination are necessary,

followed by a chest X-ray, blood tests and an echocardiogram. All of his risk factors need attention.

5. The important diagnosis to exclude is aortic dissection and extension of the dissection proximally to a coronary artery (most commonly the right coronary artery). If the pain is not suggestive of aortic dissection and the patient is perfectly well and examination is normal, the symptom may be due to backache. It is sometimes very difficult to decide, and if you are concerned that this could be a dissection, send her directly to hospital for assessment. Small aortic tears that heal up spontaneously may not result in severe symptoms or any signs. A CT or MRI scan of her aorta and back would be very helpful.

FURTHER READING

Bassand J-P, Hamm CW. ESC guidelines on the diagnosis and treatment of non-ST-segment elevation acute coronary syndromes. *Eur Heart J.* 2007; **28:** 1598–660.

Braunwald E, Antman EM, Beasley JW *et al.* ACC/AHA 2002 guideline update for the management of patients with unstable angina and non-ST segment elevation myocardial infarction: a report of the American College of Cardiology/American Heart Association task force on practice guidelines. *J Am Coll Cardiol.* 2002; **40:** 1366–74.

Handler C, Coghlan G. *Living with Coronary Disease.* London: Springer; 2007. ISBN-10:1-84628-550-X.

Thygesen K, Alpert JS, White HD on behalf of the Joint ESC/ACCF/AHA/WHF Task Force for the Redefinition of Myocardial Infarction. Universal definition of myocardial infarction. *Eur Heart J.* 2007; **28:** 2525–38.

Yeghiazarians Y, Braustein JB, Askari A *et al.* Unstable angina. *NEJM.* 2000; **342:** 101–14.

Claudication and peripheral vascular disease

NINE

Clinical cases

1. A 78-year-old hypertensive man who smokes 20 cigarettes a day comes to see you with pain in the buttock and down the leg when he walks, stands or bends. These symptoms are not affected by walking. What do you do?
2. An 85-year-old diabetic woman with a previous myocardial infarct and a long history of angina and claudication asks you whether chelation therapy would be helpful. What advice do you give her?
3. A 47-year-old previously fit man presents with an acutely ischaemic foot. It is white, pulseless and painful. What do you do?
4. A 76-year-old man with a long history of both coronary artery and peripheral vascular disease and who had a femoro-popliteal bypass 10 years ago presents with recurrent claudication in the same leg, and absent foot pulses, but the foot is not threatened. You refer him back to the vascular surgeon, who does not think that either angioplasty or bypass is possible. What advice do you give the patient?
5. A 68-year-old smoker who has claudication comes to see you. He tells you that his neighbour takes vitamin E and various homeopathic medicines and asks whether he should do the same. What do you advise him?
6. A 76-year-old man tells you that he has a cramping pain in his left leg when he walks. The symptoms started a year ago and are now interfering with his ability to do his job. He has a palpable right femoral pulse, and weak pulses in the right leg. There are no pulses below a weak left femoral artery pulse. What is the diagnosis and what do you do?

Peripheral arterial disease: a component of widespread vascular disease

Peripheral vascular disease is part of a common, widespread, atheromatous process that affects all arterial territories – the carotid, coronary, aortic, sacral and renal arteries – although it may occur in isolation. Claudication is a prognostically important condition. It increases cardiovascular morbidity and mortality. It has a detrimental impact on a person's quality of life, restricting their activities because of unpleasant exertional pain in their legs. However, the risk of limb loss is low (less than 2%) for patients who do not have diabetes. Most patients with peripheral arterial disease die from myocardial infarction or stroke. This highlights the important clinical point that peripheral arterial disease is part of a multifocal atheromatous disease, and should be investigated and treated as a component of a patient's vascular disease condition.

> Patients with peripheral vascular disease should have comprehensive cardiovascular risk factor screening and treatment, and examination and assessment for vascular disease in other arterial territories.

Risk factors for peripheral arterial disease

Smoking is the single most important risk factor for peripheral vascular disease, increasing the risk in a 'dose-related' way by at least threefold. The majority of patients (80%) with claudication either are smokers or have smoked. Smokers should understand that their symptoms, and the serious consequences of peripheral vascular disease, will progress unless they stop smoking. Smoking cessation is fundamental to management. Other interventions are unlikely to be effective if patients continue to smoke.

Diabetes increases the risk of limb loss by threefold.

Treatment of obesity, hypertension, dyslipidaemia and diabetes, together with modification of diet, are key parts of the treatment. Exercise, combined with treatment of all risk factors, is very helpful in improving symptoms of claudication; intervention may then not be necessary.

Role of primary care clinicians in managing peripheral arterial disease

- ✧ Increase awareness of the increasing incidence of peripheral arterial disease and its consequences.
- ✧ Improve the identification of patients with symptomatic peripheral arterial disease.
- ✧ Increase rates of detection of individuals with asymptomatic disease.
- ✧ Initiate a screening programme for patients at high risk.
- ✧ Improve risk factor management of patients with peripheral arterial disease with effective smoking cessation, blood pressure control, treatment of diabetes and dyslipidaemia, weight loss and dietary advice.
- ✧ Arrange exercise testing and exercise therapy.
- ✧ Refer the patient to an exercise training clinic or to a vascular surgeon.

Diagnosis and management of all but the minority of patients with severe, complicated peripheral vascular disease (who require hospital-based diagnosis and intervention) can be done in primary care.

Prevalence

In common with vascular disease in other arterial territories, peripheral vascular disease is becoming more common because people are living longer. Cardiovascular risk factor management may simply delay the onset of the disease and symptoms. Around 20% of people aged 65–75 years have reduced leg pulses on clinical examination, but less than 50% of them have symptoms, and these may be atypical. Symptoms of arterial disease depend on the patient's activity. Peripheral arterial disease is therefore common in primary care, but may be under-diagnosed because patients and clinicians may not recognise symptoms as being due to leg muscle ischaemia.

Symptoms and risk

The pathology, risk factors and principles of management of peripheral arterial disease are similar to those for coronary heart disease. In the same way as patients with coronary heart disease may have no or negligible angina, because angina symptoms correlate inconsistently with the extent of coronary heart disease, patients with severe peripheral vascular disease may not complain of claudication. They may interpret and dismiss their symptoms as sciatica or musculoskeletal pain. At least 50% of patients with peripheral arterial disease do not have claudication and may therefore go undiagnosed. Whether or not they have symptoms, these patients have a sixfold increase in mortality within 10 years compared with patients without peripheral arterial disease.

A comprehensive evaluation for atheromatous disease in other territories should be performed before revascularisation for any arterial territory. This is particularly important prior to myocardial revascularisation, because coexisting vascular disease increases the peri-operative risk, particularly of renal failure and stroke. Similarly, coronary artery disease increases the risk of peripheral artery surgery.

Management of peripheral vascular disease necessitates:

- ✧ an anatomical and functional assessment
- ✧ exclusion of non-atheromatous causes of claudication
- ✧ a comprehensive survey and prompt and aggressive treatment of risk factors
- ✧ effective lifestyle, medical and, where necessary, revascularisation interventions.

Claudication

Symptoms

Symptoms may occur if an artery is narrowed by more than 50%. A long but less severe stenosis may also result in poor flow and claudication. Most patients (80%) with peripheral arterial disease have no or minimal symptoms. The condition is often detected during routine clinical examination, particularly in patients who present with angina, and those with cardiovascular risk factors.

Claudication is described as pain in the calf, buttock or foot, or tightness or cramp on walking that is relieved promptly by rest and worsens with exercise. It does not get better with continued walking. It is present in 15–40% of patients with peripheral vascular disease. Patients may experience cold feet and calf cramp at night, which is relieved by hanging the leg out of the bed.

Many patients present not with typical claudication but with tiredness, leg 'weakness' or fatigue with walking, and other types of leg pain.

> Patients with a variety of leg symptoms and cardiovascular risk factors should be assessed for peripheral arterial disease, because only a minority of patients with peripheral arterial disease present with typical claudication.
>
> It is important to assess the severity of symptoms by recording the claudication distance and asking whether the patient has pain at rest.

Patients may be unable to perform their normal activities, and may become deconditioned and dependent on others.

Signs

The patient's shoes and socks should be removed.

Signs of peripheral vascular disease include reduced foot pulses, arterial bruits and ischaemic skin changes with ulcers in severe disease. Look and feel for changes in skin colour and temperature, and in capillary refilling time. Feel both radial, brachial and foot pulses. The blood pressure should be checked. Feel and listen for bruits over the carotids, and femoral pulses. Feel the abdominal aorta and listen for bruits. Examine the fundi for signs of hypertension and diabetes.

Diagnosis

The ankle-brachial index is the most effective method. This involves wrapping a blood pressure cuff around the leg just above the ankle, inflating the cuff to above the systolic pressure, and then listening with a hand-held Doppler device for the return of blood flow as the cuff is deflated. Systolic pressures are measured in both the posterior tibial and dorsalis pedis arteries, and the higher of the two systolic readings is compared with the Doppler-detected systolic pressure in the brachial artery. An ankle to brachial pressure ratio of < 0.9 is diagnostic of peripheral arterial disease.

However, a normal ankle to brachial pressure ratio does not exclude the diagnosis.

An ankle-brachial index of < 0.5 is associated with a five-year survival of 63%. An ankle-brachial index of 0.7–0.9 is associated with a five-year survival of 91%. It is simple to measure, reproducible, and could be used as a screening tool in primary care.

If the ankle-brachial index is normal in the presence of clinical features of peripheral disease, the index should be re-calculated after exercise. The patient can be exercised on a treadmill, but in primary care they can be asked to stand and repeatedly raise themselves off the floor on their toes. The index will decrease with exercise in the presence of significant peripheral stenosis due to vasodilatation.

Risk factor checklist

✧ Smoking is the most common and important risk factor, and patients must be advised of the risks of smoking and the potential benefits of stopping. They should be encouraged to stop, and given every assistance with this.
✧ Hypertension.
✧ Diabetes.
✧ Lipid profile.
✧ Renal function, because peripheral vascular disease is commonly associated with renal artery stenosis and renal impairment.
✧ β-blockers may aggravate claudication symptoms and may need to be either stopped or the dose reduced.

Differential diagnosis of leg pain

✧ Venous claudication, which results in a bursting sensation that affects the whole leg and is relieved by elevating the leg. There may be a history of deep vein thrombosis.
✧ Nerve root pain, which results in a poorly localised, shock-like pain, which may affect both legs, and is relieved by sitting down or changing posture. There may be signs of lumbar spine arthritis.
✧ Inflammatory vasculitis (Buerger's disease). This affects the small and medium-sized arteries and veins of the arms and legs in young people, predominantly male smokers. There may be thrombosis of peripheral vessels leading to ulceration and gangrene. More than one limb is affected, and proximal vessels are usually normal. Referral to an expert vascular unit is required and revascularisation strategies are usually of little value. Management is based on smoking cessation, local treatment of ulcers, and antithrombotic drugs and occasionally sympathectomy. Amputation may be necessary, particularly if the patient continues to smoke.
✧ Arthritic pain that causes aching and restriction of movement of the hip and knee with weight bearing and exercise. Examination may show signs of arthritis.
✧ Spinal stenosis.
✧ Hip arthritis.
✧ Baker's cyst.

Natural history (see Figure 9.1)
The leg
The prognosis for the ischaemic leg has improved with the introduction of aggressive and effective risk factor management, and exercise prescriptions. For most patients the symptoms and prognosis improve, and they should be told this. Around 25% of patients deteriorate. Revascularisation is necessary in only a minority of patients. Major limb amputation is rarely necessary.

Overall vascular prognosis
Because peripheral vascular disease is usually a manifestation of generalised atheromatous disease and is more common in the elderly, the overall vascular prognosis is poor. Around 30% of patients will die, and a further 10% will have a non-fatal infarct. Around 60% of patients survive for five years with no vascular complications (*see* Figure 9.1).

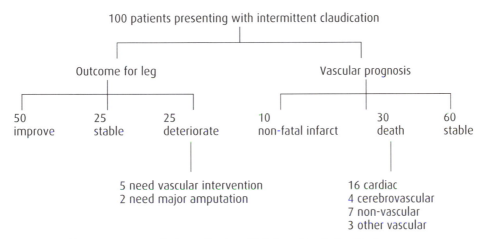

FIGURE 9.1: Five-year prognosis for patients with intermittent claudication.

Atheroembolism
Embolisation of atheromatous material from plaques may result in ischaemic infarction. This may affect the kidneys with acute renal failure, or one or both legs, depending on the source of the embolism. Patients present with acute severe pain and an ischaemic foot and/ or leg that is cold, pale and either is pulseless or has reduced pulses. If atheroembolism is suspected, the patient should be referred to a good and experienced vascular unit for prompt investigation and treatment.

Management of peripheral artery disease
All risk factors must be addressed vigorously, in conjunction with a lifelong exercise programme.

Antiplatelet medication
Aspirin
Aspirin acts by blocking the cyclo-oxygenase pathway and reducing thromboxane-induced platelet aggregation. It should be used for both primary and secondary prevention. It reduces the risk of non-fatal and fatal vascular events and decreases cardiovascular

mortality by an average of 20%. It also reduces the need for revascularisation. In addition, it improves patency rates after revascularisation performed using bypass grafting or angioplasty. All patients should be given aspirin 75 mg. Compared with placebo, aspirin prevents 19 fatal and non-fatal cardiovascular events per year for every 1000 patients treated.

Clopidogrel

This should be tried in the 10% of patients who cannot tolerate aspirin. Clopidogrel is a thienopyridine that blocks the activation of platelets by adenosine diphosphate. It has a similar side-effect profile to aspirin, and is used in patients with vascular disease for both primary and secondary prevention. Clopidogrel may be more effective than aspirin in reducing ischaemic events in patients with atheromatous disease in other arterial territories. It may be used in addition to aspirin in high-risk patients and long term after angioplasty and stent implantation. Clopidogrel prevents 24 fatal and non-fatal cardiovascular events per year for every 1000 patients treated.

Combined antiplatelet therapy

There is no evidence that combined antiplatelet therapy is superior to either drug alone.

Smoking cessation

Smoking cessation reduces the cardiovascular morbidity and mortality.

Cigarette smoking increases the risk of peripheral vascular disease fourfold, and continued smoking increases the rate of progression of disease and the likelihood of leg amputation. Smoking cessation reduces the progression of disease and the risk of cardiovascular events, including death. It is probably the single most important but possibly also most difficult intervention.

Diabetes

Diabetes is more common in patients with peripheral arterial disease. Diabetics have a fourfold higher risk of developing peripheral vascular disease compared with non-diabetics.

The HbA_{1c} should be reduced to below 7%. Tight glycaemic control, combined with correction of hypertension and other risk factors, reduces the risk of peripheral vascular disease by 34% and also reduces the risk of myocardial infarction. However, tight glycaemic control alone has been found to have little or no proven benefit in reducing the risk of amputation.

Lipids

Reducing total cholesterol and LDL-cholesterol levels has recently been shown to improve claudication symptoms and prognosis by reducing cardiovascular events. Aggressive lipid lowering using dietary interventions, exercise, statins and cholesterol-absorption blockers should be used to achieve a target LDL-cholesterol concentration of < 2.0 mmol/l and a total cholesterol concentration of < 4.0 mmol/l. All patients with peripheral arterial disease should be prescribed a statin.

Hypertension

Hypertension (blood pressure > 140/85 mmHg) increases the risk of peripheral vascular disease by threefold. All antihypertensive drugs may be used in patients with peripheral vascular disease. In the absence of bilateral renal artery stenosis, and using careful biochemical monitoring, ACE inhibitors, particularly in diabetics, are the drug of first choice and may be used for patients with peripheral vascular disease without diabetes or hypertension.

The Joint British Societies' recommendations for the prevention of coronary heart disease include a treatment target for patients with peripheral vascular disease of ≤ 140/85 mmHg, although there is no evidence that lowering blood pressure improves the prognosis of patients with peripheral vascular disease.

Patient education

The prognosis as shown above should be explained, together with the potential benefits of risk factor improvement and the consequences of inadequate risk factor control.

Exercise training

Daily vigorous walking or cycling combined with aggressive risk factor modification improves exercise performance and quality of life. Regular exercise, walking for 30 minutes at a time, improves pain-free walking time by 180%. Exercise training appears to be more effective than medication, and the benefits are noticeable within a few weeks.

There is little information from randomised controlled trials comparing exercise and revascularisation. There is some evidence that vigorous daily exercise and aggressive risk factor modification is as effective as surgery or angioplasty in improving quality of life and maximum walking distances.

Patients should be told to walk every day until they claudicate, and then to stop and start again. The benefits become apparent after a few weeks and continue for at least several months. Potential mechanisms for the benefits of exercise training include increased muscle strength, improved vascular function and dilatation, and improved muscle metabolism.

Drug treatment for claudication symptoms

Cilostazol is a phosphodiesterase type 3 vasodilator with mild antiplatelet activity. At a dose of 100 mg twice a day, it increases walking distance by 50%. It is contraindicated in heart failure. Cilostazol and naftidrofuryl improve symptoms in some patients, but there is no evidence that they affect the long-term outcome of the disease. Both drugs have gastrointestinal and cardiovascular side-effects (palpitation, angina, arrhythmias, chest pain and oedema).

There is no evidence that vitamin E, oral prostaglandins, chelation therapy, omega-3 fatty acids or any foodstuffs or complementary preparations improve outcome.

Revascularisation

This is reserved for very symptomatic patients who have not responded to exercise and drug treatment. Coexisting conditions which would limit exercise even if claudication was improved (e.g. intractable angina or respiratory disease) are a contraindication to revascularisation.

This is a rapidly developing multi-disciplinary specialty that requires the input of radiologists, vascular surgeons, cardiologists, lipidologists, secondary prevention nurses, exercise training personnel, and staff experienced in smoking cessation. There are several areas of controversy and continuing doubt surrounding the benefits of revascularisation.

Percutaneous angioplasty

Percutaneous angioplasty and (where appropriate) stenting, aided by intravascular ultrasound, is now performed for a wide variety of lesions in peripheral, renal and carotid artery disease. It is preferred in younger patients (< 50 years) because they have a higher risk of graft failure after bypass surgery. Angioplasty in suitable lesions is more cost-effective and is a less risky procedure than bypass surgery.

However, it only has short-term benefits. Stenting in peripheral arteries is not as effective as coronary stenting, due to mechanical compression, longitudinal stretching and torsion of the stent. At present, and in contrast to angioplasty and stenting for coronary artery disease, the long-term benefits with stenting, including drug-eluting stents, are not established. Laser angioplasty and adjunctive angioplasty techniques (cutting balloons, atherectomy, and brachytherapy to reduce restenosis) have not been shown to be beneficial.

The current recommendations are for angioplasty in patients with a single stenosis < 3 cm long in the common or external iliac artery, with a single stenosis or occlusions < 5 cm in the femoro-popliteal segment or with multiple lesions each < 3 cm long and not involving the distal popliteal artery.

Bypass surgery

Surgery is used in cases where the above techniques are not at present appropriate, but there is considerable variation in attitudes to bypass surgery and to which patients it should be offered. The associated morbidity (2–30%) and mortality (around 5%) have to be taken into consideration when offering a patient only the possibility of symptomatic relief for an uncertain period.

The results of bypass surgery compared with angioplasty are similar after four years. The risks of death and amputation are similar.

Advice for patients with peripheral arterial disease

- The symptoms of claudication are due to a build-up of fat in the arteries that supply blood and oxygen to the leg muscles. It is part of a generalised furring up process, which may affect other arteries.
- Patients with peripheral vascular disease are at increased risk of stroke and heart attack.
- If you have pain in your toes or you get pain in your feet at night, come to see us as soon as possible.
- If left untreated, this condition may progress to severe pain and restricted activities, and in very severe cases to amputation of the leg.
- You can do a lot to help yourself by stopping smoking, losing weight, taking daily regular exercise for 30 minutes at a time, and making sure that your blood pressure is normal and your cholesterol level is low. If you have diabetes, this needs very tight control.
- You will be prescribed various tablets, including aspirin, possibly an angiotensin-converting-enzyme inhibitor, and a statin.
- If your claudication is intolerable, we will refer you to a vascular surgeon who will do some tests to see why you have claudication, where the arterial blockages are, and whether you would benefit from a ballooning procedure or a bypass operation to improve the blood supply to your legs and feet. These tests include an ultrasound scan, imaging of your arteries with a CT scan or magnetic resonance imaging scan, and an invasive arterial angiogram.
- The ultrasound scan is painless and quick, and a probe is put over the arteries of the

legs to detect blockages in the flow of blood. For the angiogram you lie on an X-ray table and a needle is inserted into the artery in the groin of the affected leg, and radio-opaque fluid is injected into the artery. Pictures are then taken to locate and assess the severity of the arterial narrowings.

❖ Take the condition seriously, take all your tablets, and let us know straight away if your symptoms deteriorate or you develop a painful white foot. If you do, you should go to hospital immediately.

❖ Most patients can avoid the need for surgery or angioplasty if they do everything they can to look after themselves.

❖ Daily exercise, walking outside or on a treadmill or cycling, is very effective in improving your symptoms. After two months of vigorous walking you may be able to double the distance that you are able to walk.

Answers to questions about clinical cases

1. Although this patient may have peripheral vascular disease, his symptoms are not consistent with claudication. They may be due to sciatica or lumbar canal stenosis. If he has good pulses, claudication is unlikely and he should be referred to a back surgeon for evaluation. The ankle-brachial index should be recorded. He should be advised to stop smoking and should be offered buproprion and all other cardiovascular prevention advice.

2. Advise the patient that chelation therapy is not helpful and that it is expensive. Ensure that she has full cardiovascular secondary prevention, and check her medication and make sure that she is taking it. Her diabetes must be tightly controlled. She should be referred (or referred again if she has already been seen) to the vascular surgeon for investigation to see whether angioplasty would help her.

3. It is possible that this patient has had an embolus. He needs to be referred as an emergency to hospital for a diagnosis and treatment to save the leg. Possible causes include a thrombotic embolus due to atrial fibrillation, trauma to the leg arteries and (rarely) an atrial myxoma or a blood disorder. He will need urgent ultrasound and angiography and appropriate treatment. Depending on the cause, he may need long-term anticoagulation.

4. There appears to be no prospect of further revascularisation. Aggressive secondary prevention, including aspirin, possibly with clopidogrel, high-dose statins and ACE inhibitors, stopping or reducing β-blockers are important. Make sure that the patient is not diabetic or smoking. He should be strongly encouraged to take at least daily energetic exercise training on a treadmill or cycle in the hope that this will improve his symptoms. The long-term prognosis is not good, but it is important to encourage him and support him.

5. Unfortunately, vitamins and homeopathic medicines are not effective. The most sensible thing this patient can do is to stop smoking altogether, immediately. You should offer him every assistance and encouragement.

6. This patient has intermittent claudication due to stenosis or occlusion of the left superficial femoral artery. The ankle-brachial index should be measured to confirm the diagnosis. All of his risk factors should be assessed and treated (smoking, blood pressure, dyslipidaemia), and he should have aspirin 75 mg a day, in addition to statins, and antihypertensives if necessary. β-blockers are contraindicated. ACE inhibitors should be used with caution because there is a high probability that he has renal artery stenosis. An aortic aneurysm should be excluded by clinical examination and ultrasound. The patient should be encouraged to walk as far as he can every day. He could be given a trial of cilostazol. Revascularisation is indicated if his symptoms remain intolerable and if, after imaging, the lesion responsible appears to be suitable

for angioplasty with a high chance of success and low risk of complications. Imaging may be done with duplex ultrasound, computerised tomographic angiography or magnetic resonance angiography. Angioplasty may be performed as part of the digital subtraction angiography.

FURTHER READING

Burns P, Gough S, Bradbury AW. Management of peripheral arterial disease in primary care. *BMJ*. 2003; **326:** 584–8.

CAPRIE Steering Committee. A randomised, blinded trial of clopidogrel versus aspirin in patients at risk of ischaemic events (CAPRIE). *Lancet*. 1996; **348:** 1329–39.

Cassar K, Bachoo P. Peripheral arterial disease. *Clin Evid*. 2006; **15:** 164–76.

Gardener AW, Poehlman ET. Exercise rehabilitation programs for the treatment of claudication pain. A meta-analysis. *JAMA*. 1995; **274:** 975–80.

Hiatt WR. Medical treatment of peripheral arterial disease and claudication. *NEJM*. 2001; **344:** 1608–21.

Hirsch AT, Haskal ZJ, Hertzer NR *et al*. ACC/AHA 2005 guidelines for the management of patients with peripheral arterial disease (lower extremity, renal, mesenteric, and abdominal aortic): executive summary. A collaborative report from the American Association for Vascular Surgery/ Society for Vascular Surgery, Society for Vascular Medicine and Biology, Society of Interventional Radiology and the ACC/AHA Task Force on Practice Guidelines (Writing Committee to Develop Guidelines for the Management of Patients with Peripheral Arterial Disease) endorsed by the American Association of Cardiovascular and Pulmonary Rehabilitation, National Heart, Lung and Blood Institute, Society for Vascular Nursing, Transatlantic Inter-Society Consensus, and Vascular Disease Foundation. *J Am Coll Cardiol*. 2006; **47:** 1239–312.

Hirsch AT, Treat-Jacobson D, Lando HA *et al*. The role of tobacco cessation, antiplatelet and lipid-lowering therapies in the treatment of peripheral arterial disease. *Vasc Med*. 1997; **2:** 243–51.

Leng GC, Lee AJ, Fowkes FGR *et al*. Incidence, natural history and cardiovascular events in symptomatic and asymptomatic peripheral arterial disease in the general population. *Int J Epidemiol*. 1996; **25:** 1172–81.

Stewart KJ, Hiatt WR, Regenstein JG. Exercise training for claudication. *NEJM*. 2002; **347:** 1941–51.

Transatlantic Inter-Society Consensus (TASC) Working Group. Management of peripheral arterial occlusive disease: TASC document. *J Vasc Surg*. 2000; **31 (Suppl.):** S1–27.

White C. Intermittent claudication. *NEJM*. 2007; **356:** 1241–50.

Valve disease

TEN

Clinical cases

1. An 82-year-old man complains of breathlessness and giddiness when he walks uphill. What are the possible causes and what do you do?
2. A 54-year-old man complains of breathlessness two weeks after a heart attack. What is the probable diagnosis and what do you do?
3. A 76-year-old man complains of fatigue, anorexia and weight loss and night sweats for the previous four weeks. He had been seen in hospital several years ago, where he was told that he had a systolic murmur that did not need attention, and he had not thought it necessary to have this checked. What are the possible causes and what do you do?
4. A 35-year-old woman known to have Marfan's syndrome complains of severe back pain and sweating. What are the possible causes and what do you do?
5. A 39-year-old woman who came to the UK a year ago from the Middle East complains of recent onset of breathlessness and palpitation. What are the possible causes and what do you do?
6. You hear a systolic murmur in a 29-year-old woman during a routine examination. What do you do?

Valvular heart disease in primary care

In developed countries, *degenerative valve disease*, which has similar risk factors to coronary heart disease, is becoming more common as life expectancy increases. The most common forms of valvular heart disease in primary care are aortic valve thickening (*aortic sclerosis*), which may progress in the elderly to *calcific aortic stenosis*, and *mitral regurgitation* due to ischaemic damage to the papillary muscles. Mitral valve prolapse is very common. It should be considered a variant of normal, but may cause mitral regurgitation. Only rarely is the associated mitral regurgitation severe.

Aortic regurgitation and *mitral stenosis* have become less common in the UK and other developed countries.

Tricuspid regurgitation may occur in mainlining drug addicts who develop infective endocarditis. They may present with fever, weight loss and debility. In the elderly, these non-specific features may also be due to infective endocarditis.

Rheumatic heart disease is due to transmission of a group A streptococcus, and can be considered a disease of poverty. Acute rheumatic fever and rheumatic heart disease have become rare in people born in the UK compared with 50 years ago, due to better living standards with less overcrowding, antimicrobial treatment with penicillin for primary prevention, and public health measures with better hygiene. It may be the cause of valve disease, most commonly *mitral stenosis*, in adults who were born and grew up in developing countries and who have come to live in the UK.

Role of the primary care team in managing patients with valve disease

Open-access or surgery-based electrocardiography and echocardiography enable GPs, in consultation with cardiologists, to diagnose and manage valve disease. Good dental services and regular check-ups are important for patients with valvular heart disease. Patients should be continually educated about their heart condition.

The aims of monitoring patients with valvular heart disease are to evaluate symptoms and signs of valvular deterioration. Heart failure, outflow tract obstruction and coronary heart disease may cause increasing and intolerable breathlessness, dry cough, orthopnoea, ankle swelling, dizzy turns, syncope, chest pain, palpitation and fatigue. Fever, weight loss, malaise and non-specific features may be due to infective endocarditis.

GPs and practice nurses manage anticoagulation and provide advice for infective endocarditis prophylaxis. They should know when to refer patients to a cardiologist for review and consideration for intervention, the indications for infective endocarditis prophylaxis and how to investigate it, when surgery or new percutaneous treatments for valve disease are indicated, and the possible complications following valve replacement. Asymptomatic patients should be seen annually.

This interesting and important work can be done safely by GPs trained in cardiology, with support from a cardiologist. Patients may expect a similar level of care and clinical education about their condition from their GP as they would receive from a cardiologist.

> Management of low-risk valve conditions in primary care, with primary-care-based echocardiography, reduces the need for hospital follow-up.

Patients with complex valve disease, who have cardiac impairment, arrhythmia or endocarditis, are usually under review by a cardiologist. The management of advanced valve disease may be difficult because of the often very fine balance between risk and benefit, and the high morbidity associated with surgery, particularly in the elderly. The decision to intervene has to involve a comprehensive medical assessment. Patients and their families need to be able to make informed choices, and this is often difficult in the elderly with complex co-morbidity.

> GPs should have a register of patients with valvular heart disease who require regular monitoring for the potential complications of aortic stenosis, heart failure and suspected infective endocarditis. These patients should be referred promptly to a cardiologist for evaluation and investigation, because they may need valve surgery.

Acute rheumatic fever

The incidence of acute rheumatic fever is at least 1% in developing countries and 0.1% in developed countries. It mainly affects children living in poor, overcrowded communities in developing countries, with low-quality medical services and public health. It is caused by a group A β-haemolytic streptococcus, *Streptococcus pyogenes*. This infection causes a sore throat with pus and fever.

Prevalence of rheumatic heart disease

There are 470 000 new cases of rheumatic fever and 233 000 deaths due to rheumatic fever per year, but these figures probably underestimate the size of the problem.

The prevalence of rheumatic heart disease is estimated at 15.6 million worldwide. The prevalence measured by echocardiography is at least 3% in developing countries, which is substantially higher than the prevalence estimated by clinical examination alone.

Primary and secondary prevention of rheumatic heart disease

In the UK, streptococcal sore throats are generally treated with penicillin (primary prevention of rheumatic fever), so acute rheumatic fever is rarely seen in the UK. Rheumatic heart disease complicates 3% of untreated patients, and 50% of patients with previous untreated infection. There is usually a three- to four-week delay between infection and the appearance of symptoms. These include fever, large joint polyarthritis with pain and tenderness, pancarditis (aortic and mitral regurgitation, heart failure, pericarditis), and chorea in 20% of patients (with full recovery after a few months). Erythema marginatum is the red rash seen on the trunk, arms and legs in 20% of patients. Subcutaneous nodules over the elbows, knees, wrists, ankles and Achilles tendon last for a few weeks.

Diagnosing acute rheumatic fever

There are several causes of a fever and a heart murmur in children.

The diagnosis of acute rheumatic fever requires evidence of a group A streptococcal pharyngitis from a positive throat swab, or a positive antigen blood test, or a rising antibody titre.

Also, there should be two major, or one major plus two minor Jones criteria.

Major criteria for acute rheumatic fever diagnosis include:
- ⬦ polyarthritis
- ⬦ carditis
- ⬦ chorea
- ⬦ erythema marginatum
- ⬦ subcutaneous nodules.

Minor criteria for acute rheumatic fever diagnosis include:
- ⬦ fever
- ⬦ arthralgia
- ⬦ prolonged PR interval
- ⬦ elevated erythrocyte sedimentation rate (ESR) and C-reactive protein (CRP).

Treatment of acute rheumatic fever

Patients should be referred promptly to a specialist for confirmation of the diagnosis. They are treated with oral penicillin V (250 mg three times daily for 10 days) or intramuscular penicillin (a single injection of 1.2 million units). Oral erythromycin is used for patients with penicillin hypersensitivity. Aspirin 4–8 g daily for fever is used until ESR and CRP return to normal. Prednisolone is used to treat carditis. Heart failure is treated with diuretics, digoxin and ACE inhibitors.

Some authorities recommend penicillin G (benzylpenicillin) injections every four weeks for many years in people with a history of rheumatic fever, in order to prevent recurrent episodes (secondary prophylaxis). Secondary prevention is the only strategy that is cost-effective and practicable in developing countries.

Outcome of acute rheumatic fever

The possible outcomes of rheumatic heart disease are cardiac failure, stroke, endocarditis and death.

Murmurs resolve in 50% of cases, but this may take up to five years after the initial infection. Recurrent attacks are common, resulting in valvular heart disease in over 50% of patients.

Patients with rheumatic valvular disease should have long-term antibiotic prophylaxis before potentially septic procedures (i.e. dental and surgical procedures).

Presenting symptoms in patients with valve disease

Valve disease may present in a variety of ways:

✧ shortness of breath, cough, tiredness, anorexia and ankle swelling due to *heart failure*
✧ palpitation and thromboembolism due to *atrial fibrillation*
✧ fever, weight loss and emboli due to *infective endocarditis* on either a native or prosthetic valve
✧ breathlessness, angina, syncope or near syncope due to *left ventricular outflow tract obstruction* in aortic stenosis
✧ *haemolytic anaemia* in patients with a prosthetic valve.

Clinical evaluation of valvular heart disease

Clinical evaluation remains important despite the quick, safe and widely available diagnostic power of echocardiography and Doppler examination. Patients should be asked how much exercise they can manage, whether they feel more tired and breathless, and whether they have reduced their activities because of breathlessness.

Clinical examination will point to the most likely valvular problem and confirm the presence or absence of heart failure and hypertension. Check the pulse rate and rhythm and the blood pressure. Inspect and feel the carotid upstroke for signs of aortic valve disease (slow in stenosis, big pulsations in regurgitation). Systolic waves in the jugular venous pulse suggest tricuspid regurgitation, and a raised venous pressure and swollen feet and legs indicate right heart failure. Crackles in the lungs are a sign of pulmonary oedema. Look for signs of infective endocarditis, the presence of other relevant conditions (including Marfan's syndrome), pathology with organomegaly in the abdomen (malignancy, splenomegaly, liver or renal enlargement), and vascular disease (carotid bruits and an aortic aneurysm).

Echocardiography

Echocardiography with Doppler examination is available in hospitals and in community hospitals. It is also performed in some primary care centres. It provides a safe, quick and accurate anatomical diagnosis, and can be repeated when necessary to monitor the valve condition and the effects of cardiac size and function. This information is important for clinical management.

> This is the most useful test for diagnosing valvular heart disease and for assessing its severity. All patients with undiagnosed heart murmurs should have echocardiography.

Echocardiography provides data on:

✧ valve area of stenotic valves
✧ mean and peak gradient across stenotic valves

✧ grading of severity of valvular regurgitation
✧ valve structure
✧ presence of vegetations
✧ presence of intracardiac thrombus
✧ anatomical information about the valve apparatus
✧ anatomy of the ascending aorta
✧ function and size of the left ventricle, which has prognostic importance in aortic and mitral regurgitation.

Transthoracic echocardiography is performed when a transthoracic examination does not provide images of sufficient diagnostic quality. Transoesophageal echocardiography is particularly helpful for imaging posterior aspects of the heart and suspected thrombosis, vegetations and prosthetic dysfunction. It is used intraoperatively during valve repair.

Three-dimensional echocardiography is not used in routine clinical practice, but may be useful for providing information about valve structure.

Chest X-ray

A chest X-ray may show pulmonary oedema and lung pathology, which are important to evaluate if cardiac surgery is contemplated. Cardiac size is most accurately measured with echocardiography.

Fluoroscopy is occasionally useful when trying to differentiate between fibrosis and calcification.

Stress testing

Exercise testing provides an objective assessment of exercise capacity, and can be used serially to monitor a patient. Patients who have a good exercise performance, without symptoms or signs of ischaemia or arrhythmia, can be encouraged to exercise. If the test shows features of ischaemia, coronary angiography should be considered. This provides prognostic information in asymptomatic patients with aortic stenosis.

Stress echocardiography is not yet established for diagnostic or prognostic testing in patients with valvular heart disease.

Computed tomography (CT) scanning

This measures valve calcification, which is of prognostic value.

Magnetic resonance imaging (MRI)

This is rarely necessary. It provides useful anatomical and some physiological information. Accurate measurements of cardiac function, cardiac dimensions, intracardiac shunts and the severity of valve regurgitation are obtained.

Cardiac catheterisation and coronary angiography

This is done before valve replacement if coronary artery disease is suspected, and when coronary artery surgery is considered as an additional procedure. There is a 1/1000 risk of a stroke or heart attack occurring with this procedure. Coronary angiography is very rarely necessary in young patients.

Modern echocardiography and Doppler examination have reduced the need for invasive pressure measurements, particularly in mitral valve disease in young people.

Blood tests

Symptomatic patients should have haematology and biochemical testing. Blood cultures are mandatory when there are features that suggest endocarditis.

Brain natriuretic peptide blood tests are helpful. High levels indicate impaired ventricular function and cardiac enlargement, which are major predictors of an adverse prognosis. Increases in brain natriuretic peptide levels suggest cardiac decompensation.

Principles of management of patients with valve disease

- ❖ An accurate anatomical and functional diagnosis is essential. In most cases, this is obtained from clinical evaluation and echocardiography.
- ❖ All patients with significant valvular heart disease should have antibiotic prophylaxis before potentially septic procedures.
- ❖ Patients with mild valve conditions and those in whom the risks of surgery are unacceptably high may be treated medically and monitored in primary care.
- ❖ Patients with valvular heart disease should be monitored carefully and referred for a specialist opinion if their symptoms deteriorate and are thought to require intervention.
- ❖ Anticoagulation is necessary for patients with atrial fibrillation and prosthetic heart valves.
- ❖ The decision to investigate and perform valve replacement should be made on an individual patient basis with full discussion with the patient and, when appropriate, with their family. This is particularly important in the elderly asymptomatic patient. The risk of intervention has to be balanced against the early operative risks and the later risks related to rehabilitation and valve problems.
- ❖ 'Old age' is not a contraindication to valve surgery or intervention.
- ❖ Operative mortality and morbidity depend on the patient's age, co-morbidity (renal disease, liver disease, haematological problems), left ventricular function, presence and severity of coronary artery disease, presence and severity of lung disease, aortic pathology, carotid disease, pulmonary hypertension, previous myocardial infarction and previous stroke.

Surgery in patients with valve disease

Before recommending cardiac surgery, there are several difficult issues that need careful consideration and discussion between cardiologists, cardiac surgeons and anaesthetists. The GP's perspective of the patient's clinical state, quality-of-life aspirations and support network at home are also important components of the decision-making process.

Surgery for valve disease is a major procedure and carries a significant morbidity and mortality, which depend on several factors. These risks must be clearly explained to the patient.

Valve repair

Valve repair is recommended for most patients with mitral valve disease (both stenosis and regurgitation), because it allows retention of the native valve and excludes the risks associated with a prosthetic valve (lifelong anticoagulation, haemolytic anaemia, endocarditis) and the limited lifespan of a biological valve. It demands considerable surgical skills and experience.

Valve replacement

Valves may be replaced using either a prosthetic or a bioprosthetic valve.

Prosthetic mechanical valves

These have excellent durability but, because patients need lifelong anticoagulation, they are generally implanted in young patients (< 70 years) and those who require anticoagulation for other reasons.

Complications of prosthetic heart valves

Valve thrombosis

Thromboembolism and anticoagulant-related bleeding account for nearly all the problems after valve replacement. Adequate and careful anticoagulation is essential in order to reduce the risk of valve thrombosis.

The incidence of valve thrombosis is 0.1–6% per year. This is a serious complication with a high mortality. The consequences are sudden death, pulmonary oedema, syncope or embolisation. Emergency echocardiography is required. Intravenous heparin or, for large thrombi, thrombolysis is given. If this does not work or is unlikely to work, emergency valve replacement is necessary.

Infective endocarditis

Endocarditis is a very serious but less common complication. All patients with prosthetic valves should have antibiotic prophylaxis before potentially septic procedures. The incidence of infective endocarditis is 3–6% per year. Early endocarditis occurs within two months of surgery, and is due to peri-operative skin or wound infections or indwelling catheters. The patient should be referred back to hospital for diagnosis and treatment. Antibiotics should not be started unless blood cultures have been taken.

Emboli

The incidence is 1% in patients on warfarin and 4% in patients who are not anticoagulated. The risks are much higher in patients who are in atrial fibrillation, the elderly, and those with reduced left ventricular function or a mitral prosthesis. Emboli may be due to infective endocarditis. The management of thrombotic cerebral emboli is difficult. Warfarin should be stopped if the CT scan of the brain shows a bleed, and the patient should be treated with intravenous heparin and referred for a neurosurgical opinion. If the stroke is due to an embolus, anticoagulation should be given.

Haemolysis

Haemolytic anaemia is a rare complication after implantation of a prosthetic heart valve. The underlying cause (e.g. valve dysfunction, leakage, infection) should be treated, and this may require valve replacement if there is significant anaemia.

Prosthetic valves

Prosthetic valves last longer than bioprosthetic valves. Compared with a bioprosthesis, a mechanical valve is less likely to deteriorate in patients with renal failure or hypercalcaemia. If a valve fails, it must be replaced.

Prosthetic valves are preferred in patients:
- with an expected long lifespan
- who have a mechanical valve in a position different from that of the valve to be replaced
- with renal failure, on haemodialysis
- who require warfarin
- under 65 years of age for aortic valve replacement
- over 70 years of age for mitral valve replacement.

Bioprosthetic valves

Anticoagulation is not necessary for bioprosthetic valves in patients who are in sinus rhythm. Because of this they are recommended for patients over the age of 65 years because of the increased risks of bleeding in the elderly treated with warfarin. They have a lifespan of around 15 years.

Indications for a bioprosthetic valve:

⋄ elderly patients
⋄ those who cannot or will not take warfarin
⋄ patients aged over 65 years who need aortic valve replacement and do not have risk factors for thromboembolism
⋄ patients aged over 70 years who need mitral valve replacement and do not have risk factors for thromboembolism.

After valve replacement

Patients without complications are discharged within one week of surgery. They should have had a clinical assessment, patient education from the surgical team, and some may have had post-operative echocardiography, which provides useful baseline information. Patients may have a follow-up hospital outpatient appointment 6–12 weeks post-operatively.

It is recommended that all patients should be followed up for life by a cardiologist to detect early deterioration of the valve, new symptoms, features of endocarditis, and progression of disease in another valve. Annual echocardiography is advised.

TABLE 10.1: Choice of heart valve prosthesis

	Mechanical prosthesis	Bioprosthesis
Durability	Many years	Around 10 years
Anticoagulation	Yes	No, unless atrial fibrillation
Survival	No difference	No difference
Young patient (< 40 years)	Preferred	Avoid
Renal failure or hyperparathyroidism	Preferred	For poor prognosis

Percutaneous treatments for valve stenosis

Percutaneous treatments for valve disease offer the potential for lower morbidity and mortality because heart bypass surgery is not required. Patients generally prefer minimally invasive procedures if they are as effective as open heart surgery.

Percutaneous treatment for valvular heart disease is established for mitral stenosis, but is being used only in clinical trials to treat mitral regurgitation, aortic stenosis, and pulmonary regurgitation as part of congenital heart disease. It is not yet clear whether percutaneous treatments of valve disease will be of clinical value.

Mitral valvuloplasty for mitral stenosis is a safe and useful method for widening a narrowed, non-calcified and, at most, mildly regurgitant mitral valve in symptomatic patients who have no left atrial thrombus.

Bleeding risks of anticoagulation and antithrombotic treatment

All patients with a prosthetic heart valve and/or atrial fibrillation require warfarin. The risk of thromboembolism is higher in patients with a prosthetic valve in the mitral compared with the aortic position.

The practical difficulties of monitoring warfarin treatment and the risks of bleeding have to be taken into account when considering valve replacement. Tighter anticoagulation control has reduced the incidence of major bleeding (defined as the requirement for a transfusion of more than four units of blood).

An INR of 2.5–3.5 is recommended for patients with a prosthetic valve.

The following circumstances increase the risk of bleeding:

✧ elderly patients (aged over 75 years), who may be frail, forgetful, and are more likely to have coexisting medical conditions or be taking other medication that increases the risk of bleeding. They may have an increased sensitivity to warfarin, or lower dietary vitamin K levels. The doses for warfarin loading and maintenance are lower in elderly patients
✧ a history of uncontrolled hypertension
✧ excess alcohol consumption
✧ peptic ulcer
✧ poor anticoagulation control
✧ other drugs that increase susceptibility to bleeding (e.g. aspirin, non-steroidal anti-inflammatory drugs).

> Intracranial haemorrhage is the most serious bleeding complication.
> Patients who are prescribed warfarin should be warned of the risks of bruising and bleeding. INR monitoring should be performed regularly and carefully in all patients, but particularly in those at high risk.

If the INR is high, but if there is no bleeding or only minor bleeding, warfarin should be stopped or the dose reduced and the INR monitored. Oral or subcutaneous vitamin K 2–5 mg is given to patients who are bleeding, but *not* to patients with a prosthetic valve unless there is intracranial bleeding, because of the risks of thrombosis and obstruction of the valve. It is advisable to refer these patients to hospital. Fresh-frozen plasma is sometimes given.

Management of anticoagulation in patients who require dental care

Anticoagulation should not be stopped for procedures in which bleeding is unlikely or would be unimportant if it occurred.

When there is likely to be a substantial bleeding risk, aspirin should be stopped one week before the procedure and started as soon as it is considered safe by the surgeon or dentist.

Warfarin should be stopped before the procedure to reach an INR of < 1.5, and should be restarted 24 hours after the procedure.

Interim heparin to provide anticoagulation when warfarin is stopped is advisable for patients:

✧ with recent thrombosis or embolus (within the last year)
✧ in whom thrombotic problems occurred previously when anticoagulation was stopped
✧ with three or more of the following thrombotic risk factors: atrial fibrillation, previous thromboembolism, hypercoagulable state, impaired left ventricular function, mechanical prosthesis. These patients should be referred to hospital because there is currently insufficient evidence to recommend low-molecular-weight heparin.

Mitral stenosis

Pathology

Only 50% of these patients recall an attack of rheumatic fever in childhood. The resulting fibrosis, thickening, fusion and calcification of the valve cusps and valve apparatus lead to progressive narrowing of the mitral valve orifice.

The normal mitral valve area is 4 cm^2. Moderate to severe mitral valve disease is associated with a mitral valve area of less than 1.5 cm^2. This results in restricted flow of blood from the left atrium to the left ventricle, with progressive increases in left atrial pressure, pulmonary venous pressure, pulmonary oedema and breathlessness. Pulmonary venous pressure is increased further in patients with atrial fibrillation, which occurs in the majority of patients due to stretching of the left atrium. The onset of atrial fibrillation may lead to pulmonary oedema in previously stable patients.

Atrial fibrillation, together with increasing age and left atrial size, put patients at high risk of arterial embolism. All patients with mitral valve disease and atrial fibrillation should be anticoagulated unless there are important contraindications.

Symptoms

Symptoms appear most commonly, and slowly, between the ages of 40 and 50 years, but may occur at a younger age in patients from developing countries and during pregnancy, when the plasma volume increases. Shortness of breath and orthopnoea are due to pulmonary oedema and postural changes. Acute pulmonary oedema may occur with an increase in heart rate during exercise, with the onset of atrial fibrillation or with a chest infection.

Atrial fibrillation may lead to emboli. Fatigue is due to a low cardiac output in moderate to severe mitral stenosis. Chest pain is unusual, but may occur in patients with severe mitral stenosis and pulmonary hypertension. Angina is usually due to coronary heart disease. Compression of the surrounding structures by a large left atrium is uncommon nowadays in the UK because of early diagnosis and treatment.

Signs

There is a loud first heart sound, an opening snap (if the mitral valve remains pliable) and a diastolic murmur. A systolic murmur may be heard in patients with mitral regurgitation. The aortic valve may also be affected. Atrial fibrillation may occur in patients with a dilated left atrium. A malar flush (reddening of the face) is not a reliable sign.

Investigations

ECG

Atrial fibrillation; measure the ventricular response and look for signs of conduction disease (bundle branch block).

Chest X-ray

The findings depend on the severity of the stenosis and its effects on pulmonary venous pressure. The X-ray may be normal in patients with mild mitral stenosis and a well controlled heart rate. Patients with moderate or severe mitral stenosis may have pulmonary oedema, but this depends on several factors, including the heart rate, the distensibility of the left atrium, and the mitral valve gradient. In pure mitral stenosis the left atrial appendage may be enlarged but the heart shadow may be normal.

Echocardiography

Transthoracic echocardiography is the most helpful investigation in patients with mitral valve disease. It shows the extent of the pathological changes affecting the valve cusps and their apparatus.

The main aspects of echocardiography are the measurement of the mitral valve area to grade the severity of the stenosis, the structure of the valve, and whether and how much it is calcified, as well as Doppler studies to measure the gradient. In severe mitral stenosis the pulmonary artery pressure may be high.

Measurements of the valve orifice area indicate the severity of the stenosis:

✧ mild stenosis – mitral valve area > 1.5 cm^2
✧ moderate stenosis – mitral valve area < 1.5 cm^2
✧ severe mitral stenosis – mitral valve area < 1.0 cm^2.

Associated mitral regurgitation, other valve conditions and vegetations may be seen. Left and right ventricular function and dimensions are evaluated and left atrial dimensions measured. This information relates clinical features to cardiac structure and function, and provides the information necessary to decide on the optimum approach to treatment. The absence of significant calcification and mitral regurgitation suggests that percutaneous mitral valvuloplasty may be appropriate.

Transoesophageal echocardiography is performed to assess possible left atrial thrombus prior to electrical cardioversion or percutaneous mitral valvuloplasty, or when a transthoracic study is unsatisfactory.

Exercise testing
This is useful when measuring a patient's exercise tolerance, and in older patients with cardiovascular risk factors, who may show signs of ischaemia.

Cardiac catheterisation and coronary angiography
This is indicated in patients who may have coronary artery disease, and to obtain accurate haemodynamic data as part of the evaluation prior to percutaneous mitral valvuloplasty or surgery. Coronary angiography is not necessary in young patients prior to mitral valve surgery, because they are at low risk of having coronary artery disease. The mitral valve gradient at rest, after exercise, and the pulmonary artery pressure are high in patients with severe mitral stenosis.

Medical treatment of mitral valve stenosis
Mild symptoms may be controlled medically.

Diuretics improve breathlessness that is due to pulmonary venous hypertension and oedema.

Atrial fibrillation results from left atrial dilatation, and responds best to mechanical relief of valve stenosis. Uncontrolled atrial fibrillation should be controlled with β-blockers either alone or combined with *calcium antagonists* or *digoxin*. Other approaches to the treatment of atrial fibrillation (e.g. radiofrequency ablation) may need to be considered.

Anticoagulation should be considered in all patients who are in atrial fibrillation.

Because emboli may occur shortly after the onset of atrial fibrillation, it is also appropriate to anticoagulate patients who are in sinus rhythm.

Prophylactic antibiotics (phenoxymethylpenicillin 250 mg twice a day orally) are given to patients who have had rheumatic fever, until the age of 40 years or for at least 10 years after the last attack of rheumatic fever. All patients with mitral stenosis should have prophylactic antibiotics before undergoing potentially septic procedures.

Percutaneous mitral balloon valvuloplasty for mitral stenosis
This is performed in specialist units by experienced operators. The presence of left atrial thrombus must be excluded by transoesophageal echocardiography in order to avoid the risk of arterial embolism during the procedure.

The patient is sedated and the procedure performed with local anaesthetic. It involves a right heart catheterisation and puncture of the interatrial septum to allow passage of a balloon from the right to the left atrium and then through the mitral valve. The balloon is positioned across the mitral valve using X-ray visualisation, and is then inflated for a few seconds at a time (the inflated balloon obstructs the circulation) until the stenosed valve is optimally dilated. Echocardiography is used during the procedure to monitor the mitral valve changes and to check for cardiac tamponade, which is a rare and important complication. An overnight stay is required for uncomplicated cases.

Successful dilatation of the mitral valve depends on the morphology of the valve and its subvalvar apparatus. Failure occurs in 1–15% of patients. Complication rates are as follows: death, 0.4–4%; haemopericardium, 0.5–10%; embolism, 5%; severe balloon-produced mitral regurgitation, 2–10%. Emergency surgery is required in less than 1% of patients.

Ten years after the procedure, 35–70% of patients are well. Surgery is usually required within a few weeks or months if the immediate post-procedure result is not satisfactory.

Indications for percutaneous balloon mitral valvuloplasty

✧ Symptomatic patients with moderate or severe mitral stenosis, favourable mitral valve morphology (pliable valve cusps with little or no calcification or mitral regurgitation) and absence of left atrial thrombus (risk of embolism).
✧ Asymptomatic patients with moderate or severe mitral valve stenosis and pulmonary hypertension.
✧ Symptomatic patients with moderate to severe mitral stenosis and a non-pliable valve, who are considered too high risk for surgery.

Indications for surgical mitral valvotomy

✧ Symptomatic patients with moderate to severe mitral stenosis, with mitral valve morphology favourable for mitral valve repair, if balloon valvuloplasty is not available or when it is contraindicated by left atrial thrombus.
✧ Symptomatic mitral valve stenosis with a calcified, non-pliable valve that is not suitable for valvuloplasty.

Indications for mitral valve replacement

✧ Symptomatic patients with moderate or severe mitral stenosis who are not candidates for either balloon valvuloplasty or valve repair.
✧ Patients with severe mitral stenosis but minimal symptoms who have pulmonary hypertension.

Mitral regurgitation

Mitral regurgitation is the second most common valve condition in the UK (aortic stenosis is the most common). The common causes are degeneration of the valve, and ischaemic damage to the papillary muscles following myocardial infarction. Rheumatic mitral valve disease is less common in people who were born in the UK, but is an important cause of mixed mitral valve disease (combined mitral stenosis and mitral regurgitation) in people who were born and grew up in developing countries where rheumatic fever and heart disease remain common.

Pathology

Mitral regurgitation may be due to a primary valve abnormality (e.g. rheumatic valve disease, mitral valve prolapse, endocarditis) or secondary to a left ventricular problem (e.g. myocardial infarction or cardiomyopathy, where the valve cusps are normal but there is stretching of the mitral valve annulus due to left ventricular dilatation). Chronic progressive volume overload of the left ventricle leads to left atrial and left ventricular hypertrophy and dilatation, heart failure, pulmonary hypertension and death.

The presentation of *acute* mitral regurgitation is dramatic because the left atrium has not had time to adapt. The acute increase in atrial volume overload leads to sudden increases in left atrial and pulmonary venous pressure and pulmonary oedema. Surgery should be performed urgently. These patients should be referred to a cardiac surgical centre for prompt evaluation.

Chronic mitral regurgitation is well tolerated for many years because the left ventricle is initially able to adapt to the volume overload. Patients become symptomatic when left ventricular impairment develops. Symptoms are a sign of important mitral regurgitation indicating cardiac decompensation. Surgery should be performed before left ventricular dilatation occurs. The timing is difficult.

Causes of mitral regurgitation
Chronic mitral regurgitation
✧ Ischaemic papillary muscle dysfunction.
✧ Cardiomyopathy.
✧ Myxomatous degeneration of the mitral valve (mitral valve prolapse).

Acute mitral regurgitation
✧ Chordal rupture (Marfan's syndrome).
✧ Infectious endocarditis, which causes leaflet destruction, perforation and chordal rupture.

Symptoms
Symptoms depend on left ventricular function, heart rate and rhythm, pulmonary venous pressure and the activity and general medical condition of the patient. Exertional breathlessness, fatigue and orthopnoea are symptoms of significant left ventricular impairment. These patients should be treated and referred for echocardiography and specialist assessment.

Patients with chronic, slowly progressive mitral regurgitation who do little exercise may remain content and relatively asymptomatic for many years when they may develop symptoms of heart failure. Patients with acute mitral regurgitation will develop acute pulmonary oedema.

Signs
Patients with mitral regurgitation have a pansystolic murmur and possibly a displaced apex beat. A mid-systolic click and a mid- to late-systolic murmur are found in mitral valve prolapse. Pulmonary oedema and a third heart sound may be found in patients with severe or acute mitral regurgitation and left ventricular failure.

ECG
The ECG may be normal or there may be non-specific ST and T-wave changes. Left ventricular hypertrophy with or without atrial fibrillation may be seen in patients with left ventricular dilatation.

Chest X-ray
The chest X-ray may be normal or there may be non-specific ST and T-wave changes, depending on the severity and speed of onset of the regurgitation, and left ventricular function.

Echocardiography

This shows the morphology of the valve, the size and function of the left ventricle, and left atrial size, provides a semi-quantitative assessment of the severity of mitral regurgitation, demonstrates associated valve lesions, and provides an estimate of pulmonary artery pressure. Ruptured chordae or signs of endocarditis may be seen in patients with acute mitral regurgitation. The diagnosis of mitral valve prolapse is made clinically and confirmed with echocardiography.

Cardiac catheterisation and coronary angiography

This is done to identify the need for coronary angioplasty or coronary artery surgery, which may be necessary at the time of mitral valve surgery. In addition to identifying the severity and location of coronary artery disease, it provides information on left ventricular function. The severity of mitral regurgitation is assessed from left ventriculography. Right heart catheterisation measures right atrial pressure, pulmonary artery pressure, pulmonary vascular resistance and cardiac output.

Natural history of mitral regurgitation

Predictors of a poor prognosis include age, atrial fibrillation, degree of mitral regurgitation, left atrial size, left ventricular size and left ventricular function.

In asymptomatic patients, the five-year mortality rate is 15%. Around 33% of patients develop heart failure, atrial fibrillation or cardiac death within five years.

Follow-up of patients with mitral regurgitation

Asymptomatic patients with preserved left ventricular function and *moderate* mitral regurgitation should be reviewed annually, with echocardiography performed every two years.

Asymptomatic patients with severe mitral regurgitation and preserved left ventricular function should be reviewed every six months, and echocardiography should be performed every year.

Patients should be advised to report symptoms promptly.

Medical treatment of mitral regurgitation

Patients with heart failure are treated medically, and surgery is scheduled as soon as the patient is haemodynamically stable. Patients who pose an unacceptably high surgical risk due to their age, the presence of other medical conditions or very poor left ventricular function are treated medically.

Endocarditis prophylaxis should be given to all patients with mitral regurgitation.

The principles of treatment of heart failure due to mitral regurgitation are similar to those for other causes of heart failure. Diuretics for peripheral or pulmonary oedema, rhythm or rate control of atrial fibrillation with anticoagulation, ACE inhibitors and/or angiotensin II receptor antagonists, spironolactone and β-blockers may be used. ACE inhibitors are used only in patients with heart failure.

Surgical treatment of mitral regurgitation

Urgent surgery is necessary for acute mitral regurgitation. Even though some patients may tolerate the condition initially, without valve repair or replacement there is a high risk of pulmonary hypertension.

For chronic mitral regurgitation, surgical treatment is the preferred approach. The valve can be either repaired (preferably with preservation of the chordae tendinae) or replaced with a prosthetic or tissue valve. The choice of valve depends on the age of the patient and their prognosis, and the practicalities of and necessity for anticoagulation.

Mitral valve repair in expert hands is the favoured technique because it has a lower peri-operative mortality, better long-term survival, better post-operative left ventricular function and lower long-term morbidity. The decision to repair or replace the valve is made by the cardiac surgeon at the time of surgery, but information from echocardiography is helpful.

The risks are higher and the surgical results are poorer in patients with more severe mitral regurgitation who have left ventricular dilatation and poor function, and are particularly high in those with pulmonary hypertension due to longstanding severe mitral regurgitation and left ventricular impairment.

Mitral valve surgery (repair or mitral valve replacement) is indicated in:

- symptomatic patients with a dilated heart
- patients with acute mitral regurgitation – as an emergency
- symptomatic or asymptomatic patients with impaired left ventricular function or dilatation
- symptomatic patients with preserved left ventricular function and atrial fibrillation or pulmonary hypertension
- asymptomatic patients with signs of increasing left ventricular dilatation as judged by serial echocardiography.

Mitral valve surgery in asymptomatic patients

This is controversial because of the risks of surgery. There are no randomised trials to guide the management of asymptomatic patients. Surgery is not recommended in asymptomatic patients who have a normal-sized and normally functioning left ventricle. These patients should be followed up annually with echocardiography. They should be referred if there are increases in left ventricular dimensions, left ventricular impairment, if they develop atrial fibrillation, or if Doppler examination indicates pulmonary hypertension.

Surgery for associated atrial fibrillation may be performed at the same time as mitral valve repair or replacement, although radio-frequency ablation is more commonly used.

Surgery for secondary mitral regurgitation is a more complex decision and should be individualised.

Mitral valve prolapse

This is a common and generally benign cardiac condition that occurs in 10% of the adult population. It is due to the presence of abnormal and often excess collagen in the mitral valve leaflets. It is a variant of normal, rather than a valve abnormality, and is more common in tall slim females. It is not a cause of any cardiac symptom unless there is important mitral regurgitation. It is diagnosed clinically by a mid-systolic click, with a systolic murmur present if there is mitral regurgitation. The presence of a murmur is a reason for advising antibiotic prophylaxis. The signs may be variable in the same patient. Some patients have a typical body shape and are slim, have a straight back, and have a pectus excavatum or scoliosis.

Investigations

Echocardiography shows thickening (myxomatous degeneration of the valve cusps) with varying degrees of prolapse of the valve cusps into the left atrium in systole. Serial echocardiography is indicated in patients with mitral regurgitation. The ECG is normal and occasionally may show non-specific, unimportant ST and T-wave changes. Palpitation is quite common, and is unrelated to the valve condition. A 24-hour ECG recording may be helpful for identifying frequent arrhythmias. The most common ones are unifocal ventricular ectopic beats, which do not require treatment unless the patient is very symptomatic despite reassurance. Cardiac catheterisation is only indicated when surgery is being considered in patients who are likely to have coronary artery disease.

Management

The prognosis is generally excellent, and the patient should be reassured. No medical treatment is necessary. Chordal rupture resulting in a flail leaflet and severe acute pulmonary oedema is very rare, but would necessitate urgent mitral valve repair or replacement. Cerebral embolism is rare and presents as a stroke, transient ischaemic attack or amaurosis fugax. Antibiotic prophylaxis is only necessary if there is mitral regurgitation.

Percutaneous mitral valve repair is being developed to treat mitral valve prolapse. This currently requires a general anaesthetic and transoesophageal echocardiography during the procedure. Compared with a percutaneous approach, open heart surgery allows a more comprehensive inspection and repair of all parts of the mitral valve apparatus (mitral valve annulus, leaflets, chordae tendinae and papillary muscles).

Ischaemic mitral regurgitation

This is caused by ischaemic damage to the papillary muscle of the mitral valve due to myocardial infarction. It may present either as acute severe mitral regurgitation and shock, or later as chronic mitral regurgitation and left heart failure. Both types of mitral regurgitation have a poor prognosis, which is made worse by the presence of increasing age, impaired left ventricular function and coronary artery disease.

Diagnosis is by echocardiography, and coronary angiography should be performed in patients with angina and in those who are considered for mitral valve surgery.

Surgery is more complex, and has a higher mortality than surgery for valvular mitral regurgitation. Patients with ischaemic mitral regurgitation are more likely to have co-morbidity.

Surgery is indicated for *severe* ischaemic mitral regurgitation and symptoms with a left ventricular ejection fraction of > 30%, if the patient is having coronary artery surgery. The decision to repair or replace the valve is individualised in patients with *moderate* mitral regurgitation.

Mitral regurgitation due to left ventricular dilatation and heart failure

This may be due to a dilated cardiomyopathy. The clinical presentation of heart failure and the assessment with echocardiography are similar to those for patients with other types of mitral regurgitation.

The results of surgery are poor, with an operative mortality rate in the range 5–18%, a two-year survival of 70% and a five-year survival of 60% in patients with severe left ventricular impairment. These patients would usually be under the care of a cardiologist, and in the UK most of them are treated medically. Young patients may be referred for transplantation.

Aortic valve stenosis

Degenerative aortic valve disease is the most common cause of valvular heart disease in the Western world, causing significant morbidity and mortality. Mild aortic valve disease with aortic valve thickening (aortic sclerosis) is an age-related finding and very common in patients over 70 years of age. Calcific, haemodynamically significant aortic stenosis is the most common form, occurring in 7% of people aged > 65 years. Rheumatic aortic stenosis is now much less common.

Symptoms

Progressive pressure overload results in left ventricular hypertrophy and this, even in the absence of coronary artery disease (which is present in the majority of patients), may cause angina and breathlessness due to a stiff non-compliant heart muscle. Exertional syncope or dizziness occurs due to severe obstruction of the outflow tract.

Elderly patients who have giddy turns, falls or episodes of feeling light-headed may have aortic stenosis as well as other causes of these symptoms, including bradycardia, neurological disease and vestibular problems.

> Elderly patients who have falls and 'funny turns' may have aortic stenosis as well as other conditions. All possible causes need to be investigated and excluded in order to define the most appropriate management.

Signs

A loud systolic ejection murmur radiating to the neck, with a slow rising carotid artery pulse or 'shudder' are the main findings, and these suggest important aortic valve stenosis. The second heart sound, due to aortic valve closure, may be quiet in severe stenosis with calcified immobile valve cusps.

Aortic stenosis may also commonly present with heart failure. Because aortic stenosis is so common among the elderly in primary care, it is good practice to listen to the heart of all patients aged over 70 years annually.

Investigations

The diagnosis and its severity are best confirmed with echocardiography and Doppler examination.

Coronary angiography is performed in adults who are being considered for valve replacement, because of the high probability of associated coronary artery disease, particularly in the elderly. The aortic valve gradient will be spuriously low in patients with significant left ventricular impairment, so the decision to replace the valve is made after considering several factors. Measurement of the aortic valve area with echocardiography or cardiac catheterisation is important. Aortic valve replacement is effective, allows the patient to live a normal life, and should be considered in all patients with significant stenosis.

Pathology, progression and prognosis

Aortic valve calcification is the result of an active process, similar to atherosclerotic vascular disease. Around 50% of patients have coronary heart disease. It appears to be mediated by turbulence of blood and mechanical stresses, and is associated with diabetes, hypertension, hypercholesterolaemia and smoking. However, there is no evidence that treating these risk factors favourably influences the natural history of the condition.

Aortic stenosis usually presents either in the elderly, or as premature calcification of a congenitally bicuspid valve in middle age.

> Once symptoms develop, patients with aortic stenosis survive for only 3–5 years without aortic valve replacement. Diagnosis, monitoring of patients and specialist referral are therefore very important.

ECG

This may be normal even in severe aortic stenosis. Tall R-waves in the left chest leads and ST and T-wave changes reflect left ventricular hypertrophy due to increased left ventricular work.

Chest X-ray

This may be normal or it may show post-stenotic dilatation of the aorta. A penetrated chest X-ray may show aortic valve calcification, but this is now rarely necessary due to the wide availability of echocardiography.

Echocardiography and Doppler examination

Most patients are imaged satisfactorily with a transthoracic study. Transoesophageal echocardiography is only occasionally required. Echocardiography is the most useful non-invasive test, showing the anatomy and function of the aortic valve, the degree of valve calcification, the presence and severity of associated aortic regurgitation, the diameter of the aortic root, the extent of left ventricular hypertrophy, left ventricular size and function (which influences the aortic valve gradient) and other valve disease. Doppler examination will show the calculated peak gradient and thus the severity of the stenosis. It may be possible to measure the aortic valve area and thus the need for aortic valve replacement.

Exercise testing

This is contraindicated in severely symptomatic patients. It is used to assess exercise capacity, blood pressure response and signs of ischaemia which may be difficult to interpret in the presence of left ventricular hypertrophy. It is also useful for unmasking symptoms in asymptomatic patients with a severe aortic stenosis. This test is useful for measuring exercise capacity.

Computed tomography (CT) and magnetic resonance imaging (MRI)

These imaging tests are useful for imaging the aortic root before surgery. The role of multi-slice computed tomography is not yet known.

Cardiac catheterisation

Coronary artery disease is common in patients with aortic stenosis. Coronary artery surgery is indicated for significant coronary artery disease, even in patients without symptoms. Coronary artery surgery slightly increases the operative risk. Measuring the aortic gradient during cardiac catheterisation by passing a catheter across the aortic valve has been replaced in most centres by echocardiography and Doppler, because of the risks of stroke due to cerebral emboli from the calcified valve. In most cases, echocardiography and Doppler provide accurate measurements of the aortic valve gradient and the valve area.

Grading the severity of aortic stenosis

Patients with severe aortic stenosis but who do little exercise may have no symptoms.

> In severe aortic stenosis, the valve area is < 1 cm^2 and the mean pressure gradient across the valve is > 50 mmHg.
> In moderate aortic stenosis, the valve area is 1.0–1.5 cm^2 and the mean pressure gradient is 30–50 mmHg.

The gradient across the valve depends on cardiac output and blood flow. Therefore, patients with severe aortic stenosis and impaired left ventricular function may have a spuriously low transvalvular pressure gradient because the weak left ventricle is not able to generate high pressures within the ventricle, and there is low flow across the valve. Also, a moderately or mildly stenosed aortic valve may not open fully, and the calculated valve area measured by echocardiography may be spuriously low, exaggerating the severity of the lesion.

Prognosis and follow-up of aortic stenosis

Patients with moderate aortic stenosis may remain symptom free for many years. Symptoms of heart failure or left ventricular outflow tract obstruction indicate a poor prognosis largely due to sudden death. This highlights the importance of urgent referral of symptomatic patients with aortic valve stenosis for aortic valve replacement. Serial exercise testing and echocardiography are important. Six-monthly follow-up is recommended for patients who are symptom free but have a peak aortic gradient of > 50 mmHg, or who have a heavily calcified valve or a rapidly progressing gradient. Other asymptomatic patients can be reviewed annually.

> Patients with aortic stenosis should be reviewed regularly and asked about any symptoms.

Poor prognostic features include:
- age over 80 years
- atherosclerotic risk factors
- heavily calcified valve, peak gradient > 100 mmHg and rapid increase in valve gradient (this confers a mortality risk of 80% within two years)
- exercise-induced dizziness, chest pain or breathlessness.

Interventions for aortic stenosis
Balloon valvuloplasty for congenital aortic stenosis in young people
Prosthetic aortic valve replacement in a young patient with congenital aortic valve stenosis may necessitate a high-risk second operation if the valve fails or leaks because the patient and the aorta have grown. Therefore, balloon aortic valvuloplasty is preferred, and is performed in paediatric cardiac centres in young asymptomatic patients with non-calcified, pliable, significant (transvalvular gradient of > 50 mmHg) congenital aortic stenosis.

Balloon valvuloplasty in adults
Aortic valvuloplasty for aortic stenosis is a percutaneous procedure that is used only occasionally to widen (or crack open) a calcified and severely narrowed aortic valve. It is only occasionally used for elderly patients with severe aortic stenosis who, because of coexisting conditions, are considered too high risk for aortic valve replacement. The procedure has a high mortality rate and a high risk of cerebral emboli, and restenosis within one year. Complications occur in at least 10% of patients.

Percutaneous aortic valve replacement
This is technically very difficult, and is associated with a high morbidity and mortality. Surgical, open-heart aortic valve replacement is the safest and most effective approach.

Aortic valve replacement

This is the only effective treatment for severe aortic stenosis. The operative mortality is 3–5% in patients aged < 70 years and 5–15% in patients aged > 70 years. Age is not a contraindication for surgery, and the decision to operate on a 90-year-old is made on an individual patient basis, taking into account the wishes of the patient and all medical and social factors. The operative risks are higher with older patients, female patients, emergency operations, heart failure, patients with coronary artery disease and those with previous heart surgery. The prognosis after valve replacement is good if there was no pre-operative cardiac failure.

Indications for aortic valve replacement

⬦ Patients with severe aortic stenosis with symptoms.
⬦ Patients with severe aortic stenosis without symptoms at rest, but with symptoms induced during exercise testing, *or* a rapidly increasing aortic gradient, *or* a heavily calcified valve, *or* an ejection fraction of < 50%.
⬦ Patients with moderate aortic stenosis who are undergoing coronary artery surgery, aortic surgery or other valve surgery.
⬦ Patients with severe aortic stenosis who have impaired but potentially recoverable left ventricular function.

Coronary bypass surgery performed at the same time as aortic valve replacement increases the operative risk, but carries a lower risk than not performing necessary bypass surgery.

Medical treatment of aortic stenosis

This is necessary for patients who are not fit for surgery, or who decline surgery. Medical treatment does not improve survival. Cardiovascular risk factor treatment is recommended, but has not been shown to improve survival.

Diuretics are used for symptomatic pulmonary or peripheral oedema, but over-diuresis may be dangerous due to reduction in the circulating plasma volume and reduction in cardiac output.

Digoxin or other bradycardic drugs, electrical cardioversion or radio-frequency ablation may be necessary for uncontrolled atrial fibrillation.

ACE inhibitors or angiotensin II antagonists may be used for heart failure. They may need to be started in hospital in patients who are thought to develop hypotension.

β-blockers are contraindicated in patients with left ventricular impairment due to their depressant (negative inotropic) action on the left ventricle reducing cardiac output.

Endocarditis prophylaxis is recommended for all patients.

Aortic regurgitation (AR)

Pathology

Chronic aortic regurgitation causes volume overload of the left ventricle with compensatory hypertrophy and dilatation, which is often well tolerated for many years. The increased stroke volume results in hypertension, which adds a pressure overload on the heart. These changes may be reversed by timely aortic valve surgery.

Causes of aortic regurgitation

Aortic regurgitation may be due to an abnormality either of the valve cusps, resulting in mixed stenosis and regurgitation, or of the aortic root.

Acute aortic regurgitation may be due to aortic dissection associated with hypertension. It has a poor prognosis without surgical treatment.

Valve conditions that cause aortic regurgitation

- Age-related degeneration of the cusps:
  - calcific bicuspid valve
  - rheumatic heart disease.
- Infective endocarditis (acute aortic regurgitation).

Aortic root conditions that cause aortic regurgitation

- Aortic root disease associated with hypertension.
- Marfan's syndrome.
- Aortic dissection.
- Ankylosing spondylitis.

Symptoms

Patients are often symptom free until they decompensate, when they experience symptoms of heart failure.

> The onset of symptoms in aortic regurgitation is a bad prognostic sign and an indication for aortic valve surgery.

Acute aortic regurgitation causes a sudden increase in left ventricular end-diastolic pressure with pulmonary oedema and sudden breathlessness.

Signs

Patients are usually in sinus rhythm, but have visible and forceful carotid artery pulsation, a wide pulse pressure with systolic hypertension, and a very low diastolic pressure, which results in a number of physical signs. The diastolic murmur is best heard with the patient sitting forward. A systolic murmur due to the increase in forward flow may also be heard. The apex beat may be displaced if the left ventricle is enlarged.

ECG

There are voltage criteria relating to left ventricular hypertrophy with ST and/or T-wave changes.

Chest X-ray

The following signs indicate cardiac decompensation and aortic root involvement and a poor prognosis: increased heart size, aortic root dilatation in aortic root disease, calcification of the aortic valve cusps, and signs of heart failure.

Echocardiogram

This is the most useful diagnostic test, and the findings strongly influence timing of valve replacement. Echocardiography shows left ventricular size, hypertrophy and function and any associated aortic stenosis, and other valve disease that may occur in rheumatic heart disease. The proximal aortic root may be examined and measured. The necessity for and timing of aortic valve replacement are influenced by enlargement of the left ventricle and the width of the regurgitant jet shown on Doppler examination (the wider the jet, the more severe the regurgitation). The aorta should be imaged in detail in order to gain information about the feasibility of valve repair.

Cardiac catheterisation

This should be performed in patients who may have coronary artery disease (those with angina or vascular disease, cardiovascular risk factors or a family history of coronary artery disease). The severity of aortic regurgitation is assessed with aortography. It may not be necessary to perform cardiac catheterisation before aortic valve replacement in young patients (< 40 years).

Magnetic resonance imaging (MRI)

This is not routinely done but is helpful in imaging the aortic valve, cardiac chamber size, and left ventricular filling and contraction.

Prognosis of aortic regurgitation

The prognosis depends upon age, and left ventricular function and size.

✧   The prognosis of asymptomatic patients with normal left ventricular function and size and severe aortic regurgitation is good. Less than 5% of these patients die or develop heart failure.
✧   The mortality rate of symptomatic patients is more than 10% per year.
✧   Symptoms of heart failure develop in 25% of patients per year who develop left ventricular enlargement and impairment.

Surgical management

The aim of valve replacement is to prevent left ventricular impairment and associated heart failure and death. Patients with aortic regurgitation should be followed up clinically and with serial measurements of left ventricular size and function from echocardiography.

Indications for surgery for aortic regurgitation include:

✧   *acute* symptomatic aortic regurgitation – urgent surgery is indicated
✧   symptomatic patients with severe aortic regurgitation
✧   asymptomatic patients with severe aortic regurgitation and reduced left ventricular function (ejection fraction < 50%, end-systolic diameter > 50 mm, or end-diastolic diameter > 70 mm)
✧   aortic root dilatation irrespective of severity of aortic regurgitation. The threshold for surgery depends on the underlying pathology. Surgery is indicated in all patients when the aortic root diameter is > 55 mm, and for Marfan's syndrome if the root diameter is > 45 mm. The prognosis of patients with a dilated aortic root is very poor. Mortality is 10% per year if the aortic root is > 6 cm in diameter.

Aortic valve repair is possible in certain cases. The prognosis of symptomatic patients with severe aortic regurgitation and an enlarged left ventricle (end-systolic diameter > 50 mm) is poor.

Left ventricular impairment and dilatation may partly regress after timely aortic valve replacement.

The prognosis is better in young, asymptomatic patients with normal left ventricular dimensions, even if they have severe aortic regurgitation. The risk of heart failure or death is 4% per year. They should be followed up every six months clinically and with echocardiography.

Operative mortality in asymptomatic patients who have only aortic valve replacement is 2%, but in symptomatic patients who have both aortic valve replacement and aortic root surgery it is 7%, and if coronary artery surgery is performed it is higher still.

Replacement of the ascending aorta using a graft for Marfan's syndrome has a mortality of 2%. Aortic root replacement is recommended if the aortic root is > 55 mm in diameter, or less if it is increasing in diameter rapidly. Family members of patients with Marfan's syndrome should be screened.

Medical treatment of aortic valve regurgitation

Diuretics and vasodilators (ACE inhibitors and nifedipine) are used for symptom control in patients who are awaiting valve replacement. They may be used in asymptomatic patients with severe chronic aortic regurgitation without left ventricular impairment or dilatation or other indications for surgery.

Acute aortic regurgitation

This should be suspected in patients with hypertension, infective endocarditis, or Marfan's syndrome and symptoms of acute aortic dissection (acute pain between the shoulder blades, and breathlessness). This condition is rare, but demands immediate referral to a surgical centre for emergency aortic valve replacement.

β-blockers slow the progression of aortic dilatation in patients with Marfan's syndrome, and are also given post-operatively. Family members of patients with Marfan's syndrome should be screened.

Follow-up of patients with aortic regurgitation

Patients with *severe* aortic regurgitation and normal left ventricular function should have six-monthly follow-up. These patients should be followed up and referred for surgery if their left ventricle enlarges (measured on echocardiography).

Patients with *mild to moderate* aortic regurgitation and normal left ventricular function should be reviewed annually.

Patients with a dilated aortic root and those with Marfan's syndrome should be followed up annually, and more often if the aortic root enlarges. They should be referred for surgery if the aortic root enlarges rapidly.

Tricuspid valve disease

Pathology

Isolated tricuspid valve disease is very rare in primary care. Tricuspid valve regurgitation is most commonly seen as part of severe congestive heart failure or any other condition that produces pulmonary hypertension. This results in right heart dilatation and stretching of the tricuspid valve ring. Rheumatic heart disease and cardiomyopathy are the most common causes. Tricuspid regurgitation may be seen in mainlining drug addicts.

Tricuspid stenosis is very rare, and is due to rheumatic heart disease.

Symptoms

These include ankle swelling, breathlessness, abdominal distension and discomfort due to ascites, and liver enlargement.

Examination

Systolic 'V'-waves due to reflux of blood to the jugular veins during right ventricular contraction, signs of right heart failure (raised venous pressure, enlarged tender liver and peripheral oedema) and pulmonary hypertension (loud pulmonary component to the second heart sound) may be present.

Investigation

Echocardiography will provide information on both the right and left heart and valve structure and function. Trivial tricuspid regurgitation on echocardiography is very common, and is normal. Important tricuspid regurgitation is due to annular dilatation and increased right ventricular pressure due to pulmonary hypertension, or volume overload. The common causes of pulmonary hypertension are left-sided heart failure, chronic obstructive lung disease and idiopathic pulmonary arterial hypertension. Atrial septal defects cause right ventricular volume overload and dilatation.

Echocardiography will provide information about the left heart, may show vegetations due to endocarditis, features of carcinoid, measure semi-quantitatively the severity of tricuspid regurgitation, right ventricular size and function, and will provide measurement of the peak right ventricular systolic pressure as an estimate of pulmonary artery pressure by measuring peak tricuspid regurgitant velocity.

Cardiac catheterisation is required only to assess coronary anatomy prior to revascularisation or valve replacement, and to measure the pulmonary artery pressure before cardiac transplantation.

Treatment

Peripheral oedema is treated with diuretics. Medical treatment to reduce the volume and pressure overload may be sufficient in mild and moderately severe cases.

Tricuspid annuloplasty using a prosthetic ring is the preferred technique and conserves the valve.

Tricuspid valve replacement, with or without annuloplasty, is not as successful as left heart valve replacement, and patients need careful evaluation. The operative risk may be as high as 40% in patients with severe tricuspid regurgitation and right heart failure. Bioprostheses are preferred to mechanical prostheses. Reducing pulmonary artery hypertension and the pressure overload on the right ventricle is difficult, and necessitates treatment of the underlying cause.

Indications for surgery include severe tricuspid regurgitation in a patient who is undergoing left heart valvular surgery, and severe symptomatic tricuspid regurgitation with preserved right ventricular function.

Antithrombotic treatment

Valve thrombosis is most likely to occur in the first three months after the operation, and more frequent monitoring may be necessary during this early period. The INR should be above the recommended lower limit.

> Most patients go to their GP surgery for monitoring and control of their INR.
> Those who are able to do so can measure their own INR and, with support from primary care clinicians, can be taught to prescribe the appropriate dose.

Target International Normalised Ratio (INR) for mechanical prostheses

The surgical unit advises the target INR, which is written in the patient's yellow anticoagulation record book. This book shows the clinician responsible for anticoagulation, and records the daily dose of warfarin and the INR results.

Indications for anticoagulation

Anticoagulation with warfarin is recommended for:
 ❖ all patients with a mechanical valve
 ❖ all patients with established atrial fibrillation
 ❖ the first three months after implantation of a bioprosthetic valve. Some units use aspirin instead.

The recommended INR for most patients with a prosthetic valve is 3.0–3.5. It may be higher (4.0) if patients have a Starr–Edwards valve and have had previous thromboembolism, or if they have an intracardiac clot or poor left ventricular function.

The risk of bleeding increases when the INR is > 4.5, and is significant if the INR is > 6.0. Unless the patient is bleeding, an INR of < 6.0 should not be reversed, because of the risk of valve thrombosis, which is particularly likely with mitral valve prostheses.

Management of bleeding in a patient with a prosthetic valve on warfarin

Patients who have a significant bleed (gastrointestinal bleed or uncontrolled nosebleed) should be admitted to hospital urgently.

Management plan

1. Stop the warfarin.
2. Resuscitate and group and cross-match blood.
3. Consult the relevant specialists (gastroenterologist or ENT surgeon).
4. Ideally, the INR should be allowed to fall without inducing rapid decreases in this parameter using vitamin K.

Major bleeding

Give vitamin K (phytomenadione) 5–10 mg IV, and give prothrombin complex concentrate (factors II, VII, IX and X) *or* fresh frozen plasma.

INR > 8.0

If there is no bleeding or only minor bleeding, stop the warfarin. Restart warfarin when the INR is < 5.0. Small doses of vitamin K may be necessary if the patient has other risk factors.

INR 6.0–8.0

Stop the warfarin, and restart it when the INR is < 5.0.

Bleeding at the target INR

This may be due to a haematological or other pathological problem, and requires urgent referral for investigation.

Addition of antiplatelet drugs (aspirin, clopidogrel) to warfarin

This increases the risk of bleeding.

The addition of an antiplatelet drug to warfarin is indicated in the following circumstances:

✧ vascular disease (coronary artery disease, carotid disease, peripheral vascular disease)
✧ after definite embolic events despite a satisfactory INR
✧ after coronary artery stenting when aspirin and clopidogrel are necessary. They are continued for one year after insertion of a drug-eluting stent. In order to avoid the risk from a combination of warfarin and intense antiplatelet drugs, drug-eluting stents should be avoided in patients with a prosthetic valve, or those who are likely to have a prosthetic valve fitted within one year of stent implantation.

> Patients with a bioprosthesis do not benefit from long-term antiplatelet drugs unless they have another indication for antithrombotic treatment (e.g. cardiovascular disease).

Stopping anticoagulation for dental work and minor surgery
If bleeding can be controlled easily and the risk of significant bleeding is small, anticoagulation should not be stopped. The INR should be lowered to 2.0.

Stopping anticoagulation before major surgery
Warfarin will have to be stopped if the INR before surgery has to be < 1.5. Examples of this would include major gastrointestinal surgery, and major orthopaedic or neurological surgery. These patients should be admitted to hospital and transferred to unfractionated heparin. Low-molecular-weight heparin can also be used unless there is renal failure, and given twice a day.

When the INR is < 1.5, the heparin should be stopped six hours prior to surgery and restarted six hours after surgery, assuming that there is no bleeding.

Warfarin should be restarted as soon as possible to reach the target INR.

Obstructive valve thrombosis
Obstruction of a prosthetic valve prevents blood circulation and has a high mortality. It is a rare complication when there has been good anticoagulation monitoring and achievement of target INR levels. It is more likely if anticoagulation has been inadequate, in patients with infection or dehydration.

Less severe valve thrombosis is more common and presents as sudden breathlessness or features of emboli.

It carries a high mortality. Thrombolysis has a high risk because of systemic bleeding, systemic embolism and recurrent thrombosis. Urgent cardiac surgery is also a high-risk strategy.

Patients should be referred to a cardiothoracic centre as an emergency.

Urgent valve replacement is the treatment of choice. The valve should be replaced with a valve that is theoretically less thrombogenic.

Thrombolysis (fibrinolysis) is recommended:
❖ for critically ill patients who are unlikely to survive repeat heart surgery (due to age, poor cardiac function and/or co-morbidity)
❖ when cardiac surgery is not immediately available
❖ for thrombosis on the tricuspid or pulmonary valves, where the success rate is higher than for left-sided heart valves.

Non-obstructive valve thrombosis
This is diagnosed after an embolic event by echocardiography. It is most likely to occur in elderly people who are in atrial fibrillation and who have mitral valve prostheses. They may have left atrial thrombus, and may have had an infection or a period of dehydration.

A small thrombus (< 10 cm in diameter) will usually fragment with adequate oral anticoagulation. Fibrinolysis may occasionally be necessary, and surgery is only necessary if there is a persistent significant thrombus, or recurrent thromboembolism.

Heart failure after valve replacement
This is not uncommon. Causes include:
❖ non-compliance with heart failure medication
❖ valve problems (e.g. deterioration, paravalvar leak, endocarditis)
❖ myocardial infarction, arrhythmia.

Patients should be referred to a cardiologist and investigated. Treatment can be started in primary care. If endocarditis is suspected, blood cultures should be taken before starting antibiotics.

Non-cardiac surgery in patients with valvular heart disease

Patients with significant valve disease may develop problems that necessitate non-cardiac surgery.

Aortic stenosis

This is not uncommon in primary care among the elderly. The risk of surgery (orthopaedic surgery, gastrointestinal surgery) is high if there is severe aortic stenosis (aortic valve area < 1.0 cm^2). Patients should have a careful risk assessment. Those at low risk can have non-cardiac surgery.

Asymptomatic patients with severe aortic stenosis can have a low- to intermediate-risk operation without the need for aortic valve replacement.

Patients at *high risk* (> 5%) include:

✧ the elderly
✧ those with severe aortic stenosis
✧ those undergoing high-risk surgery (aortic aneurysm repair, other major vascular surgery, major gastrointestinal surgery).

Procedures with *intermediate risk* (1–5%) include:

✧ carotid endarterectomy
✧ head and neck surgery
✧ orthopaedic surgery
✧ endoscopy
✧ breast surgery
✧ cataract surgery.

> Non-cardiac surgery should not be performed in patients with important cardiac valvular disease unless it is strictly necessary.

Aortic valve replacement should be performed before non-cardiac surgery in patients who have symptoms of aortic stenosis and who are an acceptable risk for aortic valve replacement. A bioprosthesis is preferred in patients who are to have non-cardiac surgery after aortic valve replacement.

Infective endocarditis

Role of the GP

Infective endocarditis is a dangerous condition with a high mortality and morbidity. Mortality varies according to the infective organism, ranging from 50% for fungal infections to 5% for *Streptococcus viridans*. Mortality is higher with prosthetic valve endocarditis or when infection is complicated by heart failure, emboli or an abscess, which are signs of aggressive, advanced, uncontrolled infection.

Infective endocarditis is treated by cardiologists in close collaboration with a microbiologist and cardiac surgeons. Primary care clinicians should discuss with a microbiologist concerns about patients who they think may be at risk, or may have endocarditis.

Infective endocarditis: practice points for primary care clinicians

✧ Patients with high-risk cardiac conditions should have prophylactic antibiotics.
✧ The diagnosis of infective endocarditis has to be suspected by GPs and patients referred urgently to hospital for investigation and treatment. Suspicious symptoms include fever, sweats, chills, weight loss or anaemia.
✧ The GP plays a crucial part in diagnosis and treatment by *arranging blood tests before starting antibiotics* for undiagnosed fever and non-specific illness in patients at risk (i.e. those with known heart valve disease or a prosthetic heart valve, intravenous drug abusers, or those with congenital heart disease and previous attacks of endocarditis).
✧ Patients with suspected endocarditis should be referred urgently to hospital.

Causes of infective endocarditis

Infective endocarditis may affect both normal and abnormal native valves. It presents a particularly difficult and dangerous management problem when it affects prosthetic valves. Endocarditis is more commonly seen in the elderly with degenerative valve disease, in intravenous drug abusers, and preceding valve replacement and vascular procedures than after dental treatment in patients with comparatively low-risk cardiac conditions.

Community-acquired infection is caused by oral viridans streptococci (now called enterococci) and *Staphylococcus aureus*, although virtually any organism may be responsible. Hospital-acquired infection may be caused by staphylococci and methicillin-resistant *Staphylococcus aureus* (MRSA). Intravenous access site infection is a common source. Intravenous drug abuse may result in tricuspid valve endocarditis, often due to *Staphylococcus aureus*. Treatment is more difficult in patients with multi-drug-resistant organisms.

Clinical features

These are variable and depend on the type of infection, the valve(s) affected and the clinical state of the patient. Fever, weight loss and malaise are common, although fever may be absent in the elderly. Congestive heart failure due to valve regurgitation is the most frequent and important cardiac complication, and it is important to recognise it. Joint pain and back pain, neurological problems and headache are common, but peripheral signs due to microemboli are neither common nor diagnostic.

Prevention and management of endocarditis in primary care

Successful treatment of endocarditis depends on:
✧ the identification of patients who are at risk of developing endocarditis
✧ good oral health
✧ awareness of the procedures associated with bacteraemia
✧ antibiotic prophylaxis in appropriate cases
✧ prompt referral of patients with suspected infection.

Diagnosis

Infective endocarditis is often difficult to diagnose, especially in elderly patients, because the symptoms and signs in the early stages may be dismissed as part of an insignificant illness. The most common sign, namely fever, may be absent in the elderly and in immunocompromised patients. It may be particularly difficult to distinguish between infective endocarditis and an alternative cause of fever and infection in a patient with a heart murmur.

Blood cultures may be negative if the patient has recently been treated with antibiotics.

The Duke diagnostic criteria (*see* Box 10.1) are used to confirm the diagnosis. Antibiotics may have been prescribed for a throat or chest infection, and this may make subsequent microbiological diagnosis difficult. Any antibiotics that have been prescribed within the previous few weeks should be mentioned with the referral. Blood culture negative endocarditis occurs in 5% of cases and may be caused by unusual or 'demanding' organisms. Serological tests and polymerase chain reactions are also used to investigate certain infections.

The diagnosis is made by a combination of clinical features and test results (*see* Box 10.1 below). There is no single definitive criterion.

Pathological criteria	Positive histology or microbiology of pathological material obtained at autopsy or cardiac surgery.
Major criteria	• Persistent bacteraemia with two positive blood cultures (or both bottles of a single blood culture) showing typical organisms consistent with infective endocarditis (e.g. *Streptococcus viridans*), *or*
	• persistent bacteraemia from two blood cultures taken more than 12 hours apart or three positive blood cultures where the pathogen is less specific (e.g. *Staphylococcus aureus* or *Staphylococcus epidermidis*), *or*
	• positive serology for *Coxiella burnetii*, *Bartonella* species or *Chlamydia psittaci*, *or*
	• positive molecular assays for specific gene targets
	• echocardiographic visualisation of a vegetation or abscess or dehiscence of a prosthetic heart valve.
Minor criteria	• Predisposing heart condition or intravenous drug abuse.
	• Fever (< 38°C).
	• Emboli (septic pulmonary infarcts, splenomegaly, finger clubbing, arterial emboli, petechiae, purpurae, intracranial haemorrhage).
	• Immunological phenomena (glomerulonephritis with microscopic haematuria, raised C-reactive protein and ESR).

BOX 10.1: Modified Duke criteria.

Definite endocarditis is diagnosed by:
✧ pathological criteria positive, *or*
✧ two major criteria, *or*
✧ one major and two minor criteria, *or*
✧ four minor criteria.

Features that exclude endocarditis
The absence of all of the following features excludes endocarditis:
✧ previous heart valve replacement
✧ intravenous drug abuse
✧ signs of emboli

⬧ central venous access
⬧ positive blood cultures.

Echocardiography in diagnosis and management

Transthoracic echocardiography may diagnose vegetations in only 50% of cases, and therefore the fact that a vegetation is not observed should not affect the presumptive diagnosis, which should be made using the Duke criteria.

> A negative echocardiogram does not exclude infective endocarditis.

The specificity of transthoracic echocardiography is high (98%), so the absence of a vegetation in a patient in whom the diagnosis is unlikely is reassuring. Transthoracic echocardiography may be diagnostically limited in 20% of patients, and prosthetic valves are difficult to image.

Transoesophageal echocardiography should be performed:
⬧ when the transthoracic study is not of diagnostic quality
⬧ in patients who have a prosthetic heart valve
⬧ when the diagnosis is at least moderately likely but the transthoracic study is normal
⬧ in patients who may have complications (e.g. valvular regurgitation, an abscess).

Who should be referred to hospital?

All patients with suspected endocarditis should be referred to hospital.

Treatment

Treatment should be started immediately after sending off three sets of blood cultures. In patients who have been unwell for more than a few weeks it is reasonable to wait a day or two to confirm the microbiological diagnosis and select appropriate antibiotics before embarking on a long course of intravenous treatment. This is a combination of intravenous antibiotics for at least two and usually six weeks in hospital, but some patients with antibiotic-sensitive infection due to oral streptococci, who respond within a few days, may be discharged from hospital back to primary care to complete treatment on oral antibiotics. Patients who are suitable for completion of treatment at home should be haemodynamically stable, have no evidence of cardiac complication (e.g. important valve abnormality), and capable and compliant with treatment. Patients with indwelling central intravenous lines may be managed in primary care with suitable clinical support.

Surgery

Cardiac surgery with valve replacement is sometimes necessary in resistant cases where there is a persistent fever, signs of heart failure or severe valvular regurgitation, abscess formation or septic emboli. Surgery carries a high risk in these ill patients, with mortality of around 15% because of the poor clinical condition of the patients and the ongoing infection.

Antibiotic prophylaxis

The aim is to prevent endocarditis in patients with cardiac lesions which predispose them to endocarditis during procedures that result in bacteraemia. Tooth brushing or flossing and chewing may be more potent causes of a bacteraemia.

The current recommendations for antibiotic prophylaxis are to be reviewed by the National Institute for Clinical Excellence following the publication of new guidelines published by the British Society for Antimicrobial Chemotherapy. They have resulted in confusion among patients and dentists, and are not endorsed by the European and British Cardiac Societies.

These new guidelines advise that in view of the lack of evidence that prophylactic antibiotic therapy is effective in preventing endocarditis, and because it is known that bacteraemia in everyday life associated with dental sepsis is of greater magnitude than that resulting from dental procedures, prophylactic antibiotics should be restricted to patients who are at high risk. The guidelines identify these high-risk patients as those:

✧ who have previously had an episode of endocarditis
✧ with prosthetic heart valves
✧ with a surgically constructed systemic or pulmonary artery shunt or conduit.

These groups do not include patients who have previously been advised to have antibiotic prophylaxis.

Despite a similar lack of evidence for the value of prophylaxis for non-dental procedures, these guidelines advise antibiotics before some but not all gastrointestinal, urogenital, gynaecological and upper respiratory procedures in all patients at risk of endocarditis.

Although infective endocarditis is seldom associated with dental procedures, currently any dental work that is known to induce gum bleeding and professional cleaning is included as a potentially septic procedure requiring antibiotic prophylaxis (*see* Boxes 10.2 and 10.3). In addition, there are patients with low-risk cardiac lesions (e.g. pulmonary valve stenosis, atrial septal defect) in whom the risks associated with antibiotics (i.e. allergic reactions, development of antibiotic resistance) may be greater than the risk of endocarditis. The balance of risk to benefit is particularly relevant for urological procedures. At present it is recommended that the current guidelines published in the *British National Formulary* are followed.

- Dental procedures known to induce gum bleeding.
- Surgical operations involving the gut or respiratory mucosa.
- Rigid bronchoscopy.
- Oesophageal procedures.
- Cystoscopy.
- Gall-bladder surgery.
- Urological procedures.
- Gynaecological procedures.

BOX 10.2: Procedures for which antibiotic prophylaxis is currently recommended.

- Atraumatic dental procedures.
- Flexible bronchoscopy.
- Cardiac catheterisation.
- Gastrointestinal endoscopy.
- In the absence of infection:
  — insertion or removal of intrauterine contraceptive device
  — urethral catheterisation
  — dilatation and curettage, sterilisation.

BOX 10.3: Procedures for which antibiotic prophylaxis is not recommended.

Advice for patients

- Not all murmurs are important. Many of them are harmless.
- A heart valve problem is not the same as having a heart attack.
- Some people who have a heart valve problem have normal heart arteries.
- Some people are born with a slight but harmless difference in the shape of their valve, which produces a noise when we listen to their heart. This noise is called a murmur.
- Not all people who have had rheumatic fever know that they have had it.
- Not all people who have had rheumatic fever have heart valve problems.
- Not all people with rheumatic heart disease affecting their heart valves remember having had rheumatic fever.
- Not all heart valve problems are due to rheumatic fever.
- A replacement heart valve is made of either metal (mechanical valve) or may come from a pig (biological or tissue valve).
- You will need to take warfarin long term to prevent clots forming on the valve. You will need regular blood tests to make sure that you are on the right dose. You should not take aspirin or certain arthritis tablets if you take warfarin, because you may bleed from the tummy. Other tablets may interfere with the warfarin. If you cut yourself, the bleeding may take a long time to stop. If it does not stop within a few minutes, go straight to your nearest accident and emergency department.
- Anticoagulation with blood thinners is not necessary if you have a tissue valve.
- Mechanical valves last 'for ever.' Tissue valves usually last for around 10 to 15 years, but this varies a lot.
- Sometimes it is possible to repair rather than replace a leaky mitral valve. This may only be known when the surgeon does the operation and examines the valve.
- As with any surgery and anaesthetic, particularly in patients over 80 years of age or those who have other heart conditions (e.g. arterial diseases) or other medical problems (e.g. kidney disease), valve replacement is risky.
- As with any surgery, the surgeon together with the cardiologist and anaesthetist will discuss your case and decide whether an operation is really necessary. They will usually tell you the risks of surgery in your case, but these are only estimated risks. Everyone is different.
- Women of childbearing age should see a cardiologist for assessment.
- Valve disease may be detected for the first time during pregnancy.
- All patients with valve disease should be seen regularly by a cardiologist, and should have a heart ultrasound examination and clinical assessment.
- People who have certain types of narrowing of the mitral valve may be suitable for stretching of the valve using a balloon.
- Some people with heart murmurs should take antibiotics before seeing their dentist or undergoing other procedures. The antibiotics are given to reduce the chance of infection in the blood lodging on the valve. These guidelines are changing. Come in to see us so that we can keep you up to date about them.
- You may never need to have anything done to your valve. It is quite possible that even though you have a heart valve condition, you will live as long as if you didn't have one, and will be able to do everything you want.
- Some patients, even those over 80 years of age, may need to have the valve repaired or replaced and, together with the heart doctor, we will keep an eye on you to see how you get on.
- If you become breathless or feel dizzy or get chest pain, come to see us as soon as possible.
- Having a heart murmur does not necessarily prevent you from doing sport, travelling, or eating and drinking what you want.

Answers to questions about clinical cases

1. The possible causes are complete heart block, aortic valve stenosis and other medical causes, including anaemia, cerebrovascular disease with possible lung pathology or hypertensive heart disease. On examination, look for signs of aortic valve disease, hypertension, anaemia, chronic lung disease and heart failure, and measure the heart rate. Check the patient's ECG for signs of bradycardia, heart block and left ventricular hypertrophy. Request an echocardiogram and, if this is normal, a chest X-ray and some blood tests. Prompt referral to a cardiologist is necessary if the patient has significant aortic valve disease, and if he has heart block he should be sent to hospital immediately.

2. The likely diagnosis is heart failure. Look for signs of heart failure and mitral valve regurgitation, and check the patient's blood pressure. Ask him what drugs he was prescribed and what he is taking. Causes can include poor drug compliance, inadequate treatment, further infarction and heart failure, mitral regurgitation or a left ventricular aneurysm. Arrange a chest X-ray to look for pulmonary oedema, and echocardiography to assess left ventricular function and size and mitral regurgitation. Check the patient's renal function and blood count. Explain to him the reasons for his breathlessness, the importance of drug treatment (which will need modification), and the fact that he will need to be referred to a cardiologist for further assessment and investigation. This should include coronary angiography with a view to revascularisation.

3. The possible causes are infective endocarditis, malignancy, infection and hypothyroidism. All of these possibilities need investigation with blood tests, blood cultures (before antibiotics are started), X-rays, ECG and echocardiography. The patient will need to be referred to the appropriate specialist after preliminary clinical assessment. Infective endocarditis is now often community-acquired, and there may be no history of dental work or other septic procedures.

4. Aortic dissection is the most important cause to exclude, because of its common association with certain forms of Marfan's syndrome. If the symptoms and signs suggest this, the patient should be referred immediately to hospital. The diagnosis may be made by transoesophageal echocardiography, magnetic resonance imaging and CT scanning. If the aorta is normal, other causes of backache should be investigated. The sweating may be due to pain rather than a fever.

5. Palpitation suggests a cardiac rather than a respiratory infective cause. Ask the patient about congenital heart disease, infections (rheumatic heart disease) and her functional capacity. Examine her heart rate and rhythm and her blood pressure, and listen to her heart. Congenital heart disease is possible, but she would probably know about this. Atrial fibrillation is a common consequence of mitral valve disease, and results in sudden pulmonary oedema and breathlessness. An ECG and echocardiogram should provide the diagnosis. The patient should be treated with diuretics for pulmonary oedema. If she is in atrial fibrillation, she should have drugs to control the ventricular response and warfarin. It may be possible to convert her medically to sinus rhythm. She should be referred to a cardiologist for assessment and further management. If she has mitral stenosis, it is likely in view of her age that she may be suitable for percutaneous mitral valvuloplasty.

6. This may be either benign or a sign of undiagnosed structural heart disease. Benign systolic murmurs in the absence of structural heart disease are common, and are due to a high cardiac output resulting from stress, anxiety, exercise or thyrotoxicosis. Feel the carotid upstroke. A normal upstroke does not exclude valvular heart disease. A systolic murmur and a jerky upstroke suggest hypertrophic cardiomyopathy. An ejection systolic murmur and a slow rising upstroke suggest aortic stenosis, and

this would most probably be due to congenital aortic stenosis in a young patient. A pansystolic murmur suggests mitral valve regurgitation, most probably mitral valve prolapse. Echocardiography is important, and will provide the diagnosis or exclude structural heart disease. If the patient is well, without a fever and clinical suspicion of endocarditis, no other tests are necessary. It would be worthwhile re-examining the patient later, when she is relaxed.

FURTHER READING

Baddour LM, Wilson WR, Bayer AS *et al.* Infective endocarditis: diagnosis, antimicrobial therapy, and management of complications: a statement for healthcare professionals from the Committee on Rheumatic Fever, Endocarditis and Kawasaki Disease, the Council on Cardiovascular Disease in the Young, and the Councils on Clinical Cardiology, Stroke, and Cardiovascular Surgery and Anesthesia, American Heart Association, endorsed by the Infectious Diseases Society of America. *Circulation.* 2005; **111:** e394–434.

Beynon RP, Bahl VK, Prendergast D. Infective endocarditis. *BMJ.* 2006; **333:** 334–9.

Bonow RO, Carabello BA, Chatterjee K *et al.* ACC/AHA 2006 guidelines for the management of patients with valvular heart disease. A report of the American College of Cardiology/ American Heart Association Task Force on Practice Guidelines (Writing Committee to revise the 1998 guidelines for the management of patients with valvular heart disease) developed in collaboration with the Society of Cardiovascular Anesthesiologists. *J Am Coll Cardiol.* 2006; **48:** e1–148.

Carapetis JR. Rheumatic heart disease in developing countries. *NEJM.* 2007; **357:** 439–41.

Coats L, Bonhoeffer P. New percutaneous treatments for valve disease. *Heart.* 2007; **93:** 639–44.

Gould FK, Elliot TSJ, Foweraker M *et al.* Guidelines for the prevention of endocarditis: report of the Working Group of the British Society for Antimicrobial Chemotherapy. *J Antimicrob Chemother.* 2006; **57:** 1035–42.

Horstkotte LM, Follath F, Gutschik E *et al.* Task Force Members on Infective Endocarditis of the European Society of Cardiology, ESC Committee for Practice Guidelines (CPG), Document Reviewers. Guidelines on Prevention, Diagnosis and Treatment of Infective Endocarditis: executive summary. The Task Force on Infective Endocarditis of the European Society of Cardiology. *Eur Heart J.* 2004; **25:** 267–76.

Iung B, Baron G, Butchart EG *et al.* A prospective survey of patients with valvular heart disease in Europe: the Euro Heart Survey on Valvular Heart Disease. *Eur Heart J.* 2003; **24:** 1231–43.

Vahanian A, Baumgartner H, Bax J *et al.* Guidelines on the management of valvular heart disease. The Task Force on the Management of Valvular Heart Disease of the European Society of Cardiology. *Eur Heart J.* 2007; **28:** 230–68.

Arrhythmias

ELEVEN

Clinical cases

1. A 32-year-old woman complains of palpitations. She describes missed beats and extra beats when she is resting in bed and watching television. What is the probable cause and how do you manage her?
2. A 78-year-old hypertensive woman complains of short episodes of palpitations and dizzy turns but no loss of consciousness. What is the most likely diagnosis and what do you do?
3. A 38-year-old man complains of occasional palpitations without any other symptoms, lasting for a few minutes. What do you do?
4. A 65-year-old man complains of episodes of sudden loss of consciousness. Three months ago he was treated for heart failure complicating a myocardial infarction. What is the probable cause and what do you do?
5. An 86-year-old woman becomes confused, breathless and giddy. What are the likely causes and what do you do?
6. A 17-year-old girl with recurrent dizzy turns is brought to see you by her parents. She has had palpitations. Examination is normal. What do you do?

Role of primary care clinicians in the management of arrhythmias

GPs play an important part in the management of cardiac arrhythmias with regard to both diagnosis and monitoring. They are responsible for liaising with cardiologists and deciding when referral is necessary. Management of some arrhythmias is difficult and confusing, even for cardiologists.

All arrhythmias require electrocardiographic diagnosis and a thorough clinical evaluation.

The roles of primary care physicians in managing patients with arrhythmias are to:

- identify patients whose symptoms are due to arrhythmias and refer them when necessary
- identify which patients can be managed safely in primary care
- manage commonly occurring arrhythmias
- manage common precipitants of arrhythmias
- monitor and supervise anticoagulation for patients in atrial fibrillation
- appreciate the value and limitations of 12-lead and 24-hour ambulatory electrocardiography and other cardiac investigations in the investigation of arrhythmias
- recognise when patients who have pacemakers or other devices require urgent referral to a cardiac centre.

GPs should also be aware of the rapidly advancing non-pharmacological methods for treating arrhythmias. It is important to remember that these devices and procedures have to be carefully selected for individual patients.

- Cardiac resynchronisation therapy has had a major impact on the management of patients with heart failure and left bundle branch block.
- Radio-frequency ablation offers high rates of success in the treatment of atrial flutter, supraventricular tachycardia, Wolff–Parkinson–White syndrome, and certain forms of ventricular tachycardia.
- Pacing prevents syncope due to complete heart block and symptomatic bradycardia.

❖ Implantable cardiac defibrillators are indicated for patients with severe left ventricular dysfunction resulting from myocardial infarction, whether they have ventricular tachycardia or not, and in certain patients with a dilated or hypertrophic cardiomyopathy.

Clinical experience and the results of trials and observational studies are helping to define the indications for new interventional techniques and devices. The field of electrophysiology has become a major and growing cardiac specialty. GPs should know which centre and specialist to contact for complex problems.

General principles of arrhythmia management in primary care

Dizziness and syncope are important symptoms in patients with palpitations, and are more likely to occur in individuals with ventricular arrhythmias, bradycardia due to complete heart block and tachycardias with impaired cardiac function.

Both the decision to treat and the treatment depend on the symptoms, the cause of the arrhythmia, its location in the heart, precipitating factors (e.g. stress, ischaemia, anaemia, alcohol, infection, thyroid abnormalities, drugs) and its prognostic importance. Most patients will require echocardiography to assess cardiac structure and function, and testing for reversible ischaemia.

For example, ventricular ectopic beats in a young fit person with a normal heart are common and, although troublesome, are almost always benign. They do not require treatment unless the patient is very symptomatic. β-blockers can make them worse by slowing the heart rate by suppressing the sinus node.

Atrial fibrillation becomes increasingly common with age, and may not give rise to symptoms. However, it may lead to heart failure. The outcome of treatment with rate control is similar to that for rhythm control. Other tachyarrhythmias are much less common.

Symptomatic bradycardias due to heart block require pacing. Heart block may not cause syncope or near syncope, and in a sedentary elderly patient it may present with heart failure.

Trends in the management of tachyarrhythmias

Most patients are treated with anti-arrhythmic drugs. These are not completely effective because they can induce arrhythmias due to their pro-arrhythmic effects.

Radio-frequency ablation is mainly used to treat atrial flutter, and symptomatic supraventricular tachycardias due to Wolff–Parkinson–White syndrome and other accessory pathways.

Implantable cardioverter defibrillators (ICDs) are used to treat cardiac arrest due to ventricular tachycardia or ventricular fibrillation, and are implanted prophylactically in patients with heart failure. Cardiac resynchronisation therapy (CRT) is the use of a pacemaker to pace both the right and left ventricles in patients with heart failure and left bundle branch block. The pacemaker resynchronises cardiac depolarisation and contraction in patients with left bundle branch block, thereby improving cardiac output. Some cardiac resynchronisation devices also have a defibrillation facility because patients with weak hearts often get ventricular tachycardia or fibrillation. These devices are effective in improving the quality of life and reducing hospital admission rates, and their use is increasing.

Common arrhythmias
Supraventricular tachycardias (SVT)

These are classified as either regular or irregular according to the rhythm of the ventricular response. Most of them rely on a re-entry mechanism with the tachycardia initiated by an ectopic beat. The diagnosis indicates the location of the circuit.

Atrioventricular node re-entry tachycardia (AVNRT)

The re-entry circuit is in the atrioventricular node, and this is the most common cause (90% of cases) of narrow, complex, regular supraventricular tachycardias (see below). It commonly presents in early adulthood. Sinus rhythm can often be re-established using vagal manoeuvres. Episodes increase in frequency with age, and are often less well tolerated with advancing age.

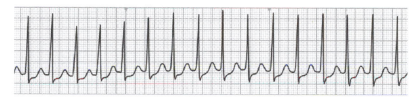

FIGURE 11.1

Atrioventricular re-entry tachycardia

The re-entry circuit is an accessory pathway connecting the atrium with the ventricle (bundle of Kent in Wolff–Parkinson–White syndrome). It may present at any age and is a regular tachycardia. These may present as narrow or broad complex tachycardias, but during sinus rhythm there is usually broadening of the QRS with shortening of the PR interval. These arrhythmias may be associated with an increased risk of sudden death.

Atrial flutter

In atrial flutter there is a single re-entrant loop within the atria, the rate of the flutter waves ranges from 240 to 320 bpm, but conduction to the ventricle is almost always limited by the AV node. As 2:1 block is most common, the presentation is of a narrow complex tachycardia with a rate of 150 bpm (see below). The circuit is often very stable, and spontaneous termination is unusual. If prolonged, the damage to the atria often leads to atrial fibrillation.

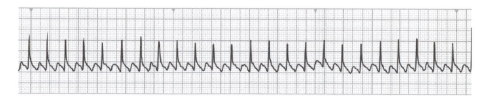

FIGURE 11.2

Atrial fibrillation

The re-entry circuits are restricted to the atrial muscle. This is the most common sustained arrhythmia, and its prevalence is rising as the proportion of elderly people increases (see below). It is associated with scarring, dilatation or stretching of the atrial muscle.

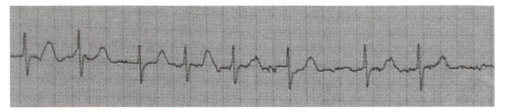

FIGURE 11.3

Ventricular ectopic beats and non-sustained supraventricular tachycardia

Ventricular ectopic beats and short runs of ventricular tachycardia are common. These are found on 0.8% of standard 12-lead ECGs, increasing in frequency with age. Six hours of Holter monitoring will show ventricular ectopic beats or non-sustained supraventricular tachycardia in 60% of middle-aged men. The risk of sudden death is not increased in the absence of heart disease. Where heart disease is present, the level of increased risk is dependent on the severity of the underlying heart disease. By contrast, ventricular arrhythmias induced by exercise are usually associated with increased risk.

Ventricular tachycardia (VT)

Although there are several different types of ventricular tachycardia, the diagnostic details are of interest only to electrophysiologists. From a general care perspective, all broad complex regular tachycardias should be assumed to be ventricular tachycardia, unless one can clearly identify P-waves before each QRS complex (sinus tachycardia with bundle branch block), as shown below.

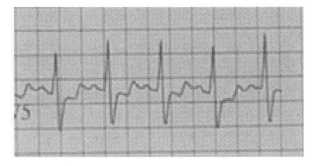

FIGURE 11.4

Because ventricular tachycardia (see below) is associated with loss of atrial transport and discordant ventricular contraction, cardiac output is much lower for any given heart rate. Presyncope or loss of consciousness is thus much more likely with ventricular tachycardia, and often occurs with rates of less than 200 bpm.

As with atrial fibrillation, ventricular tachycardia is much more likely to occur in patients with significant myocardial damage. Therefore, VT should be the diagnosis to exclude if dealing with regular palpitations associated with autonomic symptoms, or presyncope in patients with previous myocardial infarction or heart failure.

However, the diagnosis that one fears missing is ventricular arrhythmia in otherwise apparently healthy individuals, especially athletes. Fortunately, this is very rare. A family history of sudden premature death, an observation of long QT on an ECG or coved ST segments in V1–V3 should lead to formal evaluation and specialist referral.

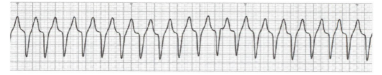

FIGURE 11.5

Arrhythmias and symptoms

Palpitations are a common cardiac symptom presenting in primary care, defined as an awareness of the heart beat. Arrhythmias may also present with chest pain, syncope or 'dizzy turns', or breathlessness.

> An ECG recorded during symptoms is required to diagnose the cause of palpitations.

Symptoms are generally unreliable for diagnosing arrhythmias. They depend on the haemodynamic consequences of the arrhythmia, which are a result of the type of arrhythmia, its anatomical origin, duration, the resulting heart rate, the underlying cardiac function, coexisting valve abnormalities and the age, medical condition and activities of the patient. However, recent-onset palpitations, with sudden onset and offset and/or associated autonomic upset or chest pain, are suggestive of pathologically significant arrhythmias as opposed to sinus tachycardia (gradual offset), ectopics (missed beats) or well-tolerated supraventricular tachycardia (long history).

> If the patient complains of palpitations, it is important to ask them what they mean by this.

Palpitations are an awareness of the heart beat, and this may be due to a forceful regular beat due to anxiety, or to an arrhythmia. Some patients may use the term 'palpitations' to mean breathlessness or chest pain.

Asking patients to tap out the rhythm of their palpitations is usually confusing and difficult even for musically trained patients, and provides unreliable information for making management decisions.

Patients with arrhythmias may be symptom-free. Atrial fibrillation with a ventricular rate of 100 bpm in an elderly patient with impaired left ventricular function, or in a patient with hypertrophic cardiomyopathy, may have serious haemodynamic effects resulting in heart failure or collapse, whereas it may be unnoticed by a fit person. Ventricular tachycardia related to a myocardial infarct scar may cause death or collapse. A heart rate of 30 bpm in a sleeping athlete is not unusual and would not be expected to result in symptoms, but if it is due to complete heart block it might result in syncope or heart failure.

Principles of drug treatment of arrhythmias

✧ Anti-arrhythmic drugs may result in proarrhythmia, particularly in patients with structural heart disease, coronary heart disease and left ventricular hypertrophy.
✧ Most anti-arrhythmic drugs are negatively inotropic and may precipitate heart failure in susceptible patients.

❖ Anti-arrhythmic drugs should be used only in patients with severe symptoms or a risk of tachycardia-induced left ventricular dysfunction.

❖ There is no evidence that prolonged suppression of atrial or ventricular ectopic beats with anti-arrhythmic drugs prevents sudden death. β-blockers may increase the frequency of ectopic beats occurring in the setting of sinus bradycardia, and precipitate symptomatic bradycardia, particularly in the elderly.

❖ Haemodynamically significant arrhythmias are difficult to treat, are associated with a high mortality, and respond better to device therapy than to drugs in general.

❖ Anti-arrhythmic drug side-effects are more likely to occur in those patients with hypokalaemia and renal and/or hepatic impairment, and in the elderly. Electrolytes and creatinine levels should be checked as part of the clinical assessment. Measurement of drug levels is only occasionally necessary.

❖ Important bradycardia may occur with the combination of a β-blocker with any anti-arrhythmic drug, particularly verapamil or digoxin, although these combinations are occasionally prescribed for patients with uncontrolled atrial fibrillation.

❖ Anti-arrhythmic drugs may occasionally cause ventricular tachycardia, ventricular fibrillation and, rarely, torsade de pointes, which is usually associated with widening of the QRS complex and prolongation of the QT interval. Anti-arrhythmic drugs should be stopped if significant ECG changes occur.

❖ Patients with symptomatic, regular, narrow complex supraventricular tachycardia or intolerable atrial fibrillation should be referred to a cardiologist.

❖ The drug data sheet and the *British National Formulary* should be consulted before anti-arrhythmic drugs are prescribed.

❖ A very large number of drugs should be avoided in those patients with long QT syndrome.

Anti-arrhythmic drugs should generally be prescribed only after a precise diagnosis of the arrhythmia and any underlying heart disease has been made. The benefits, risks and duration of treatment should be carefully considered and explained to the patient.

Non-drug treatment of arrhythmia
Radio-frequency ablation

This procedure involves inserting small electrodes intravenously into the right heart (and occasionally the left heart via the interatrial septum) under local anaesthesia and sedation. X-ray guidance or, more recently, non-fluoroscopic, computer-generated, electroanatomical maps are used to guide electrode positioning. Radio-frequency energy is used to ablate (kill) tissue, leaving it electrically inert. During this procedure, some patients experience warmth or chest pain. Depending on the problem, the procedure may last for several hours if complex pathways are being dealt with, and an overnight stay is usually recommended. The procedure has an associated risk of heart attack, stroke or death of around 0.1%, and a risk of local complications (pneumothorax if the subclavian vein is used), bleeding or femoral vein damage of around 1%.

Results of ablation for supraventricular tachycardia

Ablation (destruction) of part of the re-entry circuit facilitating tachycardia results in high cure rates (over 98%) for supraventricular tachycardia, Wolff–Parkinson–White syndrome and atrial flutter.

Symptomatic patients with supraventricular tachycardia, Wolff–Parkinson–White syndrome and atrial flutter should be referred to an electrophysiology centre for evaluation.

The success rate of radio-frequency ablation in treating atrial fibrillation is only 50%. Compared with treating SVT or atrial flutter, there is a higher procedural complication rate because a trans-septal puncture (passing the catheter across from the right to the left atrium) is required to ablate and 'isolate' the cuff of pulmonary vein. Most atrial fibrillation starts from ectopic beats originating from the junction of the pulmonary veins and the left atrium. Radio-frequency ablation for atrial fibrillation is offered to patients with intolerable atrial fibrillation despite medical treatment. Most atrial fibrillation in primary care is managed with anticoagulation and rate control.

Non-pharmacological management of ventricular tachycardia (VT) and ventricular fibrillation (VF)

These conditions are rare in primary care. Ventricular tachycardia and fibrillation may present as 'failed sudden death', brief changes in conscious level or palpitations. Most commonly they result from an arrhythmia focus in a scarred and weak left ventricle due to myocardial infarction or a cardiomyopathy. Occasionally, ventricular tachycardia may be benign when it originates from the right ventricular outflow tract.

An *implanted cardioverter defibrillator (ICD)* reduces the risk of sudden cardiac death in patients at high risk. These devices have revolutionised the management of ventricular arrhythmias and the prevention of sudden death in those at risk. Before implantation it is important to ensure that medical therapy for any associated heart disease has been optimised, and that the patient has a high probability of otherwise surviving with good functional status for at least one year.

Indications for ICD implantation
- Patients presenting with cardiac arrest, failed sudden death or haemodynamically unstable ventricular tachycardia, except those with a 'curable' condition (ablation of bypass tract for Wolff–Parkinson–White syndrome) or a transient cause (within 48 hours of myocardial infarction).
- Patients who have had a myocardial infarction at least 40 days previously, with New York Heart Association (NYHA) class II or III limitation and an ejection fraction of less than 30–40%, or with NYHA class I limitation and an ejection fraction of less than 30–35%.
- Patients with dilated cardiomyopathy, NYHA class II or III, and an ejection fraction of less than 30–35%, or NYHA class I with unexplained syncope or sustained VT and poor left ventricular function.
- Hypertrophic obstructive cardiomyopathy (HOCM) associated with failed sudden death, haemodynamically unstable ventricular tachycardia, family history of sudden death, unexplained syncope, left ventricular wall thickness > 30 mm, or abnormal blood pressure response to exercise.
- Arrhythmogenic right ventricular dysplasia (ARVD) associated with ventricular tachycardia or ventricular fibrillation, extensive disease on echocardiography, or a family history of sudden death or unexplained syncope.
- Brugada syndrome associated with ventricular fibrillation or spontaneous ST elevation in V1, V2 or V3, plus syncope or ventricular tachycardia.
- Long QT syndrome (LQTS) associated with failed sudden death, syncope or ventricular tachycardia despite β-blockade, or high-risk features (QTc > 500 ms).

The devices provide bradycardia support like a normal pacemaker, but also recognise important ventricular arrhythmias and deliver a shock until normal rhythm is restored.

They are similar to a pacemaker in size. They are implanted under local anaesthesia and tested with the patient fully anaesthetised. The batteries last for three to six years depending on the number of shocks delivered. The complications include infection, pneumothorax, inappropriate shocks (which may result in major psychological disability) and lead failure. Some patients find it difficult to tolerate repeated shocks and the unpleasant sensation that they experience in their chest.

Although the modern devices are simpler to implant, device checks, follow-up and problem solving require highly skilled and experienced technical back-up.

Ablation treatment for ventricular arrhythmias

Radio-frequency ablation of ventricular arrhythmias originating from the right ventricular outflow tract and a focal point in the left ventricle may be treated with ablation. Patients with myocardial scarring who remain symptomatic despite having an implantable cardioverter defibrillator may benefit from ablation of foci of arrhythmias in the ventricle.

Ventricular ectopic beats and non-sustained supraventricular tachycardia can also often be managed by ablation. Especially where these arise from the right ventricle (left bundle morphology), this can be particularly helpful in patients with intractable symptoms that are unresponsive to drug therapy, or in cases where the patient does not wish to take long-term therapy. This is, however, a symptomatic therapy.

Adjunctive anti-arrhythmic drug treatment

This may be necessary in order to reduce arrhythmia and symptoms in patients who have an implantable cardioverter defibrillator or who have had ablation.

Management of sinus tachycardia

This is common, particularly in younger patients and during pregnancy. It is generally benign, often linked to anxiety and less commonly related to anaemia or thyrotoxicosis. It must be distinguished from other causes of a fast heart rate. It may be related to drug therapy, particularly inhaled β-agonists used to treat airways obstruction, over-the-counter cold cures containing sympathomimetic agents, and illicit recreational drugs. Treatment involves excluding these causes together with an explanation of the condition to the patient with the aid of an ECG recorded during an attack. Drugs are not indicated.

Management of atrial and ventricular ectopic beats

Patients may describe 'missed' and 'extra' beats or a temporary difficulty in catching their breath. When benign, ectopic beats occur with a slow resting heart rate and disappear as the heart rate increases with exercise, and patients find this reassuring and therapeutic. Ectopic beats are more common in patients with left ventricular hypertrophy due to hypertension, resting bradycardia due to regular exercise or hypertrophic heart muscle disease.

History

A thorough history forms part of both the investigation and management of ventricular ectopic beats and non-sustained ventricular tachycardia. One should ensure that there is no prior history of heart disease, syncope or associated haemodynamically significant palpitations. In addition, one should ask about drug treatments and exposure to toxins (e.g. alcohol, caffeine, cocaine), and ascertain whether there is a family history of premature sudden death.

A standard ECG should be evaluated for evidence of heart disease (Q-waves, prolongation of the QRS, T-wave inversion in leads V1–V3) and ion-channel abnormalities (QTc > 440 ms [long QT syndrome] or < 300 ms [short QT syndrome], or ST elevation in leads V1–V3 [Brugada syndrome]).

Investigations
24-hour ambulatory ECG
Twenty-four-hour ambulatory electrocardiography will show the frequency and number of ectopic beats, and is useful for establishing the diagnosis. The recording shows the patient that their symptoms are real but benign, and that they have been taken seriously. Echocardiography may be used to measure left ventricular wall thickness and function in ventricular arrhythmias.

Exercise testing
Exercise testing may be used to demonstrate that ventricular arrhythmias are suppressed by exercise and therefore benign. It should generally be performed where there is at least an intermediate likelihood of ischaemic heart disease.

Drug treatment of atrial and ventricular ectopic beats
β-blockers are not advised because, by slowing the heart rate, they may increase the number of bradycardia-related ectopic beats as well as having other side-effects. Exceptions to this rule are exercise-induced or ischaemia-associated ectopic beats, which can respond symptomatically.

Flecainide or propafenone can be used if symptoms are very distressing, if there is no previous history of myocardial infarction.

Ablation may be successful if symptoms are very distressing or if non-sustained ventricular tachycardia is so continuous as to risk left ventricular impairment.

> Ectopic beats are benign and do not require treatment or investigation unless they are associated with underlying structural heart disease or induced by exercise. Treatment directed toward suppression of the ectopic beats does not change the prognosis.

Management of atrial fibrillation
This is the most common important arrhythmia seen in primary care, affecting 2% of the population in the UK. Its prevalence increases with age, and it is becoming more common. It is due to electrical re-entry circuits in the atrial muscle or the muscle of the pulmonary veins. Most patients are treated with drugs. The treatment for persistent atrial fibrillation remains controversial.

Risks of atrial fibrillation
Patients with atrial fibrillation have a sixfold increased risk of stroke and a twofold increased risk of death.

Atrial fibrillation is a major cause of:
✧ palpitations
✧ heart failure due to cardiac dilatation, tachycardia and loss of atrial contraction
✧ thromboembolism due to thrombus formation in the left atrial appendage. Embolic

strokes resulting from non-valvular atrial fibrillation are more severe than ischaemic strokes, and are associated with a higher mortality. It is important that anticoagulation is considered in all patients (see below).

Permanent atrial fibrillation

Atrial fibrillation is classified as permanent if it has been present for more than one year, if it cannot be terminated with drugs or electrical cardioversion, or when electrical cardioversion is not indicated.

Clinical evaluation of atrial fibrillation (from the Joint American College of Cardiology, American Heart Association and European Society of Cardiology guidelines)

The following should be ascertained, and determine management:
⬧ symptoms
⬧ clinical type of atrial fibrillation
⬧ date of onset (patients may be symptom-free)
⬧ frequency, duration, precipitating factors and modes of termination
⬧ response to anti-arrhythmic drugs
⬧ presence of underlying cardiac or reversible medical conditions.

Clinical features

The average age of patients with atrial fibrillation is 75 years, and the majority are older than 65 years. Around 10% of people over 75 years of age are in atrial fibrillation.

Most patients have symptoms, but these are very variable and depend on the type and duration of atrial fibrillation, the ventricular response rate, and the age and clinical status of the patient. For example, in a patient with a stiff left ventricle due to hypertrophic cardiomyopathy, whose cardiac output depends on left atrial contraction, acute atrial fibrillation may cause collapse. Elderly sedentary patients may be symptom-free and the arrhythmia may be detected by chance. It may present with palpitations, breathlessness due to congestive heart failure, syncope due to either a fast or slow heart rate or, alarmingly, with emboli. It is important to find out whether the patient is symptomatic and how much they are affected by atrial fibrillation. The decision to consider drug treatment or radio-frequency ablation is determined largely by the patient's symptoms.

Ask about alcohol consumption, caffeine intake (although this is not a common cause of atrial fibrillation), fever, pericarditis, recent heart surgery and thoracotomy, recent flu or upper respiratory tract infection, and radiation treatment for breast cancer or other chest malignancy.

On examination, look for signs of thyrotoxicosis, anaemia, excess alcohol consumption, heart failure, mitral valve disease, chest infection, breast lumps, lymphadenopathy and liver enlargement. Record the blood pressure.

In atrial fibrillation, the heart and pulse rate are completely irregular and this results in a discrepancy between the apex and radial heart rate. Low-volume cardiac contractions may not be palpable at the wrist.

Investigation of atrial fibrillation
Essential tests
⬧ ECG confirmation in all cases, and heart rate. Look for left ventricular hypertrophy, prior myocardial infarction, delta waves, bundle branch block, and QT interval in patients on anti-arrhythmic drugs.
⬧ Echocardiography to assess valve lesions, ejection fraction, left ventricular hypertrophy,

wall motion abnormalities, intracardiac clot, left atrial size, pericardial disease and pulmonary hypertension.

✧ Bloods: full blood count, electrolytes, renal and liver function and thyroid function.

Additional tests which may be helpful

✧ Twenty-four-hour ECG monitoring if the average heart rate is not controlled below 100 bpm, or if the heart rate is very slow with pauses of > 2.5 seconds. This would usually cause presyncope or syncope. β-blockers or digoxin, or other drugs that cause bradycardia should be stopped or the dose reduced. Usually a pacemaker will be required to treat the bradycardia, particularly if the atrial fibrillation is a manifestation of sinus node disease.

✧ Exercise testing will help to evaluate the heart rate response to exercise, and may unmask subclinical ischaemia. Flecainide is contraindicated if there is ischaemia.

✧ Chest X-ray to investigate chest infection or pneumonia.

Anticoagulation or antithrombotic treatment in atrial fibrillation

✧ Using warfarin, anticoagulate all patients with sustained (> 30 seconds) atrial fibrillation shown on an ambulatory ECG recording.

✧ If the annual stroke risk is less than 2%, or there is lone atrial fibrillation in male patients under 75 years of age or female patients under 65 years, treat with aspirin only.

✧ If the annual stroke risk is greater than 6%, anticoagulate unless there is a major contraindication (clinical or practical).

Situations where the annual risk of stroke is greater than 6% and anticoagulation is recommended

✧ Metal valve.
✧ Mitral stenosis.
✧ Previous cerebrovascular accident/transient ischaemic attack or embolism.
✧ Two or more moderate risk factors: age > 75 years, hypertension, diabetes, heart failure, or ejection fraction < 35%.

Grey area where either aspirin or warfarin may be appropriate

If the stroke risk is 3–5% (the patient may have only one moderate risk factor), discuss the risk–benefit ratio with the patient.

Anticoagulation will reduce the risk of stroke by 60% (from 5% down to 3%), but there will be an annual risk of a major bleed of 1%.

Anti-arrhythmic drugs (AADs) used to convert atrial fibrillation to sinus rhythm and maintain sinus rhythm

There is a group of anti-arrhythmic drugs with proven efficacy in converting atrial fibrillation to sinus rhythm and maintaining sinus rhythm. They include dofetilide, flecainide, propafenone and amiodarone.

Other anti-arrhythmic drugs, including disopyramide, procainamide and quinidine, are less effective. Digoxin and sotalol are not recommended for converting atrial fibrillation to sinus rhythm, and should not be used for this purpose.

Anti-arrhythmic drugs that are used as pharmacological converters in atrial fibrillation can be divided into those agents which also provide rate control (amiodarone) and those that may require additional rate-controlling therapy during use (flecainide, propafenone and dofetilide).

Amiodarone can be used in virtually all patients, but is generally considered second line

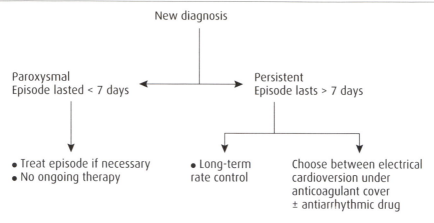

FIGURE 11.6: Rate and rhythm management of first diagnosis of atrial fibrillation.

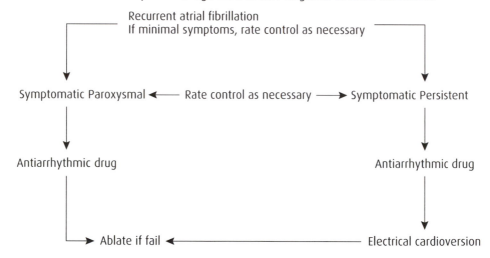

FIGURE 11.7: Mangement of recurrent atrial fibrillation.

because of its toxicity. The exception is heart failure patients, in whom only amiodarone and dofetilide have been shown to be safe.

Flecainide and propafenone may cause ventricular arrhythmias in patients with coronary heart disease, so they should not be used in these subsets of patients with atrial fibrillation.

Sotalol should be avoided in cases where there are contraindications for β-blockade and where the QT interval is prolonged (> 450 ms), or there is a risk of prolongation (e.g. left ventricular hypertrophy and hypokalaemia).

Principles guiding management

Rate control is as good as rhythm control for most patients.

Conversion to sinus rhythm will most probably occur spontaneously or with drug treatment in the first 48 hours, and does not require anticoagulant cover within this time frame.

Conversion to sustained sinus rhythm becomes increasingly difficult over time, and is unlikely after one year in atrial fibrillation.

Relapse after cardioversion is most likely to occur in the first two weeks.

Cardioversion is associated with an increased risk of thromboembolic events, especially in the first week after conversion. If atrial fibrillation persists for more than 48 hours, then three weeks of anticoagulation before and four weeks of anticoagulation after cardioversion is required. Alternatively, transoesophageal echocardiography documentation of absence of thrombus should be followed by ensured adequacy of anticoagulation for four weeks.

All patients who have had sustained atrial fibrillation remain at increased risk of thromboembolic events. There is no clear evidence that this risk diminishes over time despite remaining in sinus rhythm. Anticoagulation should be considered equally in those who have had one episode of atrial fibrillation and those who have been in this rhythm for many years.

The only clear exception is where a transient cause has now resolved (e.g. acute myocardial infarction, alcohol binge, myocarditis, pericarditis, pulmonary embolism or pneumonia).

Patients at low risk who can self-medicate with a 'pill in the pocket'

There has been a recent change in recommendations for the management of attacks of paroxysmal atrial fibrillation in low-risk patients. The aim is to allow patients to treat themselves with an anti-arrhythmic tablet so that they can avoid the need to go to hospital. Patients must first be evaluated and structural heart disease excluded. Attacks should be infrequent (less than four per year). They should not become hypotensive and should be able to tolerate their attacks. They should understand when to take the medication, which they would have taken as a trial in hospital for a previous attack. They should be told to take the tablet if their attack has not resolved spontaneously within 30 minutes. When the attack starts they should sit or lie down until the attack resolves. If the attack does not resolve within four hours, or if they feel light-headed or have any other symptom, they should go to hospital.

They should be given either flecainide (300 mg) or propafenone (600 mg) during an attack. On the first occasion when this is tried they should be observed in hospital. Currently, neither drug is licensed for patients to use in this way. This approach is not recommended for patients who are taking prophylactic anti-arrhythmic drugs, because of possible interactions. If the tablet converts them to sinus rhythm, they can be given a supply of tablets to take as a 'pill in the pocket' in order to abort further attacks. Patients should be advised to go to hospital if an attack does not respond to an appropriate dose of drug.

Prognosis of atrial fibrillation

The prognosis of atrial fibrillation depends on its cause and the patient's age, their underlying cardiovascular status and other medical conditions.

It has a good prognosis in young fit individuals with no cardiovascular disease ('lone atrial fibrillation'). Similarly, atrial fibrillation usually resolves without consequences within a few days of an alcohol binge, acute pericarditis or cardiac surgery. It is usually persistent and associated with haemodynamic impairment and an increased risk of thromboembolism in patients with a dilated cardiomyopathy due to chronic alcohol consumption, viral myocarditis or other causes, mitral valve disease or coronary heart disease.

Permanent atrial fibrillation in the elderly is associated with a poor prognosis due to the risk of stroke (which is largely preventable with warfarin) and heart failure.

Testing the INR in primary care

Responsibility for the management of anticoagulation is increasingly being devolved to primary care, and this has great advantages for patients. There are a number of instruments available for testing the INR, and they have been shown to be as reliable as laboratory measurements. Self-measurement and control of anticoagulation is safe and may become common practice in the same way that diabetic patients measure and control their blood sugar levels.

Antithrombotic treatment (aspirin or clopidogrel) should be used in patients who are at low risk of stroke, those who do not wish to take warfarin, those for whom it is logistically difficult to monitor the International Normalised Ratio (INR), and patients in whom warfarin is contraindicated. Clopidogrel is a platelet inhibitor with a risk of bleeding similar to that for aspirin (2%). It is used in patients who cannot tolerate aspirin, and has a half-life of several days.

No anticoagulation is required for patients with supraventricular tachycardia or atrial fibrillation of more than 48 hours' duration.

Anti-arrhythmic treatment options

- ✧ Flecainide, 200–300 mg orally or 150 mg slowly IV. This is successful in around 75% of patients if given within 24 hours of the start of the attack.
- ✧ Dofetilide (dose depends on renal function, age and weight).
- ✧ Propafenone, 450–600 mg orally.
- ✧ Amiodarone (first-line treatment in patients with heart failure), 100–400 mg daily.

Pacing for atrial fibrillation

Dual-chamber pacing with pacemaker software is designed to recognise and pace the heart at specified rates and to reduce the frequency of attacks of palpitation in symptomatic patients with bradycardia-dependent atrial fibrillation. 'Prevent AF' pacing is appropriate for those patients who may develop symptomatic bradycardia at a later stage. Patients require aspirin and may need anti-arrhythmic drugs.

Rate control is achieved using anti-arrhythmic drugs (digoxin, β-blockers, diltiazem, verapamil, or combinations of these).

Occasionally in patients whose ventricular rate remains fast despite drug treatment, atrioventricular node ablation may be necessary. This isolates the atria (which continue to fibrillate) electrically from the ventricles (which contract at their intrinsic rate of around 30 bpm). The atrioventricular block thus created is irreversible, and a permanent pacemaker is almost always necessary and implanted as part of the procedure.

Electrical cardioversion
Indications for cardioversion

- ✧ After failed anti-arrhythmic drug treatment in patients with paroxysmal atrial fibrillation and a fast ventricular rate complicated by heart failure, angina, hypotension or unacceptable symptoms, particularly in patients with acute myocardial infarction or diastolic dysfunction (e.g. hypertrophic cardiomyopathy) and during pregnancy.
- ✧ To prevent ventricular fibrillation in patients with Wolff–Parkinson–White syndrome in whom atrial fibrillation occurs with a rapid ventricular response and haemodynamic instability.
- ✧ For patients with persistent atrial fibrillation when early recurrence after cardioversion is unlikely.

✧ To restore sinus rhythm in patients who are having their first attack of atrial fibrillation.
✧ Repeated cardioversion with prophylactic drug therapy is indicated for patients who revert back to atrial fibrillation after successful cardioversion without drug therapy.

The procedure

Most cardiologists recommend that an anti-arrhythmic drug should be taken both before cardioversion, to improve the likelihood of success, and for at least a few weeks after the procedure, to reduce the likelihood of reversion back to atrial fibrillation. Outpatients are admitted to hospital starved. The heart rhythm is monitored with an ECG, the patient is given a short general anaesthetic and cardioversion is performed. Patients generally leave hospital after a few hours, but should not drive home or go to work until the following day.

Management after cardioversion

Patients should be reviewed after a week. If they are in sinus rhythm, their anti-arrhythmic drug(s) and anticoagulation should be continued because of the continued possibility of recurrent atrial fibrillation. They should be reviewed again one month later to assess their need for long-term anticoagulation or antithrombotic and anti-arrhythmic drugs, which may be stopped in those at low risk of recurrence. These drugs may need to be continued in patients with risk factors for recurrent atrial fibrillation.

Patients may continue to experience mild palpitation and have 24-hour ECG evidence of recurrent, paroxysmal atrial fibrillation, which does not result in haemodynamic upset. This may be viewed as an incomplete but satisfactory result. These patients can be reassured and require intermittent review to assess whether the attacks have become troublesome and require different treatment.

For patients who have reverted back to atrial fibrillation at any stage, it may be appropriate to try cardioversion again, possibly using a different anti-arrhythmic drug but continuing anticoagulation. Alternatively, if there is little likelihood of long-term successful cardioversion, the patient should be treated with rate control and anticoagulation. Occasionally, non-pharmacological treatments for atrial fibrillation are used for symptomatic patients, and these patients should be referred to a cardiologist.

Atrial flutter

This often occurs with atrial fibrillation, and is associated with similar conditions in elderly patients.

Treatment of atrial flutter

Drug treatment using amiodarone or flecainide may reduce recurrence rates but permits fast ventricular rates and heart failure. It is often better to use digoxin combined with β-blockers to slow the ventricular rate.

Catheter ablation of atrial flutter is more successful than drug treatment, can be performed quickly with a low risk of complications, and in many patients is probably the treatment of first choice.

Anticoagulation in atrial flutter

Although generally perceived as lower risk than atrial fibrillation, the risk of thromboembolic events is similar in patients with atrial flutter, and a similar approach to that described above for atrial fibrillation should be used to determine the need for long-term anticoagulation.

Treatment of acute attacks of supraventricular tachycardia (SVT)

Vagal manoeuvres (e.g. sucking ice, coughing or straining against a closed glottis), slow conduction through the atrioventricular node and may be effective. In young patients without a bruit in the carotid, massaging the upper carotid for five seconds may terminate the attack. Eyeball pressure is no longer recommended, as this can damage the retina. Patients should be taught how to do a Valsalva manoeuvre if they get attacks of SVT.

Adenosine administered intravenously is highly effective. It is administered in hospital, as ECG monitoring and access to resuscitation equipment are mandatory. Patients may develop atrial fibrillation, asystole, chest pain or bronchospasm. Adenosine is injected as a 3 mg bolus. If this does not work, a further 6 mg is injected after two minutes. If there is still no response, a further 12 mg is injected. Most patients respond to this regime. Indeed, no response to adenosine makes the diagnosis of SVT less likely. The patient feels very flushed and unwell for a few seconds and should be warned about this before treatment. Adenosine is contraindicated in allergic asthma, as mast-cell degranulation, which is merely unpleasant for most people, can provoke prolonged bronchospasm in these patients.

Verapamil, β-blockers and digoxin are long-acting drugs and are used mainly for prophylaxis for supraventricular tachycardia rather than for treating acute attacks. Verapamil and β-blockers should be used only after consultation with a cardiologist because of the risk of serious hypotension and bradycardia.

Radio-frequency ablation is an effective treatment for frequent attacks of supraventricular tachycardia. Ablating one arm of the circuit near the atrioventricular node is highly successful, and most patients with frequent attacks are now referred for ablation. Working near the atrioventricular node there is a small risk of damage to the latter, in which case permanent pacing is required.

Management of ventricular tachycardia

This is not a primary care task. All patients with ventricular tachycardia should be evaluated by a cardiologist. However, there are some points of interest, in particular why some patients are still treated with drugs, and what drugs one should avoid in patients with specific problems.

Management of underlying heart disease

In most cases of ventricular arrhythmia there is associated heart failure, impaired ventricular function or ischaemic heart disease. Optimal management of the underlying heart disease is pivotal to improving prognosis and quality of life.

Management of electrolyte abnormalities

In practice this means avoiding hypokalaemia, although magnesium may be important in some circumstances (long QT), and significant calcium abnormality is best avoided.

Amiodarone and sotalol are the preferred drugs. However, both prolong the QT interval, so β-blockade is more common adjunctive therapy in these groups. Flecainide and propafenone are now less commonly used, as they may increase mortality in the setting of ischaemic heart disease. Drug therapy alone may be used in patients with good left ventricular function and non-haemodynamically significant ventricular tachycardia, with the exceptions outlined above for hypertrophic cardiomyopathy, QT abnormality, Brugada syndrome and arrhythmogenic right ventricular dysplasia (ARVD). In most other instances these drugs are used in patients who have an implantable cardioverter defibrillator (ICD), but in whom symptomatic ventricular tachyarrhythmias continue to cause problems (the ICD will only deal with life-threatening events, and even then reducing the frequency of such events can be important for improving quality of life).

Amiodarone

This is a useful and effective anti-arrhythmic drug. It is more effective than propafenone and sotalol for maintaining sinus rhythm in patients with paroxysmal or persistent atrial fibrillation. It is usually used as a second-line drug because it has significant side-effects in 20% of patients, and complex pharmacokinetics resulting in a long half-life of around two months. It has comparatively little negative inotropic activity, so is used as a first-line drug in patients with impaired left ventricular function and significant arrhythmias.

Indications

◇ All tachyarrhythmias of any origin.
◇ Ventricular arrhythmias in patients with structural heart disease (e.g. hypertrophic cardiomyopathy).
◇ Prior to elective electrical cardioversion and afterwards to maintain sinus rhythm.

Contraindications

◇ Severe thyroid abnormalities.
◇ Severe conduction abnormalities if there is no pacemaker back-up.

Interactions

Amiodarone is strongly protein bound and raises the plasma concentration of warfarin, digoxin and phenytoin. The doses of these drugs should be reduced in order to avoid side-effects, and the INR/prothrombin time should be checked more frequently. Amiodarone prolongs the QT interval, increasing the probability of torsade de pointes, so should not be prescribed with class Ia and III anti-arrhythmic drugs, antipsychotics, tricyclic antidepressants, antihistamines, antimalarials or bradycardic agents.

Dose

Amiodarone should be administered at a dose of 200 mg three times a day for one week, 200 mg twice a day for the second week and then 200 mg per day. The dose may need to be reduced in elderly or small patients. The minimum effective dose should be used in order to avoid side-effects, and a weekly dose of 300 mg (100 mg on alternate days) may be sufficient.

Side-effects

Sensitivity to sunlight, resulting in erythema and burning, is not a major problem for patients living in the UK, but patients should be warned to cover up and to use a high-protection barrier cream in sunny weather, and should be advised not to sunbathe, especially if they are fair skinned.

Amiodarone contains iodine, and both hypothyroidism and hyperthyroidism may occur even after prolonged use. Interpretation of thyroid function tests is difficult, because they may be abnormal even if the patient is euthyroid. Thyroid function tests should be checked before starting treatment, six-monthly thereafter, and again after stopping treatment. Regular clinical assessments are recommended. Amiodarone-induced thyroid abnormalities usually resolve within three months of drug withdrawal.

Pulmonary fibrosis, although rare, may be fatal even if it is recognised early. It is diagnosed with a chest X-ray, and usually resolves within a few months after drug withdrawal. Amiodarone should be used very cautiously in patients with lung disease.

Deranged liver function tests may resolve spontaneously. If they do not, the drug should be stopped.

Microdeposits in the eyes are benign, rarely affect vision and do not necessitate drug withdrawal.

Peripheral neuropathy and myopathy are rare and may not be reversible. Impotence may also occur.

Sotalol

This has class II and III actions and shares the indications and contraindications of other β-blockers and class III drugs.

Indications

* Supraventricular and ventricular arrhythmias.
* As for other β-blockers.

Dose

Sotalol should be administered at a dose of 40 mg twice a day, increased gradually if necessary to 160 mg twice a day. The dose should be reduced in patients with renal impairment.

Side-effects

Torsade de pointes is the most important side-effect, and caution should be exercised when prescribing it in patients with predisposing factors, congestive heart failure or exacerbation of chronic obstructive airways disease.

Flecainide

This is a sodium-channel blocker that can be given both orally and intravenously. Tablets may be used to treat acute non-life-threatening arrhythmias.

Flecainide is useful for treating supraventricular tachycardias. It can also be used as a 'pill in the pocket' for treating paroxysmal atrial fibrillation.

Indications

* Atrioventricular node reciprocating tachycardia (AVNRT) causing supraventricular tachycardia (SVT).
* Wolff–Parkinson–White syndrome.
* For conversion of paroxysmal atrial fibrillation to sinus rhythm.
* Sustained ventricular tachycardia.
* Symptomatic ventricular ectopic beats.

Dose

Flecainide should be administered at a dose of 50–300 mg per day in two divided doses.

Contraindications

* Heart failure.
* Unpaced heart block, bundle branch block, sinus node disease and bradycardia.
* One study showed a doubling of mortality or non-fatal cardiac arrest when flecainide was used to treat asymptomatic ventricular ectopic beats after myocardial infarction. Therefore, it should not be used in patients with prior myocardial infarction or those with known coronary artery disease. It should be used with caution in elderly patients because of their risk of having clinically unrecognised coronary artery disease.
* There is no evidence that flecainide increases the risk of sudden death in patients with supraventricular tachycardia.

Side-effects

These include ventricular tachycardia, congestive heart failure, conversion of atrial fibrillation to atrial flutter, and slowing flutter rate permitting 1:1 conduction.

Propafenone

Indications, contraindications and side-effects

These are similar to those for flecainide.

Dose

Propafenone should be administered at a dose of 150–300 mg three times a day.

Torsade de pointes

This is an uncommon and dangerous form of ventricular tachycardia, which is diagnosed on an ECG if the QRS complex appears to be twisting around a baseline. It may readily degenerate to ventricular fibrillation and cardiac arrest. It results from prolongation of the QT interval. There is a genetic predisposition in some cases (see section on long QT syndrome below). There are several causes, including any anti-arrhythmic drug that prolongs the QT interval, and interactions between anti-arrhythmic drugs and other drugs, including antidepressants, antihistamines and antibiotics (e.g. intravenous erythromycin). Hypokalaemia, hypomagnesaemia, hypocalcaemia and bradycardia are predisposing factors.

Treatment of torsade de pointes involves admitting the patient to hospital as an emergency to deal with the possibility of cardiac arrest, stopping the offending drug(s), and correction of predisposing biochemical abnormalities. Infusion of magnesium sulphate is usually effective. A β-blocker (but not sotalol) and atrial or ventricular pacing may be effective in treating any predisposing bradycardia. Some of the predisposing conditions and drug causes of torsade de pointes are listed in Boxes 11.1 and 11.2.

Female sex
Hypokalaemia
Bradycardia
Heart failure

BOX 11.1: Risk factors for torsade de pointes.

High risk (> 1%)	Disopyramide, quinidine, sotalol, procainamide, dofetilide, ajmaline
Lower risk	Amiodarone, cisapride
	Clarithromycin, erythromycin, pentamidine
	Domperidone, chlorpromazine, haloperidol, thioradazine methadone

BOX 11.2: Drugs that cause torsade de pointes.

Specific conditions associated with increased risk of ventricular arrhythmias

Long QT syndrome

The most common ion channelopathy is long QT syndrome, which occurs once in every 5000 people. The condition presents in young people who may have unexplained blackouts due to ventricular tachycardia, or palpitations. Some patients die suddenly. The diagnosis can usually be made from an electrocardiogram. Young adults with palpitations or blackouts should be referred to a cardiologist or a neurologist, depending on the clinical picture. Some genetic channelopathies can be diagnosed by genetic testing.

Treatment of long QT syndrome

✧ β-blockers block the effects of adrenaline and are usually effective, reducing the risk of sudden death.
✧ Implantable cardiac defibrillators (see above for indications).

Advice to patients with ion channelopathies

Patients with long QT syndrome should be advised to stop excessive exercising and to avoid certain drugs (*see* Box 11.2 above). These include:

✧ class I and III anti-arrhythmic drugs; macrolide, quinolone, antifungal agents; antimalarial drugs
✧ tricyclic antidepressants, phenothiazines (chlorpromazine), and the newer antidepressants (citalopram, fluoxetine)
✧ antimigraine tablets
✧ over-the-counter medications containing sympathomimetics, bronchodilators, and all adrenaline-like drugs
✧ illicit drugs, particularly cocaine, are very dangerous in susceptible people, and death in drug addicts may be due to ventricular fibrillation induced by drugs with sympathomimetic properties in vulnerable individuals
✧ all close blood relatives of a person who has died of sudden arrhythmic death syndrome should be referred to a specialist centre for investigation. Only 50% of relatives show evidence of a genetic problem, because the victim may have had a mutation or the family members may be carriers but have no signs of disease.

Brugada syndrome

This is a rare condition that mainly affects young men from South-East Asia. Patients may have no symptoms or blackouts or palpitations. Sudden death may occur, often during sleep. There are characteristic ECG appearances with broadening of the QRS complex and elevation of the ST segment. Drugs are not usually effective, and patients may be advised to have an implantable cardiac defibrillator fitted.

Arrhythmogenic right ventricular dysplasia (ARVD)

This is a rare condition that predominantly affects young men. The ECG usually shows T-wave inversion in leads V1, V2 or V3, associated with some prolongation of the QRS (> 110 ms). Ventricular arrhythmias are common, especially if the involvement of the right ventricle is significant. If severe, abnormalities are generally apparent on echocardiography and can be associated with heart failure. In other cases only microscopic abnormalities are found. Indications for ICD implantation are given above.

Management of bradycardia in primary care

Bradycardia may be defined as a heart rate slower than 60 bpm while the patient is awake. However, this is such a common finding as to be diagnostically useless. Only if the heart rate is slower than 50 bpm should one seriously consider a haemodynamically well patient to be bradycardic. The heart rate may fall to a rate of around 40 bpm during sleep, particularly in young people and atheletes. Bradycardia is mainly due to degenerative disease affecting the sinus node and atrioventricular node.

Sinus node disease

This is common in primary care and is associated with coronary heart disease, hypertension, cardiomyopathy, anti-arrhythmic drugs, hypothyroidism, and infection in patients with predisposing conditions. In contrast to the sinus bradycardia seen in athletes, the heart rate in patients with sinus node disease does not increase with exercise (this is known as chronotropic incompetence).

Sinus node disease may present as 'tachy-brady' (or 'sick sinus') syndrome, which is the presence of intermittent sinus bradycardia and paroxysmal atrial tachycardias, often including atrial fibrillation. It is a common cause of syncope and palpitations.

The diagnosis is made with a combination of ECG and 24-hour ambulatory ECG recording. For patients with occasional episodes, loop recorders or trans-telephonic rhythm monitors may be used. Patients place the device over their heart during an attack and transmit the recording to hospital over the telephone. Implantable event recorders are occasionally utilised, and are used for patients with undiagnosed syncope thought to be due to a cardiac arrhythmia.

Management of sinus node disease

No treatment is necessary in symptom-free patients without atrial fibrillation, because their prognosis is good.

Pacing for sinus node disease

Sinus node disease is the most common indication for pacing in the UK. It is important to have evidence demonstrating that symptoms relate to bradycardia before implanting a pacemaker. Atrial rather than single-chamber ventricular pacing is recommended, because it reduces the incidence of permanent atrial fibrillation and thromboembolism. Dual-chamber pacing (electrodes positioned in both the right atrium and right ventricle) is only indicated in patients who have or are likely to develop atrioventricular node disease.

Patients should be referred for implantation of a pacemaker if they have:
⬧ symptomatic bradycardia
⬧ paroxysmal atrial fibrillation requiring anti-arrhythmic drugs but causing symptomatic bradycardia
⬧ symptomatic chronotropic incompetence.

Rate-responsive pacing, in which a sensor in the pacemaker determines the heart rate depending on the activity of the patient, improves the physiological response to exercise.

Atrioventricular node disease

Stokes–Adams attacks, which are attacks of syncope due to complete heart block, were first described by examination of the jugular venous pulse and observation of skin colour changes, nearly 200 years ago.

There are three degrees of heart block.

First-degree heart block

The PR interval is > 0.2 seconds and there is a delay in conduction within the atrio-ventricular node.

First-degree heart block does not result in symptoms, is benign, and no treatment is necessary.

Second-degree heart block

There are two types, which have different implications and management. The block is in the atrioventricular node.

Type I (Wenckebach) second-degree atrioventricular block

Typically, the ECG shows progressive lengthening of the PR interval until a P-wave is not conducted to the ventricles and the sequence starts again. There are other atypical patterns.

This condition is benign if there is no other conduction disorder, patients are usually symptom free and pacing is not indicated.

Type II (Mobitz) second-degree atrioventricular block

The PR interval is constant, but P-waves are intermittently not conducted to the ventricles, resulting in pauses equal to two P-P intervals. This condition is usually associated with bundle branch block. Pacing is indicated even in symptom-free patients, because the majority of patients progress to complete heart block.

Third-degree (complete) atrioventricular block

The P-waves are dissociated from the QRS complexes because they reflect independent electrical activity. Congenital complete heart block is seen with narrow QRS complexes at a rate of 50 bpm, which increases with exercise, because the block is in the atrioventricular node. Acquired complete heart block affects the His-Purkinje tissue below the atrioventricular node. This results in a wide QRS complex with a rate of 30 bpm. When associated with syncope there is a risk of sudden death, and immediate permanent pacing is usually mandatory. The only exceptions are where this is due to drug toxicity, myocarditis or acute myocardial infarction. In these cases temporary pacing until the underlying cause has been resolved can be considered.

Bundle branch block

The QRS complex exceeds 120 ms on the ECG.

Right bundle branch block is usually benign. No treatment is required. Echocardiographic assessment of the right ventricle should be considered, as right bundle branch block may be associated with right ventricular strain (as in atrial septal defects and pulmonary hypertension).

Left bundle branch block is usually associated with heart disease (hypertension, cardiomyopathy or coronary heart disease), a small proportion of patients may progress to complete heart block, and its prognosis depends on the underlying cardiac condition.

Sudden death

The incidence of sudden death – death within one hour of the onset of symptoms – is around 300 000 patients each year in Europe. This represents around 10% of all deaths, and nearly half of all cardiac deaths. Around 50% of cardiac deaths have had no prior diagnosis of heart disease, and therefore truly occur 'out of the blue.' However, the incidence of sudden death is low in the general population, at one in 100 000 in those aged under 30 years, and 0.1–0.2% for all ages.

Risk factors for sudden death

Many factors have been shown to be associated with an increased risk of sudden death, including increasing age, cigarette smoking, obesity, hypertension, left ventricular hypertrophy, left bundle branch block and undertaking high-level physical activity. A positive family history of sudden death is a strong risk factor except in families with long QT syndrome and Brugada syndrome, where other features are stronger predictors (see section on ICD indications above).

Assessing the risk of sudden cardiac death

Sudden death in young people may occur during sport and are an understandable cause of anxiety for the bereaved family. It is important to evaluate the risk of sudden death in the relatives. In addition to the history and examination, relevant investigations include the following:

◆ ECG: look for evidence of infarction (Q-waves), conduction disorders (QRS > 120 ms), left ventricular hypertrophy, long QT (QTc > 440 ms), short QT (QTc < 300 ms), coved ST elevation in leads V1–V3 (Brugada syndrome), and T-wave inversion in leads V1–V3 (this may indicate arrhythmogenic right ventricular dysplasia).
◆ Exercise testing: for those with an intermediate likelihood of ischaemic heart disease.
◆ 24-hour Holter monitoring: for arrhythmic substrate.
◆ Echocardiography for reduced left ventricular ejection fraction, aortic stenosis, hypertrophic cardiomyopathy and right ventricular abnormalities (arrhythmogenic right ventricular dysplasia).

> The National Service Framework on arrhythmias recommends that all family members of an individual with sudden unexpected cardiac death syndrome should be referred to an arrhythmia specialist for evaluation of their risk.

Sudden death in children and young adults

This is a rare condition, but GPs may occasionally have to see parents who have been bereaved by this dramatic and tragic event.

Causes of sudden death in children and young adults

◆ Heart disease, including hypertrophic and dilated cardiomyopathy, arrhythmogenic right ventricular cardiomyopathy, congenital heart disease (e.g. Fallot's tetralogy), myocarditis, connective tissue disease and conduction disease (e.g. Wolff–Parkinson–White syndrome).
◆ Medication (cocaine, illegal drugs and, less commonly, some over-the-counter drugs used in excess).
◆ Prolonged epileptic fits, pulmonary embolism, asthma.

Advice for patients

◆ Palpitation is the symptom that occurs when you are aware of your heart beat. It is usually harmless and nothing to worry about. If you get dizzy turns, feel faint or actually lose consciousness, see us or preferably go to the accident and emergency department.
◆ Palpitation may be due to a fast regular pulse, missed beats or added beats.

- Palpitation is not the same as a heart attack. Occasionally, palpitation may be a consequence of a heart attack.
- The best way to diagnose the heart rhythm abnormality that is causing your palpitation is by recording an ECG during an attack, usually with a 24-hour recording unless you are having an attack near an ECG machine! The recording might be normal, but this is very important information.
- Atrial fibrillation is common. Some people are not bothered by it, while others are. Your heart rhythm is completely irregular.
- Although it is not dangerous, atrial fibrillation poses a risk of blood clots moving around in the bloodstream. This is why we advise you to take warfarin, a blood thinner. This will mean that you need to have regular blood tests to make sure your blood is not too thin and not too thick. Another problem of being in atrial fibrillation, or fibrillating, is that the heart may enlarge and become weak.
- Occasionally, we try to electrically 'shock' people with atrial fibrillation back to a normal rhythm (cardioversion). This involves a short general anaesthetic. The shock is not always successful, and even if it is, your heart rhythm may go back to atrial fibrillation at any stage.
- If you have only short episodes of atrial fibrillation, a junior aspirin may be all that you need. We use different types of heart rhythm tablets.
- Supraventricular tachycardia (SVT) is due to a fast regular heart beat. It may be brought on by alcohol, but most often occurs for no obvious reason. This makes it difficult to predict and prevent.
- It may be possible for you to stop an attack of supraventricular tachycardia or slow it down by rubbing firmly over the neck artery. We will teach you how to do this. Sucking ice cubes may also help.
- Taking tablets when and if necessary or all the time to prevent these attacks is also useful.
- Catheter ablation is an effective and safe procedure that is used to treat patients with supraventricular tachycardia. It is less successful in treating atrial fibrillation and ventricular tachycardia.
- Ventricular tachycardia is more serious. It is most commonly caused by scarring of the heart muscle after a heart attack, but may also occur in patients with an abnormal and weak heart muscle. You may be treated with tablets. There is a new pacemaker-type device available called a cardioverter defibrillator. This monitors your heart rhythm and rate and delivers a shock to your heart if your heart rhythm goes out of sync.
- If you have a very slow heart rate you may need to have a pacemaker implanted. This is done using a local anaesthetic and involves staying overnight in hospital.
- The cardiologist will tell you the dos and don'ts about your pacemaker if you have one fitted.
- If you have dizzy turns or have lost consciousness, this could be due to a fault in your natural pacemaker. This is an area of special cells in your heart that sends electrical impulses to your heart so that it beats and squeezes blood around your body. A faulty pacemaker can be diagnosed with an electrocardiogram (ECG) in the surgery, or we may send you to the hospital for a 24-hour ECG test.
- If your natural pacemaker is not working you will need an artificial one. A pacemaker may also be necessary if a patient has both fast and slow heart rhythms. These patients need a pacemaker to act as an accelerator pedal and drugs to act as a brake. A pacemaker is implanted by a cardiologist at the hospital under local anaesthesia. It is a little uncomfortable, and you will feel the metal pacemaker box under your skin. The small operation takes about an hour and you will need to stay in hospital overnight. The pacemaker only cuts in to stimulate your heart to beat when your heart rate is slow.

- The battery lasts for around six years, but this depends on how often you use it. The battery can be exchanged with a new one quite easily, again under local anaesthetic. Infection of the pacemaker wound occasionally occurs. If this happens, see us or contact the pacemaker clinic. The pacemaker will be checked every six to 12 months.

- With a pacemaker you can and should lead a normal life. Your fainting and dizzy turns will not occur. You are not allowed to drive for one week after the pacemaker has been implanted. You can then start driving again so long as you no longer have any dizziness. You must tell the DVLA that you have a pacemaker. Holders of a passenger-carrying vehicle (PCV) or large goods vehicle (LGV) licence are not allowed to drive for six weeks after the pacemaker implant.

- Tell the airport security screening staff that you have a pacemaker. Keep mobile phones on the opposite side to that where the pacemaker was implanted.

- If at any time you feel unwell, dizzy or light-headed, tell us.

Answers to questions about clinical cases

1. The most likely cause is atrial and/or ventricular ectopic beats. It is important to try to capture the arrhythmia on an ECG or 24-hour ECG recorder to prove the diagnosis. Assuming that the patient has no cardiac history, no other cardiac symptoms and no abnormality on examination, no other investigations are necessary. It is helpful to explain the mechanism of the ectopic beats and their relationship to a slow heart rate. Echocardiography should be performed if there is any suggestion of structural heart disease, and a normal echocardiogram is reassuring and indicates that any ectopic beats recorded are very unlikely to be of prognostic importance. Anxious patients find this particularly reassuring, and this reduces the likelihood of further consultations for the same symptoms.

2. The most likely diagnosis is paroxysmal atrial fibrillation. This patient needs the assessment described above, and should be referred to a cardiologist.

3. This patient should be assessed clinically, and if this shows no abnormality he should have an ECG. A normal ECG does not exclude the possibility of supraventricular tachycardia due to atrioventricular node re-entry or a bypass tract, although the latter is less likely. The patient should be referred to a cardiologist for a 24-hour ECG in an attempt to capture the arrhythmia, because he may have silent short attacks. He should also have echocardiography.

4. The most likely cause is ventricular tachycardia related to a possible left ventricular scar or aneurysm resulting in 'failed sudden death.' Check the patient's medical treatment. If possible he should be on aspirin, an ACE inhibitor or angiotensin II blocker, spironolactone, a β-blocker and a diuretic. Check his electrolytes and ECG. A 24-hour ECG recording will be done in hospital. He should be referred urgently to a cardiologist, preferably in a specialist centre that provides electrophysiology. He will require coronary angiography, possible revascularisation, and will need to be considered for an implantable cardioverter defibrillator combined with biventricular pacing.

5. Examination is important, and if this shows bradycardia, the most likely explanation is heart block, which is easily diagnosed by ECG. The patient should then be referred urgently for pacemaker implantation. Other possible causes include anaemia, hypothyroidism, cerebrovascular disease, infection and malignancy, and these should be excluded if no cardiac cause is found.

6. The symptoms are probably due to a cardiac arrhythmia. Take a full drug history and, if necessary, without her parents present, ask the patient about illicit drug use. Perform an ECG and look for abnormalities in the PR interval, QRS complex and QT duration.

Whatever the result, she should be referred for an urgent cardiology appointment and thorough investigation.

FURTHER READING

American College of Cardiology/American Heart Association/European Society of Cardiology. Guidelines for the management of patients with atrial fibrillation: executive summary. *Eur Heart J.* 2006; **27:** 1979–2030.

Fuster V, Ryden LE, Asinger RW *et al.* American College of Cardiology/American Heart Association guidelines for the management of patients with atrial fibrillation: executive report. *J Am Coll Cardiol.* 2002; **38:** 1231–65.

Hylek E, Go AS, Chang Y *et al.* Effect of intensity of oral anticoagulation on stroke severity and mortality in atrial fibrillation. *NEJM.* 2003; **349:** 1019–26.

Markides V, Schilling RJ. Atrial fibrillation: classification, pathophysiology, mechanisms and drug treatment. *Heart.* 2003; **89:** 939–43.

National Collaborating Centre for Chronic Conditions. *Atrial Fibrillation: national clinical guideline for management in primary and secondary care.* London: Royal College of Physicians; 2006; http://rcplondon.ac.uk/pubs/book/af/index.asp.

Pedersen OD, Bagger H, Keller N *et al.* Efficacy of dofetilide in the treatment of atrial fibrillation-flutter in patients with reduced left ventricular function: a Danish investigation of arrhythmia and mortality on dofetilide (diamond) study. *Circulation.* 2001; **104:** 292–6.

Wyse DG, Waldo AL, DiMarco JP *et al.* A comparison of rate control and rhythm control in patients with atrial fibrillation. *NEJM.* 2002; **347:** 1825–33.

Coronary heart disease in women

TWELVE

Clinical cases

1. A 68-year-old obese woman complains of breathlessness when shopping and doing housework. She has well controlled type 2 diabetes and smokes 15 cigarettes per day. What do you do?
2. An 86-year-old woman with previously well controlled angina returns from holiday and tells you that she can now walk only 20 yards before experiencing chest pain, which she also experiences at night when lying in bed and after tea. What do you do?
3. A 28-year-old woman comes to see you complaining of stress-induced chest pain. Her mother died at the age of 49 years, apparently from a heart attack. What do you do?
4. A 48-year-old woman with a family history of coronary heart disease wants to know whether she should go on to hormone replacement therapy to reduce her risk of a heart attack. She has no menopausal symptoms. What advice do you give her?
5. An 86-year-old woman who has angina comes to see you with her husband and son. They want to know whether she would be better off having coronary angioplasty or coronary artery bypass surgery. What advice do you give her?

Historical attitudes and beliefs in the management of coronary heart disease in women

Cardiovascular disease accounts for 38% of deaths in women, whereas breast cancer accounts for 4% of deaths. For many years, medical students were taught that women were at lower risk of coronary heart disease than men, and coronary heart disease was thought to be a 'male disease.' Even now, women may believe erroneously that they are at greater risk of developing breast cancer than coronary heart disease, and so may not adopt a 'healthy heart lifestyle.'

Historically, epidemiological studies and clinical research studies on coronary heart disease focused mainly on men. Physicians and cardiologists considered coronary heart disease to be much less common in women than in men, so the possible diagnosis was less likely to be investigated, particularly with coronary angiography. Junior doctors in accident and emergency departments were less likely to consider myocardial infarction as a cause of chest pain in a woman. Acute coronary syndromes may be undiagnosed in women if heart disease is not considered by the patient, her family or her doctor to be a possible cause of her symptoms.

This would result in the under-diagnosis of coronary artery disease in women. These attitudes are still prevalent in some cultures, although they are not easily quantified.

Partly because of these attitudes and beliefs, women with coronary heart disease tend to present late, and this reduces the efficacy of treatments for myocardial infarction. At the time of presentation, possibly because they present at an older age compared with men, women are more likely to have more co-morbid conditions, including diabetes mellitus, hypertension, dyslipidaemia and heart failure.

The situation has changed and it is now more widely recognised that women are as likely to have coronary heart disease as men, and they should be managed in the same way. There should be no differences in the way in which male and female patients are investigated or treated, although it is important to understand the potential complexities when interpreting the results of certain tests.

Difficulties in diagnosing coronary heart disease in women

Part of the difficulty in diagnosing coronary heart disease is that the diagnosis may not be considered. Compared with anginal symptoms in men, such symptoms in women are more likely to be atypical. Rather than typical central chest discomfort that occurs during exercise and is relieved by rest, women more commonly report back pain, breathlessness, a burning sensation in their chest, abdominal discomfort, nausea and fatigue.

> Coronary heart disease should be considered in women with chest discomfort or breathlessness who have one or more cardiovascular risk factors, even if they do not have 'typical' angina.

Electrocardiography and exercise testing are also more difficult to interpret in women, and more likely to give rise to 'false-positive' results.

Gender differences in coronary heart disease

Coronary heart disease affects males and females equally. Whereas mortality from vascular and coronary heart disease appears to be decreasing in men, it is increasing in women, and this presents a major challenge to primary care clinicians. The prevalence of hypertension, smoking and obesity is higher in males, but these risk factors are becoming more common in women. In Europe, smoking is now more common among young women.

It is possible that there is a real increase in the incidence of coronary heart disease in women, partly due to their changing role in Western society, their work and family commitments and the associated stresses.

The prevalence, presentation and management of coronary heart disease and certain risk factors differ in women. Diabetes and low high-density-lipoprotein (HDL)-cholesterol levels exert a relatively greater atherogenic effect, and the menopause is also a cardiovascular risk factor.

> Women are much more likely to die from heart disease than from breast cancer.
>   One in three women die from coronary heart disease, which is the most common cause of death in women.
>   In women the risk of coronary heart disease rises after the age of 45 years.
>   Two-thirds of women never fully recover after myocardial infarction.

Gender differences in myocardial infarction

Women appear to be at higher risk of stroke and reinfarctions but not of death.

Gender differences in lipids

Total cholesterol and low-density-lipoprotein (LDL)-cholesterol

The levels of total cholesterol and LDL-cholesterol are lower in pre-menopausal women than in men. These levels increase after the menopause, peaking between the ages of 55 and 65 years, approximately 10 years later than in men. HDL-cholesterol levels are higher in post-menopausal women than in pre-menopausal women.

Age and hypercholesterolaemia

The impact of hypercholesterolaemia as a cardiovascular risk factor varies with a woman's age. A cholesterol level of > 6.1 mmol/l confers a relative risk of coronary heart disease of 2.4 in a woman under 65 years of age, but of only 1.1 in a woman aged over 65 years. However, there are no significant gender differences relating to homozygous familial hyperlipidaemia. The myocardial infarction rate is lower in women with the heterozygous form.

High-density-lipoprotein cholesterol levels

Levels of HDL-cholesterol are higher in women, both before and after the menopause, and appear to exert greater protection against coronary heart disease risk than in men.

A low level of HDL-cholesterol is an independent predictor of coronary heart disease in both men and women. A low HDL-cholesterol level appears to be a better predictor of coronary risk in women than high levels of LDL-cholesterol.

Low-density-lipoprotein cholesterol levels

LDL-cholesterol levels increase slightly with age. Raised levels increase the risk of coronary heart disease by threefold in younger women (under 65 years of age) but not in older women.

Triglyceride levels

High triglyceride levels are an independent risk factor for both men and women, but high levels appear to exert a comparatively greater atherogenic effect in women. The reasons for this are unclear.

Combined dyslipidaemias

The risks of coronary heart disease and its consequences are synergistic, and are greater in both men and women where the usual combination and interactions of lipid abnormalities exist.

Hypertension

Hypertension is unusual in young women, and usually coexists with other cardiovascular risk factors. The diagnosis must be confirmed by 24-hour ambulatory recordings where necessary, after a comprehensive general medical examination, before a diagnosis is made and medication is prescribed.

The prevalence of hypertension increases after the menopause.

Compared with normotensive women, hypertensive women have a 3.5-fold higher risk of developing coronary heart disease. However, compared with hypertensive men their risk is lower.

Smoking

Smoking increases the risk of peripheral vascular disease by sevenfold and the risk of coronary artery disease and myocardial infarction by fivefold. Although the proportion of male and female adult smokers has decreased over the last three decades, smoking among female teenagers has increased. Women who smoked more than 15 cigarettes per day and used 'high-dose'-oestrogen oral contraceptives (now rarely prescribed) were found to have a 20-fold increase in coronary heart disease risk. Passive smoking increases coronary risk in both men and women by 30%.

Diabetes

Type 2 diabetes is associated with a higher atherogenic risk in women than in men (2.6-fold vs 1.8-fold greater risk), but the reasons for this are unclear. Type 2 diabetes increases coronary risk by threefold in women and by twofold in men compared with non-diabetic subjects. Diabetes reduces the protection afforded by the pre-menopausal state.

Obesity

This is a major and increasing health problem in both young people and adults, and is associated with other cardiovascular risk factors, including hypertension, insulin resistance, diabetes, hyperlipidaemia and physical inactivity. Slight obesity increases coronary risk by sixfold. It is not clear whether obesity is more common in girls than in boys.

Physical inactivity

Physical inactivity is associated with other cardiovascular risk factors. Regular physical activity reduces cardiovascular risk by at least 50%. The reduction in coronary risk is related to the intensity, duration and frequency of physical exercise, which reduces stress and anxiety and enhances well-being. People who exercise regularly tend to have a healthy lifestyle and are less likely to have associated risk factors.

Inflammatory markers

C-reactive protein (CRP) is an acute-phase protein. Levels of CRP increase with age and are higher in smokers. High levels of CRP may be predictive of coronary events. CRP levels are high in post-menopausal women with cardiovascular events, but this may reflect the ischaemic inflammatory process rather than the genesis of the event. It has been suggested that part of the benefit of regular exercise is that it reduces vascular inflammation.

The menopause

Menopause is a transition, with lengthening of the cycle length. Post-menopausal status is defined as occurring when there have been no periods for one year. Most women become menopausal between the ages of 40 and 58 years. Menopausal symptoms include hot flushes, night sweats, vaginal dryness and sleep disturbance. Only a minority of women in the UK consult their GP about menopausal symptoms.

Hormone replacement therapy is the most effective treatment for menopausal symptoms.

Women who present with coronary heart disease are around 10 years older than men, and 20 years older when they have their first myocardial infarct. Coronary heart disease risk increases after the menopause, whether this is a natural 'early' menopause, or medically induced. This increased risk is attributed to lower oestrogen levels in women. The menopause is associated with various unfavourable changes in lipids, glucose and thrombotic tendency. There are increases in total cholesterol, LDL-cholesterol and triglyceride levels, glucose levels increase and insulin sensitivity decreases, fibrinogen levels increase and vascular endothelial dysfunction may occur.

Hormone replacement therapy, cardiovascular disease and general health

Experimentally, oestrogen improves lipid profiles by reducing LDL-cholesterol levels and increasing HDL-cholesterol levels. Observational studies have suggested that post-menopausal hormone replacement therapy reduces the risk of coronary heart disease, but this has not been confirmed in randomised trials.

> Long-term hormone replacement therapy is not recommended for the prevention of chronic disease, because of the increased risk of stroke, gall-bladder disease and deep vein thrombosis.

Recently, post-menopausal therapy has been shown to cause small increases in coronary events, stroke, pulmonary embolism and breast cancer. Two of each of these events occurs as a result of treating 1000 women for one year.

Hormone replacement therapy and increased risk of stroke

Both oestrogen alone and oestrogen plus progestin increase the risk of stroke by 40% and increase the relative risk by 1.4. Therefore, a woman with a 10% baseline risk has a 14% risk with hormone replacement therapy. For a woman with a 30% baseline risk of stroke, the risk would increase to 42% with hormone replacement therapy.

Progestin combined with oestrogen appears to be associated with a higher risk of coronary events, pulmonary embolism and breast cancer than oestrogen alone. Combined therapy in women aged over 65 years is associated with an increased risk of breast cancer and dementia.

The absolute risk associated with hormone replacement therapies is smaller in younger women with a lower risk of vascular disease.

> Oestrogen should be avoided in women who have vascular disease or who are at high risk of cardiovascular disease, breast cancer, uterine cancer or venous thromboembolism, and those with active liver disease.

One serious event occurs per 100 women treated for five years. In addition, although hormone replacement therapy improves the severity and frequency of flushing by 80%, it does not improve quality of life (depression, insomnia, sexual function and cognition) in asymptomatic patients. Although women with flushing are generally young and usually require treatment for only a year, a sizeable proportion of women require long-term treatment. The absolute risk of hormone replacement therapy will therefore be much lower when it is used in these patients. The estimated risk is one serious adverse event per 1000 women treated for one year.

> Hormone replacement therapy is contraindicated in women with a history of deep vein thrombosis or pulmonary embolism, breast cancer, coronary heart disease, stroke or dementia.

Before a woman starts hormone replacement therapy, her cardiovascular risk should be estimated on the basis of the following risk factors:

✧ family history of cardiovascular disease
✧ weight, height (for BMI calculation) and waist measurement
✧ blood pressure
✧ smoking history
✧ lipid profile, fasting blood glucose and urinalysis
✧ exercise testing should be performed in women with known or suspected coronary heart disease. In symptom-free women who are at intermediate cardiovascular risk, the absence of ischaemia identifies women at low cardiovascular risk.

Hormone replacement therapy should be started at a low dose, increased gradually until symptoms resolve, and then reduced every six months to assess whether it needs to be continued. Hormone replacement therapy can be stopped in most women after two years. If symptoms recur, the treatment should be restarted. The dose can be reduced after another six months to test whether symptoms recur.

Hormone replacement therapy is not recommended for asymptomatic post-menopausal women. Hot flushes disappear in two-thirds of women within a few years, but may continue for many years in some individuals.

Aerobic exercise (e.g. swimming, running, cycling, vigorous dancing, fast walking, rowing) may help with flushes. Women should be advised to drink only modest amounts of tea, coffee and alcohol.

There is no evidence that non-prescription therapies (acupuncture, yoga, Chinese herbs, dong quai, evening primrose oil, ginseng, kava, black cohosh, soy isoflavones or red clover extract) improve hot flushes. Vitamin E reduces the number of flushes, but only very slightly.

Oral contraceptives and heart disease
Oral contraceptives should not be prescribed to women over 35 years of age if they have cardiovascular risk factors.

Approach to diagnosis of women with suspected coronary heart disease
Women should be managed in the same way as men. They should be given similar advice on primary and secondary cardiovascular prevention. Women with diabetes are at particularly high risk and should be managed accordingly.

Diagnostic tests
Exercise testing may give rise to a 20% false-positive rate in women, but the reasons for this are unclear. This may dissuade a physician from investigating a woman for possible coronary heart disease, although this principle may not deter the physician from requesting a mammogram, which may have a similar false-positive rate in fibrocystic breast disease.

Despite its reduced accuracy in women, exercise testing should be used as the preferred stress test for investigating ischaemia in patients at intermediate coronary risk as well as for the other indications.

Stress echocardiography may be useful in patients who cannot exercise, and when interpretation of the ECG is complicated by left bundle branch block and other repolarisation changes.

Nuclear imaging is complicated in women because breast tissue often obscures the inferior surfaces of the heart, and this reduces its accuracy. The inherent concerns of injecting radioactive pharmaceuticals and the long duration and expense of the tests need to be weighed against what is at best a marginal benefit in women with resting electrocardiographic abnormalities.

There are insufficient data comparing the diagnostic and prognostic value of electron beam computed tomography in men and women. The technique is experimental, expensive, not available on the NHS, and adds no useful or incremental information to conventional clinical risk estimations.

Coronary angiography remains the only investigation that provides accurate anatomical information on coronary artery anatomy and atherosclerotic disease. It is indicated in patients who cannot exercise, when the results of stress testing suggest the presence of coronary artery disease, or when obstructive coronary artery disease needs to be excluded in order to define management. Complications are generally no more frequent in women than in men.

Cardiovascular medical therapy

Apart from pregnancy and breastfeeding, there are no major differences when considering cardiovascular medication in women.

When starting treatment in women with a low body mass index, the lowest recommended drug doses should be prescribed, and these may be gradually increased if necessary.

Dihydropyridine calcium antagonists used for hypertension may be unacceptable in women who develop significant peripheral oedema.

Cardiac surgery and myocardial revascularisation

Although there was concern that the short- and long-term results of coronary artery and valve surgery and coronary angioplasty were worse in women, this is no longer thought to be the case. It may have been due to a variety of other patient characteristics, including age, severity of disease at presentation, body size and coexisting disease.

Gender is not a factor when considering cardiac surgical or percutaneous interventions. The results of angioplasty and stenting using drug-eluting stents and adjunctive antiplatelet drugs (glycoprotein IIb/IIIa inhibitors) for the treatment of angina and myocardial infarction have improved outcomes for men and women equally.

Advice for patients

* Heart disease affects women just as much as it affects men. However, it affects women at an older age.
* If you are a woman aged between 45 and 64 years, you have a one in nine chance of having some form of cardiovascular disease. One in three women aged over 65 years has some form of cardiovascular disease, including furring up of the heart arteries and high blood pressure.
* You are just as likely as a man to have a high cholesterol level.
* Almost half of all heart attacks occur in women.
* Women who have had a heart attack are more likely to die in the first two weeks after it than are men. Around 40% of women die in the first year after a heart attack, but this depends on a number of factors, including age, the presence of risk factors, and the state of the heart arteries and the heart muscle.
* It used to be thought that hormone replacement therapy reduced the risk of the heart arteries furring up, but this is no longer believed to be the case. Indeed, HRT may increase the risk of heart disease in healthy women after the menopause. The

risks of a problem are higher in women aged over 60 years who have risk factors for cardiovascular disease. HRT does not protect women from heart disease, and should not be taken solely for this reason. The main reason for taking HRT is to relieve severe flushing.

✦ If you smoke you are at increased risk of having a heart attack. If you are aged over 35 years and you also smoke, you should stop the oral contraceptive pill and use another method of contraception.

✦ The risk associated with the oral contraceptive pill is even higher in women who also have a high blood pressure. These women are at increased risk of heart attacks and stroke. If you have high blood pressure you should not be taking the pill. Women without high blood pressure need to have their blood pressure checked both before starting the pill, and during treatment in case their blood pressure goes up while they are on it. The pill may need to be stopped if their blood pressure goes up and stays up.

✦ It is not yet known whether women with diabetes and/or high cholesterol levels are at increased risk of heart attacks or stroke, but we would like to keep an eye on your blood sugar and cholesterol level while you are taking the pill.

✦ The new third-generation oral contraceptive pill is more likely to cause clots in the leg veins, and these newer oral contraceptive pills should not be the first choice in new users. You should not take any type of oral contraceptive pill if you have had a deep vein thrombosis.

✦ If you smoke, you should stop. This is the most important thing you can do to help yourself. If your partner, children or close family members smoke, encourage them to stop as well. If you have young children, try your hardest to make sure that they do not start smoking.

✦ If you are overweight, it is important for you to lose weight and take regular exercise. Eat a low-fat diet. We will be happy to check your blood pressure and cholesterol levels. This is particularly important if you have other cardiovascular risk factors.

✦ As a mother, you should encourage your family to lead a healthy lifestyle.

✦ If you are stressed, which is common in women because they have to juggle work with family life and running the home, and you want to talk about this, please let us know and we will listen and help.

✦ If you have chest discomfort or you become breathless when you exercise, come and see us. We might arrange for you to see a heart doctor or arrange some tests at the hospital, but this depends on the likelihood of you having heart disease. Stress tests may provide confusing results in young women who have a low probability of having heart trouble.

✦ Some doctors recommend taking a small aspirin (75 mg per day with a meal) if a woman is aged over 50 years and has risk factors for heart disease. You should take aspirin if you have furring up in any artery or if you have had a heart attack, stroke, bypass surgery or angioplasty. You should not take aspirin if you are definitely allergic to it or have had bleeding from the gut related to aspirin.

✦ A floppy mitral valve – 'mitral valve prolapse' – is more common in slim women than in men. It is a harmless condition in which the inflow valve to the main pumping chamber of the heart flops back into the collecting chamber when the heart muscle contracts. Usually this is of no consequence, but if you have a heart murmur, this means that blood is leaking back into the collecting chamber. Although it is not dangerous, you should take antibiotics before you undergo any dental work or a gynaecological procedure or operation or delivery.

Answers to questions about clinical cases

1. Asthma, chronic bronchitis, anaemia, hypothyroidism and obesity need to be considered and assessed clinically and investigated. This patient may have angina, and if she can exercise you should arrange for her to have an exercise test. If not, a stress echocardiogram might be helpful. If coronary artery disease is suspected, and the symptoms are not severe, she should be prescribed aspirin and GTN, which she should take both prophylactically and also to abort spontaneous attacks of angina. She may need to be referred to a cardiologist if she does respond or if there is evidence of important ischaemia, as both of these suggest significant coronary artery disease. She should be advised and helped to stop smoking and to lose weight, and her other cardiovascular risk factors should be reviewed.

2. Unstable angina is the most likely diagnosis, and this patient should be referred urgently to hospital for a specialist opinion. Her anti-anginal medication should be reviewed and increased if possible. Exercise testing will add little diagnostic or prognostic information. Coronary angiography, preferably with a view to coronary angioplasty because of her age, is indicated if her symptoms do not respond to medical treatment. However, the possibility that she may need coronary artery surgery should also be discussed with the patient and her family.

3. Despite her family history or premature coronary heart disease, it is unlikely that this patient has coronary heart disease. However, if she has symptoms that suggest angina, she should have an exercise test, and if this shows ischaemia, she should be referred for a specialist opinion. If she has a low absolute coronary risk and her symptoms do not suggest angina, other causes of chest pain should be considered and investigated.

4. There is no evidence that HRT reduces the risk of cardiovascular disease. HRT is not recommended to women unless they have menopausal symptoms.

5. There is no evidence that one form of myocardial revascularisation is superior for women. The choice of approach should be guided by the patient's cardiologist in consultation with the cardiac surgeon. The safest and most effective treatment should be recommended based on a comprehensive clinical assessment, including technical considerations (the coronary anatomy and the type of lesions in the coronary artery) and a fundamental analysis of whether any form of revascularisation is necessary in this particular case at the moment.

FURTHER READING

Peterson S, Peto V, Scarborough P *et al.* for the British Heart Foundation Health Promotion Research Group. *Coronary Heart Disease Statistics 2005.* Oxford: British Heart Foundation; 2005; www.heartstats.org/temp.CHD_2005_Whole_spdocument.pdf.

Hormone replacement treatment

Grady D. Management of menopausal symptoms. *NEJM.* 2006; **355:** 2338–47.

Grady D, Herrington D, Bittner V *et al.* Cardiovascular disease outcomes during 6.8 years of hormone therapy: Heart and Estrogen/Progestin Replacement Study follow-up (HERS II). *JAMA.* 2002; **288:** 49–57.

Hays J, Ockerne JK, Brunner RL *et al.* Effects of estrogen plus progestin on health-related quality of life. *NEJM.* 2003; **348:** 1839–54.

Herrington DM, Reboussin DM, Brosnihan B *et al.* Effects of estrogen replacement on the progression of coronary artery atherosclerosis. *NEJM.* 2000; **343:** 522–9.

Hlatky MA, Boothroyd D, Vittinghoff E *et al.* Quality-of-life and depressive symptoms in post-menopausal women after receiving hormone therapy: results from the Heart and Estrogen/ Progestin Replacement Study (HERS) trial. *JAMA.* 2002; **287:** 591–7.

North American Menopause Society. Recommendations for estrogen and progestogen use in peri- and post-menopausal women: October 2004 position statement of the North American Menopause Society. *Menopause.* 2004; **118 (Suppl. 2):** 163–5.

Preventive Services Task Force. Post-menopausal hormone replacement therapy for primary prevention of chronic conditions: recommendations and rationale. *Ann Intern Med.* 2002; **137:** 834–9.

Royal College of Obstetricians and Gynaecologists, Scientific Advisory Committee. Alternatives to hormone replacement therapy for the management of menopausal symptoms; www.rcog.org. uk/index.asp?PageID=1561.

Heart disease in pregnancy

THIRTEEN

Clinical cases

1. You hear a new systolic murmur in a 20-year-old, symptom-free, pregnant woman at a routine antenatal check (20 weeks). What do you do?
2. A 33-year-old woman who had corrective heart surgery for tetralogy of Fallot in early childhood comes to see you because she is pregnant and is delighted. She wants to know the risk of her baby having heart disease. What do you tell her?
3. A 28-year-old woman with Marfan's syndrome and normal blood pressure wants to have 'natural childbirth.' What do you advise her to do?
4. A 33-year-old woman who is taking warfarin for an aortic valve replacement inserted eight years previously is 12 weeks pregnant and wants reassurance from you that all is well and will continue to be so. What do you tell her?
5. A 23-year-old woman who has Eisenmenger's syndrome comes to see you because she has recently become engaged and she and her future husband want to start a family. What advice do you give her about pregnancy?

Heart disease during pregnancy

Valvular heart disease is the most common form of acquired heart disease in pregnancy but, overall, congenital heart disease is the most common form of heart disease in pregnant women.

Most girls and young women with congenital heart disease reach childbearing age and want to become pregnant. Most of them have a residual haemodynamic problem despite intervention or surgery in infancy or childhood. When they become pregnant, they pose difficult management problems because of the haemodynamic changes during pregnancy and the increased loads on the heart with an increased risk of heart failure. It is likely that there will be an increase in the number of patients with congenital heart disease who become pregnant.

> Patients with cardiac disease should be identified before pregnancy and treated if necessary.

Maternal risks

Cardiac disease complicates 0.5% of pregnancies in the UK and Europe, and is more common in developing countries. Higher maternal age and the increased likelihood of women with congenital heart disease surviving into adulthood account for the increase in the proportion of pregnant patients with heart disease.

Women with congenital heart disease are at increased risk of having a baby with congenital heart disease.

In the UK, the incidence of maternal death during pregnancy is one in every 10 000 pregnancies. Most deaths are due to severe aortic stenosis, cyanotic heart disease, pulmonary hypertension, peripartum cardiomyopathy and left ventricular failure, myocardial infarction or aortic dissection.

Women with pulmonary hypertension have a 50% risk of dying during pregnancy, mainly during or soon after delivery. They are a particularly high-risk group. They should be advised not to get pregnant, and if they do, to have a termination of pregnancy, which carries a 7% risk. Other adverse events include stroke, pulmonary oedema and arrhythmia. These risks depend on the structural heart abnormality and the ability of the cardiovascular system to adapt to pregnancy.

Patients with non-cyanotic heart disease with left to right shunts and only slightly high pulmonary vascular resistance usually do well. This good prognostic group includes patients with small atrial septal defects, small ventricular septal defects, mild valvular stenosis or regurgitation.

Fetal risks

There are increased risks to the fetus in a mother with heart disease and cyanosis. Intra-uterine growth restriction, premature birth, intracranial haemorrhage and fetal death are more common in patients with congenital heart disease. The risk of fetal death may be as high as 80%.

Congenital heart disease occurs in 0.8% of newborn infants around the world. Around 85% of these infants survive into adulthood. Around 250 000 adults in the UK have grown-up congenital heart disease (GUCH). These patients are managed in specialist centres. Pre-conception and post-conception counselling is usually provided in multi-specialist clinics where the expertise of an obstetrician, cardiologist, paediatrician, anaesthetist and specialist in fetal medicine is available. In complex congenital heart disease, offspring mortality is high due to the high rate of premature delivery and recurrence of congenital heart disease. With appropriate evaluation and monitoring in centres with expertise, most affected pregnant women will have a successful pregnancy.

The role of primary care clinicians in the management of pregnant women with heart disease

The majority of patients with congenital heart disease are diagnosed before pregnancy. Only a minority of patients are diagnosed with structural heart disease during pregnancy. The majority of pregnant patients with important heart conditions will be managed jointly by the primary care team, the obstetrician, the cardiologist and the midwives. Patients who are identified as being at low risk can be managed in a similar way to pregnant women without cardiac disease. Those at high risk have to be managed carefully because maternal death has major implications for all of the other members of the bereaved family.

Non-pregnant women of childbearing age with a high-risk cardiac condition may want to discuss the risks of pregnancy with their GP or a cardiologist. This is a difficult task because of the medical uncertainties in each case and the often intense emotional, social and ethical issues. GPs need to be able to advise patients about the risks of pregnancy in individual cases. There are risks to the mother, the fetus and also the rest of the family.

The pregnant patient with a cardiac condition often consults the GP for advice and guidance. Patients should be able to make an informed decision about the risks of pregnancy.

GPs and primary care clinicians involved in the care of patients who are contemplating pregnancy and of pregnant patients with heart disease should understand:

✧ how the cardiovascular system adapts during pregnancy and how these normal changes can cause symptoms and signs
✧ which cardiac conditions are safe and which ones put the mother and fetus at risk
✧ which cardiac tests are safe and which ones should be avoided
✧ which medications are safe and which ones should be avoided

✧   the scheduling of assessments during pregnancy
✧   when to refer patients to specialist centres
✧   the problems that may occur during pregnancy, after delivery and in the postpartum period
✧   how to advise patients about future pregnancies, family planning and contraception
✧   the prognosis of heart disease in women and how this may impact upon their family.

Principles of management of patients with cardiac disease during pregnancy

✧   Provide women with advice about good cardiac and general health before pregnancy.
✧   Provide women with contraception until a pregnancy is wanted.
✧   Provide specialist evaluation with a baseline echocardiogram to define the anatomy and haemodynamics of the lesion.
✧   Determine the risk of pregnancy to the mother and the fetus.
✧   Liaise with the cardiologist and obstetrician.
✧   Assess the need for antibiotic prophylaxis.
✧   Assess the need for percutaneous intervention (valvuloplasty) or surgical intervention (repair or replacement).
✧   Avoid teratogenic drugs, replacing any contraindicated medications with safe alternatives.
✧   Evaluate the patient clinically and functionally (use exercise testing to obtain an objective measurement).
✧   Provide frequent monitoring (at least three-monthly) during and after pregnancy with follow-up echocardiography.
✧   Optimise the patient's cardiac condition using bed rest and oxygen when necessary.
✧   Postpartum, provide monitoring of haemodynamics, anaemia and the patient's psychological state.
✧   Review the need for intervention.

Individualised management

The management of pregnant women with cardiac disease is individualised because it is not appropriate to perform randomised trials. Therefore, compared with other cardiovascular conditions, there is no good evidence base. Much of the information that guides management is based on case reports or series from one or more centres. It is difficult to compare cases with those reported because the patients would not have identical cardiac anatomy or haemodynamic characteristics, nor would the skill mix of the obstetric and cardiology staff be identical.

Physiological and haemodynamic changes during pregnancy and delivery

Cardiac output increases by 50% due to increased placental circulation and hormonal effects by 20 weeks. Blood volume increases by 50%, resulting in dilutional anaemia. The resting heart rate increases by 10 bpm. These changes account for the common features of a systolic murmur and palpitations. Despite the increase in cardiac output, blood pressure should remain normal or low due to a fall in systemic vascular resistance and increased production of prostaglandins. These changes occur early in pregnancy, peaking in the second trimester and plateauing in the third trimester. In the third trimester, the enlarging uterus pushes the heart up, anteriorly and to the left.

During labour and delivery, there are further increases in cardiac output, heart rate, blood pressure and systemic vascular resistance. Blood pressure and cardiac output increase during delivery, and these increases are influenced by the mode of delivery, which is important in women with hypertension and those at risk of heart failure. During each uterine contraction the cardiac output increases by 34% and blood pressure increases by 12%. Blood reaching the circulation from the uterus increases the cardiac output in the early postpartum period, so pulmonary oedema may only occur after delivery. The haemodynamic changes that occur during delivery and in the postpartum period usually resolve within one week of delivery.

Clinical evaluation of cardiac disease during pregnancy

Pregnant patients with heart disease may complain of breathlessness, palpitations, fatigue or swelling of the feet. These symptoms, which are common in patients with a normal heart during a normal pregnancy, must be carefully evaluated. Other symptoms, including orthopnoea, resting dyspnoea, angina, sustained palpitation and paroxysmal nocturnal dyspnoea, are serious and not normal, and indicate underlying heart disease.

Previous cardiac procedures and operations are important and should be included in referral letters to hospital specialists. The results of previous chest X-rays, echocardiograms and exercise stress tests are helpful. Some patients with valve disease are diagnosed only after they become pregnant.

Physical findings include a slight increase in heart rate, and systolic murmurs due to increased flow across the aortic and pulmonary valves. There may be venous hums over the supraclavicular fossae, and arterial bruits over the mammary arteries. Diastolic murmurs are abnormal.

Signs of pre-eclampsia, sustained hypertension and oedema, particularly of the fingers, are abnormal and require investigation.

Clinical findings in a normal pregnancy	
Symptoms	• Fatigue
	• Decreased exercise tolerance
	• Palpitation
	• Swollen feet and legs
	• Orthopnoea
Signs	• Systolic murmur

Haemodynamic effects of pregnancy in specific cardiac conditions

The haemodynamic effects of pregnancy on the mother depend on the underlying anatomical and physiological abnormality and vary during pregnancy, at delivery and postpartum. A valve lesion that was tolerated before pregnancy may deteriorate with the increased haemodynamic demands.

Pulmonary artery pressure increases during the period just before and after delivery, so patients with pulmonary hypertension are at highest risk at this time. Patients with Eisenmenger's syndrome may deteriorate and become more cyanosed, hypoxic and breathless during pregnancy because of increased right to left shunting resulting from systemic vasodilatation and right ventricular overload.

The increase in cardiac output, particularly at and after delivery, puts a strain on both ventricles. Heart failure may occur in patients with right or left ventricular outflow tract obstruction (aortic or pulmonary valve stenosis) or a weak heart muscle (cardiomyopathy, after corrective surgery for congenital heart disease).

The increase in blood pressure during delivery poses a risk of aortic dissection, aortic aneurysm, rupture and dissection in patients with a weak aortic wall due to Marfan's syndrome.

The increase in heart rate increases the transmitral gradient in mitral valve stenosis.

Classification of maternal and fetal risk

In women with cardiovascular disease, pregnancy should ideally be planned and the risks identified *before* conception, although this is not always possible. After conception, close collaboration and clear communication between primary care and hospital specialists is important, and reduces patient anxieties and complications.

In women with known cardiac abnormalities, the risk of a potential pregnancy should be evaluated and possible options for corrective surgery and medical treatment explored and explained. Pregnancy is not recommended for patients with high-risk conditions, and termination of pregnancy should be considered in these cases.

In the less common situation where a cardiac abnormality is first detected during pregnancy, there is a more urgent need to evaluate the structural and haemodynamic consequences of the cardiac condition and its potential risks to the mother and fetus, so that management can be planned.

The risk of congenital heart disease in offspring

A baby born to a mother with congenital heart disease has a 3–12% risk of having congenital heart disease compared with a baby born to a mother without congenital heart disease. The risk of fetal cardiac disease is less than one in 1000 if the fetus has a normal nuchal thickness. Fetal echocardiography is offered to women with a strong family history of congenital heart disease.

Maternal life expectancy

Life expectancy is excellent for most patients with congenital heart disease, and depends on the cardiac abnormality, previous interventions and the haemodynamic status.

Contraception and termination of pregnancy

Women with congenital heart disease should be offered contraceptive advice.

Patients at low risk

In the absence of symptoms, cyanosis, pulmonary hypertension, significant cardiac impairment or significant arrhythmias, pregnancy is usually safe and well tolerated. Normal spontaneous vaginal delivery is usually possible in patients with low-risk conditions.

Arrhythmias, deterioration of left ventricular function and progression of pulmonary hypertension may occasionally occur. Patients who have had cardiac surgery without prosthetic valves generally do well. The frequency of clinical assessments and the need for cardiac investigations are determined individually.

Low-risk lesions

◇ Small left to right shunts:
  — atrial and ventricular septal defects, patent ductus arteriosus.
◇ Insignificant left ventricular outflow tract obstruction:
  — mild aortic valve stenosis
  — hypertrophic obstructive cardiomyopathy.
◇ Pulmonary valve stenosis. Patients with severe valve stenosis may be considered for percutaneous valvuloplasty, ideally before conception, although this may be necessary during pregnancy.
◇ Patients who have had valve replacements with non-prosthetic valves.

Patients at moderate risk

Patients at moderate risk should be evaluated in a specialist centre and their care shared between the GP and the hospital team.

Moderate-risk lesions

◇ Moderate mitral stenosis.
◇ Aortic coarctation.
◇ Unrepaired tetralogy of Fallot.

Patients at high risk

Structural and haemodynamic conditions that put the mother at high risk include:
◇ poor functional class (WHO class III or IV) before pregnancy
◇ cyanotic heart disease (e.g. uncorrected tetralogy of Fallot)
◇ significant right to left shunt without cyanosis
◇ exercise-induced hypoxaemia ($< 85\%$)
◇ previous stroke, transient ischaemic attack or pulmonary oedema before pregnancy or during pregnancy
◇ pulmonary arterial hypertension (mean pulmonary artery pressure > 25 mmHg at rest, diagnosed by cardiac catheter)
◇ weak aortic wall (Marfan's syndrome)
◇ severe aortic stenosis (aortic valve area < 1.5 cm^2) or mitral valve stenosis (mitral valve area < 2.0 cm^2)
◇ severe left ventricular impairment (left ventricular ejection fraction $< 40\%$).

The event rate in the presence of more than one of these risk factors is 75%, in the presence of one condition it is 27%, and with none it is 5%.

Risk stratification

Patients who are considered to be an acceptable risk will be monitored carefully before, during and after pregnancy, with particular attention to drug treatments.

Low-risk patients can be monitored and managed by their GP, and reassured that pregnancy is safe.

Patients at moderate risk can be managed by their GP, but in close collaboration with the specialist centre.

Management of high-risk patients

If possible, non-pregnant high-risk women should have percutaneous or surgical repair of their heart lesion before pregnancy. When valve replacement is necessary, tissue valves are generally preferred to prosthetic valves in order to avoid the need for anticoagulants during pregnancy.

Most cardiologists and obstetricians recommend termination of pregnancy in pregnant women with a high-risk cardiac condition. The risks of early termination are lower than the risks of continuing the pregnancy.

For women who decide to continue with their pregnancy, rest, prompt treatment of heart failure, and frequent, vigilant, clinical monitoring are necessary. Hospital admission may be necessary if the patient deteriorates, becomes hypoxic or develops arrhythmias. The woman will be counselled about the risks of pregnancy to herself and the baby. Her cardiac condition will be evaluated and treatment and filling pressures optimised.

Patients with hypertension and/or pre-eclampsia should be admitted to hospital for bed rest, antihypertensive treatment and consideration of early delivery. Precautions against thromboembolism should be taken particularly before and after Caesarean section, and in patients who are resting in bed.

> Pregnancy and childbirth are usually safe in patients with congenital heart disease without significant haemodynamic impairment, and in patients with mild valve disease and normal left ventricular function.
>
> Women with known or suspected heart disease should be referred to a cardiologist in collaboration with their obstetrician.

Indications for cardiology referral during pregnancy

- ✧ Patients with high-risk cardiovascular conditions.
- ✧ Unexplained or new cardiac symptoms or signs.
- ✧ Heart failure.
- ✧ Troublesome palpitations.
- ✧ Hypertension.
- ✧ Patients with structural heart disease or previous cardiac surgery.
- ✧ Marfan's syndrome.
- ✧ Patients with previous thrombotic disease.
- ✧ Anxious patients who want reassurance from a cardiologist.

Cardiac investigations during pregnancy

Radiology should be avoided during pregnancy, particularly during the first trimester, unless there is a sound clinical reason for it. Chest radiography with abdominal shielding may occasionally be necessary. CT scanning is contraindicated.

Echocardiography is used to evaluate patients with murmurs, heart failure and known structural heart disease. It is safe and provides useful diagnostic information.

> Pregnant women with anything other than a trivial heart murmur should be referred for echocardiography.

The ECG may show non-specific ST and T-wave changes. If it is recorded during palpitations, the ECG may be helpful in showing sinus rhythm or an arrhythmia, most commonly ectopic beats, which are almost always benign. A 24-hour ECG recording is safe, and is useful for the evaluation of palpitations. ECG recordings are safe.

Exercise stress testing is rarely needed during pregnancy. It can be dangerous because it may cause fetal bradycardia.

Stress echocardiography is occasionally used to assess valvular heart disease or cardiac function.

Cardiac magnetic resonance imaging is safe during pregnancy.

Cardiac catheterisation is very rarely needed during pregnancy. The high doses of radiation used are very dangerous to the fetus, and there is a very high risk of fetal abnormalities. This procedure should be avoided unless the mother is having a myocardial infarction or other acute coronary syndrome and angioplasty is being considered. Acute valvuloplasty for previously undiagnosed or sudden deterioration of mitral or aortic stenosis is only very rarely necessary, and is also very dangerous to the fetus because of the high radiation doses used.

High-risk cardiac conditions for the fetus

✧ Maternal functional class before pregnancy greater than Class II of the New York Heart Association.
✧ Maternal cyanosis.
✧ Severe aortic stenosis (aortic valve area < 1.5 cm^2) or mitral stenosis (mitral valve area < 2.0 cm^2).
✧ Mother who smokes or who has smoked recently.
✧ Treatment with anticoagulants.
✧ Mother aged < 20 or > 35 years.

Acquired heart valve disease

Congenital valve disease, sometimes associated with other acquired cardiac defects (e.g. rheumatic valve disease, prosthetic valve replacements, mitral valve prolapse and regurgitation, or previous endocarditis), is the most common type of valve disease in pregnancy.

Most patients will be diagnosed before conception, and the risks of potential pregnancy and delivery can be discussed when appropriate. Referral to both cardiac and obstetric specialists is recommended if pregnancy is contemplated.

All patients with valve disease should be referred for a cardiac evaluation including echocardiography to characterise and quantitate the valve abnormality. Those at high risk will need counselling about the risks of pregnancy, and careful monitoring by cardiologists and obstetricians in a centre with expertise. Occasionally, percutaneous or surgical intervention will be necessary before conception.

Patients with significant mitral valve stenosis should be considered for mitral valvuloplasty before conception, and again during pregnancy, if they remain symptomatic despite medical treatment.

Serial echocardiographic studies are often necessary because the effective gradient increases during pregnancy, and it is difficult to predict the haemodynamic effects of pregnancy in individual cases. Women who were very fit before pregnancy may deteriorate suddenly with an increase in heart rate and blood volume.

Aortic and mitral regurgitation are generally well tolerated in patients without symptoms, because the degree of valve regurgitation decreases during pregnancy as the systemic vascular resistance falls.

Mitral stenosis

This is the most common form of acquired valve disease in pregnant women, and is due to rheumatic fever. Patients from countries where rheumatic heart disease is relatively common should be examined carefully for mitral valve stenosis, and if the latter is suspected they should be referred. Echocardiography and Doppler studies will provide the diagnosis.

Rheumatic mitral valve stenosis is more common in women who were not born in the UK. It is important that this condition is diagnosed before conception. It may present during pregnancy with pulmonary oedema, due to the increased left atrial pressure resulting from the increase in heart rate and blood volume.

Any cause of an increase in heart rate (fever, infection or anaemia) may result in symptoms of breathlessness.

Patients should be reviewed monthly from 20 weeks. Bed rest and oxygen in hospital are recommended for symptomatic patients. Diuretics to reduce the tendency to pulmonary oedema, and β-blockers to slow the heart rate may be necessary. Endocarditis must be excluded. Antibiotics to prevent recurrence of rheumatic fever should also be considered.

The prognosis of patients with rheumatic mitral valve stenosis is determined mainly by the degree of stenosis, which if severe (< 1.0 cm^2) may result in sudden pulmonary oedema and maternal and fetal distress and death.

Percutaneous mitral valvuloplasty should be considered in suitable patients with important mitral valve stenosis if they develop pulmonary oedema or are likely to do so at any stage during pregnancy, delivery or postpartum. The aim is to treat the mother by relieving pulmonary oedema and restoring optimal placental blood flow. Open surgical valvotomy should ideally be avoided.

Aortic stenosis

This is rare, and is usually due to a congenitally bicuspid valve. Except in severe cases (aortic valve area < 1.0 cm^2), asymptomatic aortic stenosis is usually well tolerated unless the patient is symptomatic at rest or on minimal exertion. A small number of patients experience angina or heart failure, but the severity of the lesion may have been underestimated.

Medical management of symptoms consists of bed rest, oxygen, β-blockers and gentle diuresis for volume overload.

Aortic valvuloplasty may be necessary for tight aortic stenosis, and poses a lower risk than surgical valve replacement. Percutaneous aortic valve replacement performed by experts in a specialist centre may have a role.

Valve replacement should be performed before pregnancy. Pregnancy may result in heart failure in patients with moderate aortic valve stenosis, although maternal mortality in these cases is very unusual.

Pulmonary stenosis

This may be an isolated lesion or part of tetralogy of Fallot. This is usually well tolerated and can be treated if necessary by pulmonary valvuloplasty.

Aortic or mitral regurgitation

Long-standing left heart valve regurgitation lesions do not usually pose a problem until labour and delivery, due to the increase in venous return and systemic vascular resistance. Heart failure may occur in the postpartum period, so GPs should be aware that a woman with either of these lesions may have pulmonary oedema and may need diuretics.

Acute aortic regurgitation may occur in women with Marfan's syndrome or endocarditis. This requires emergency referral to a specialised centre with cardiac surgery and obstetric care for assessment. Valve replacement and repair of the aorta may be necessary.

Tissue prosthetic heart valves

There is no consistent evidence that bioprosthetic heart valves deteriorate more quickly during pregnancy. Management of women with a tissue valve is similar to that of women with a native valve lesion.

Mechanical prosthetic heart valves

Anticoagulation is the main problem in women with a mechanical prosthesis. Thrombosis of the valve is more likely during pregnancy, because the latter is a prothrombotic state, so more frequent monitoring and higher levels of anticoagulation are necessary.

Anticoagulation during pregnancy

Warfarin is teratogenic, particularly in the first trimester, when the risk of the fetus developing an abnormality, including intracerebral haemorrhage, is 5–10%.

Heparin is much less teratogenic because it does not cross the placenta. It is less reliable in reducing the risk of thrombosis, although the risk of thrombosis on an aortic mechanical prosthesis is lower than that on a mitral prosthetic valve.

There is no one method that is clearly superior, although there is a current general view that heparin should be used from week 36 until delivery. The key point is to ensure that the patient is adequately anticoagulated, whichever type of heparin is used. Either continuous intravenous unfractionated heparin through an indwelling central line, or subcutaneous unfractionated or low-molecular-weight heparin is used.

The options for anticoagulation during pregnancy are:
1. heparin for the first trimester, then warfarin until week 36, and then switching back to heparin
2. heparin throughout pregnancy
3. warfarin until week 36, and then heparin.

Cyanotic heart disease

The fall in systemic vascular resistance, particularly during exercise, increases right to left shunting with increasing hypoxaemia. Maternal mortality is 2%. The risk of complications, which include infective endocarditis, heart failure and arrhythmias, is around 30%. The fetal prognosis is poor, with a 50% risk of spontaneous abortion, 40% risk of premature delivery and a high risk of small-for-dates babies. Even in the best centres, the probability of a live birth is only 44%.

Eisenmenger's syndrome

This is a right to left shunt, most commonly due to a large ventricular septal defect. Patients have pulmonary hypertension with equal pressures and resistances in the pulmonary and systemic circulations. At rest the shunt is bidirectional. Exertion decreases the systemic vascular resistance and this increases the right to left shunt, with arterial desaturation and fatigue. The pulmonary blood flow cannot increase with increased exercise and increased demands, so exercise results in increased arterial desaturation due to increased right to left shunting.

The maternal mortality risk is over 50%. Most deaths are due to thromboembolism or pre-eclampsia. Pregnancy should be discouraged, and termination may be necessary.

Echocardiography and Doppler estimation of the pulmonary artery systolic pressure is not accurate. All patients with suspected or known pulmonary hypertension should be referred to a cardiologist.

Fetal assessment

There is a risk of around 10% of congenital heart disease in the fetus of an affected mother. If the mother has a congenital bicuspid aortic valve, the fetal risk of this abnormality is nearly 20%.

The possibility of fetal heart disease should be investigated in pregnant women. Referral to a specialist centre for consideration for termination of pregnancy or early delivery should be undertaken in women at high risk. Survival rates for babies delivered at 32 weeks are high (> 95%), but they are low (< 75%) in babies delivered before 28 weeks.

Management of arrhythmias during pregnancy

Arrhythmias, most commonly atrial and ventricular ectopic beats, are common in healthy people and usually only of importance if they increase during exercise. They may be more frequent during pregnancy, due to haemodynamic, hormonal and emotional factors, particularly in patients with structural heart disease. Important supraventricular and ventricular arrhythmias are rare in healthy pregnant women. Supraventricular arrhythmias may be seen in women who have scarring in their atria from previous surgery.

Specialist referral and 24-hour ECG recordings may be necessary for patients with unpleasant symptoms, or when the diagnosis is in doubt.

Because of the risk of teratogenicity with any drug used during pregnancy, particularly during the first trimester, anti-arrhythmic drugs should be avoided unless the patient has severe symptoms or haemodynamic consequences of the arrhythmia. Most anti-arrhythmic drugs are negatively inotropic and must be used cautiously in patients with impaired cardiac function.

Digoxin may be used to slow the ventricular rate in atrial fibrillation. Disopyramide, metoprolol and verapamil may be used to treat supraventricular arrhythmias. Amiodarone should be used only for important arrhythmias and after other drugs have been tried unsuccessfully. Long-term use may result in neonatal thyroid abnormalities.

Atrioventricular node ablation for frequent haemodynamically significant supraventricular tachycardia may be necessary during pregnancy. Permanent pacemaker implantation for serious symptomatic bradycardia is rarely necessary. Both procedures may be carried out with lead shielding of the uterus and restricted use of X-ray screening.

Infective endocarditis

This is rare during pregnancy. It should be considered in women with predisposing cardiac conditions who develop fatigue, fever, anaemia, heart failure or new murmurs, with signs of emboli. Check the C-reactive protein, the ESR, full blood count and biochemistry. Three sets of blood cultures should be done *before* starting antibiotics. Prompt specialist referral, as soon as the diagnosis is suspected and before antibiotics, is sensible and safe. Patients with infective endocarditis are admitted to hospital and treated with six weeks of antibiotics, with at least two weeks of intravenous antibiotics. Oral antibiotics can be used for the remaining four weeks in patients with streptococcal infections that are sensitive to oral and well tolerated antibiotics. Otherwise, antibiotics are given intravenously for six weeks.

Antibiotic prophylaxis during pregnancy

This is the same as for non-pregnant patients undergoing dental or other potentially septic procedures that are likely to cause a Gram-positive bacteraemia. The guidelines can be found in the *British National Formulary*.

Antibiotic prophylaxis is indicated before surgical delivery and cardiac surgery in all women with valve disease, intracardiac shunts, prosthetic valves and previous endocarditis.

Even though the risk of endocarditis during normal delivery is very low, antibiotic prophylaxis is indicated in women with prosthetic heart valves and shunts and a history of previous endocarditis. It is discretionary for normal delivery in women with rheumatic heart disease and those with mitral regurgitation due to mitral valve prolapse. Gentamicin levels must be checked because of the risks of fetal deafness.

Peripartum cardiomyopathy

This is an uncommon form of dilated cardiomyopathy that is diagnosed by the presence of new heart failure or, less commonly, by emboli or arrhythmias occurring in a previously healthy woman. Patients with pre-existing dilated cardiomyopathy usually deteriorate and present before the last month of pregnancy. Echocardiography is diagnostic, showing a dilated, poorly contracting heart. Most cases resolve, although not necessarily completely, with medical treatment. Severe cases may need to be monitored in intensive care and supported with oxygen, inotropes, an aortic balloon pump and ventricular assist devices. Cardiac transplantation is reserved for the very worst refractory cases, but donor hearts are difficult to obtain.

Patients with persistent symptoms and a dilated heart have a poor prognosis, and further pregnancies are not recommended. There are no guidelines regarding further pregnancies in patients who make a complete recovery. Repeat episodes are possible but unlikely.

Dilated cardiomyopathy

Pregnancy is not recommended in patients with dilated cardiomyopathy, because of the high risk to the mother and fetus. Termination of pregnancy is advised if the left ventricular ejection fraction is < 50% and the heart is dilated. If the patient refuses termination, admission to hospital is recommended for symptomatic patients. Close and regular clinical and echocardiographic monitoring is recommended, and patients should be advised to avoid vigorous exertion.

Hypertrophic cardiomyopathy

The systolic murmur of hypertrophic cardiomyopathy may be first diagnosed during pregnancy and attributed to the pregnancy. The condition is diagnosed by echocardiography and ECG.

Patients without a family history should be reassured that they are at low risk of sudden death. Patients with diastolic impairment are at risk of haemodynamic deterioration if they develop atrial fibrillation, and DC conversion and anticoagulation with heparin are required. Digoxin to control the ventricular rate in atrial fibrillation is contraindicated only if there is a significant left ventricular outflow tract gradient. Transoesophageal echocardiography is used to identify patients with left atrial thrombus prior to cardioversion. Symptomatic patients may be treated with rest, β-blockers and diuretics.

Marfan's syndrome

Marfan's syndrome affects one in 5000 of the population. There is often a family history. It is due to a defect in collagen synthesis and affects the skeleton, eyes and cardiovascular system in 80% of patients.

In its mild form with only trivial mitral valve prolapse, pregnancy and delivery are usually trouble free, with a less than 1% risk of heart failure, infective endocarditis or aortic dissection, although patients should be monitored carefully, particularly during the final trimester and during delivery.

Rarely, in patients with severe mitral regurgitation and those with aortic involvement with a dilated, weakened aortic root, Marfan's syndrome presents a potentially dangerous condition during pregnancy. Patients with severe mitral regurgitation may need mitral valve repair in early pregnancy. The last trimester and particularly delivery, with the associated hypertension, may be hazardous in patients who have significant aortic disease. Death may occasionally occur due to aortic dissection or ruptured aortic aneurysm. β-blockers are used to lower and blunt the systolic pressure surges, and should be continued during pregnancy.

Women with Marfan's syndrome should be referred for a cardiovascular and aortic assessment. The heart, blood pressure and aortic diameter should be assessed and monitored throughout and after pregnancy.

Coarctation of the aorta

Hypertension must be tightly controlled to lower the risk of aortic dissection, aortic rupture or subarachnoid haemorrhage from a berry aneurysm which may be associated with aortic coarctation.

Hypertension may be controlled with verapamil. Atenolol and propranolol have been associated with low birth weight. Diuretics may decrease placental perfusion, and ACE inhibitors are contraindicated. The combination of a thiazide and methyldopa is the safest combination.

Answers to questions about clinical cases

1. The murmur is probably benign and associated with the physiological changes of pregnancy. You should explain this to the patient and discuss the merits of echocardiography, which, if normal, would be reassuring and would provide useful information for her future management.
2. The maternal and fetal prognoses depend on the presence of residual shunt, right ventricular outflow tract obstruction, right and left ventricular function and pulmonary hypertension. This patient will probably be under the care of a cardiologist. Assessment should include her functional class, the precise anatomical and haemodynamic status, and presence of hypoxaemia. Pregnancy risk is low after successful correction of tetralogy of Fallot. If the patient is not already under the care of a cardiologist, she should be referred.
3. This woman should be referred to a centre with the necessary expertise and experience in aortic imaging and blood pressure assessment. Patients with a normal aortic root and no significant cardiac involvement tolerate pregnancy well, and are at low risk. In the presence of aortic root dilatation, there is an increase of approximately 1% in maternal mortality and 20% in fetal mortality. Patients with a significantly dilated root should be advised of the 10% risk of death and offered the option of termination. It is possible that stenting for disease affecting the thoracic aorta may allow pregnancy to continue. β-blockers and rest are advised for all.

4. The risks associated with pregnancy are small. The problems relate to anticoagulation. Warfarin carries a 5% risk of teratogenicity if used in the first trimester, but is the most effective and most convenient form of anticoagulation. Unfractionated heparin does not cross the placenta, and osteoporosis and thrombocytopenia are rare side-effects. Warfarin is recommended during the second and third trimesters, and should be replaced by heparin at week 36 to avoid the risk of neonatal intracranial haemorrhage during delivery. At present low-molecular-weight heparin is not recommended as anticoagulation for pregnant patients with prosthetic valves. The risks of each approach should be explained to the patient.

5. Patients with Eisenmenger's syndrome or severe pulmonary hypertension without septal defects are a very high-risk group and should be strongly advised against pregnancy. Patients who become pregnant and refuse termination face a high risk of death. They should be admitted to hospital in the second trimester for bed rest, oxygen, oximetry, prophylactic heparin and fetal monitoring. These patients should be admitted to a specialist unit with expertise in caring for high-risk patients. Most maternal deaths occur during the postpartum period.

FURTHER READING

Drenthen W, Pieper PG, Roos-Hesselink JW *et al*. Outcome of pregnancy in women with congenital heart disease: a literature review. *J Am Coll Cardiol*. 2007; **49:** 2303–11.

Ginsberg JS, Chan WS, Bates SM *et al*. Anticoagulation of pregnant women with mechanical heart valves: a systematic review of the literature. *Arch Intern Med*. 2003; **163:** 694–8.

Hung L, Rahimtoola SH. Prosthetic heart valves and pregnancy. *Circulation*. 2003; **107:** 1240–6.

Siu SC, Colman JM. Heart disease and pregnancy. *Heart*. 2001; **85:** 710–15.

Siu SC, Sermer M, Colman JM *et al*. for the Cardiac Disease in Pregnancy (CARPREG) Investigators. Prospective multicenter study of pregnancy outcomes in women with heart disease. *Circulation*. 2001; **104:** 515–21.

Stout KK, Otto CM. Pregnancy in women with valvular heart disease. *Heart*. 2007; **93:** 552–8.

Task Force on the Management of Cardiovascular Diseases during Pregnancy of the European Society of Cardiology. Expert consensus document on management of cardiovascular diseases during pregnancy. *Eur Heart J*. 2003; **24:** 761–81.

Thorne SA. Pregnancy in heart disease. *Heart*. 2004; **90:** 450–6.

World Health Organization. *The World Health Report 2005: make every mother and child count*. Geneva: World Health Organization; 2005.

Sexual problems in men with cardiac conditions

FOURTEEN

Clinical cases

1. A 55-year-old man who sustained a myocardial infarction six months ago is depressed and having marital problems. What do you do?
2. A recently married couple in their seventies come to see you together. The wife is worried about starting a sexual relationship with her husband, because her previous husband died of a heart attack. What do you do?
3. A 74-year-old man develops symptoms of prostatism and impotence and is worried that the two conditions are related. What do you do?

Erectile dysfunction

This is defined as the inability to achieve and maintain an erection sufficient to permit satisfactory intercourse.

Prevalence

Some degree of erectile dysfunction is thought to affect around 50% of all men over the age of 40 years. However, this may be an underestimate because men may be embarrassed to discuss what they consider to be a personal and private matter unrelated to their heart problem.

Role of the GP in management

The willingness of men to discuss their sexual problems depends on their age, culture, religion, upbringing, marital status, the impact the problem has on their life and also their understanding of the problem and its causes. To some men it may be an occasional, irrelevant inconvenience, whereas to others it may be a major concern and source of misery. Some men may view it as a natural part of life, like balding. Older men, who may be embarking on a new relationship, may find it a major impediment to an enjoyable and fulfilling life.

It is important that GPs offer patients (particularly those with risk factors for erectile dysfunction) and their partners the opportunity to discuss erectile dysfunction in the same way as one might ask routinely about angina or breathlessness. The GP plays an important role in educating patients about the condition and reassuring them about the increasing success of treatment. These consultations demand skill and sensitivity, but are rewarded with immense gratitude from patients.

The GP's unique insight into the patient's medical and social history and domestic situation enables them to provide helpful individualised advice on the management of this common condition.

Over the last few years men have become less reticent about discussing this problem with their GP. The social stigma attached to erectile dysfunction is being gradually replaced by an understanding of the unfortunate impact it has on quality of life for the patient and his partner. This has been brought about by the efficacy and popularity of Viagra and newer related preparations and the endorsement by the NHS of the use of this treatment in certain conditions, together with greater public awareness and discussion in the media and in GP surgeries about the condition.

Risk factors for erectile dysfunction

These are similar to the risk factors for cardiovascular disease. Erectile dysfunction is more common in individuals who smoke, or who have hypertension, diabetes or hyperlipidaemia. Urological, neurological, hormonal and other medical causes, including diabetes and adverse side-effects of drugs, should be investigated and excluded.

Depression, anxiety, psychological disorders, marital conflict and work problems are other common causes and also consequences of erectile dysfunction. Patients should be referred to the relevant specialist. Cardiovascular causes should be considered after other causes have been excluded.

The association of sexual dysfunction with cardiovascular disease

A primary objective of the treatment of cardiac conditions is to allow patients of all ages to live a contented and fully active life. Sexual activity is considered by patients to be an important part of their life and something they wish to continue. Primary care clinicians should question patients about sexual activity in the same way as they might enquire about exercise, diet and other components of lifestyle in patients with cardiovascular disease. GPs should appreciate that some patients are unwilling to discuss these matters, or feel uncomfortable about doing so.

Erectile dysfunction is common in men aged over 60 years, particularly after myocardial infarction and cardiac surgery. It adversely affects their quality of life and self-esteem, and may be an important cause of marital conflict and depression, both of which are improved after successful treatment.

Sexual dysfunction and cardiovascular disease are commonly associated with each other. Erectile dysfunction is understandably common in men during and after any illness or hospitalisation.

Most men with erectile dysfunction have one or more cardiovascular risk factors, particularly diabetes, hypertension and hyperlipidaemia. It is possible that cardiovascular risk factors are as relevant in patients with erectile dysfunction as they are in the development of coronary artery disease, although a causal relationship is not as firmly established. Sexual dysfunction may be a marker of subclinical cardiovascular disease. The vigorous treatment of cardiovascular risk factors is fundamental to the management of both conditions.

Sexual activity as a trigger of acute cardiac conditions

Sexual activity is generally safe and is encouraged as part of a normal healthy lifestyle in male and female patients with heart disease.

Cardiac symptoms, including breathlessness and angina, acute decompensation of heart failure, acute coronary syndromes and acute myocardial infarction (and, more tragically, sudden death) may be experienced for the first time during sexual activity. Increases in heart rate and systolic blood pressure during intercourse lead to a sudden increase in myocardial oxygen demand, and theoretically can trigger atheromatous plaque rupture and infarction. Sudden decreases in heart rate and blood pressure result in sudden reductions in coronary blood flow and myocardial oxygen supply, and can trigger angina.

Left ventricular work and myocardial oxygen consumption are determined by the product of heart rate and systolic blood pressure during peak exertion. This can be reduced by modifying the mechanics and dynamics of sexual activity.

Is sexual activity dangerous in cardiac patients?

Sexual activity is safe in the majority of cardiac patients. It is contraindicated only in high-risk patients, who can usually be identified clinically without the need for cardiac investigations.

Cardiac risk associated with sexual activity and medication for erectile dysfunction

The annual risk of myocardial infarction in a healthy man is 1%. This increases to a risk of 1.01% as a result of sexual activity, and this risk increases 10-fold to 1.1% in a man with coronary heart disease, which is equivalent to 20 chances in a million.

Patients at low cardiac risk

These include individuals with controlled hypertension, mild angina, full recovery and no or minimal symptoms after myocardial revascularisation, full recovery two weeks after myocardial infarction and non-significant valvular disease. Patients at low risk (i.e. those who are able to run up two flights of stairs or able to complete 12 minutes of the Bruce treadmill protocol or the WHO cycle protocol without symptoms or ischaemia, and who have a normal haemodynamic response) can be safely encouraged to resume or continue full, unrestricted sexual activity.

Most patients with erectile dysfunction and cardiovascular disease are in the low-risk group.

Patients at high cardiac risk

These include individuals recovering from recent (less than one week previously) myocardial infarction, severe heart failure, recent (less than two months previously) sternotomy for cardiac surgery in order to avoid compression or rotation strain to the sternum and costochondral joints, cardiac conditions resulting in severe breathlessness and/or angina during intercourse (e.g. unstable angina, decompensated heart failure, obstructive cardiomyopathy, severe aortic stenosis), uncontrolled hypertension and significant arrhythmias, including bradycardia (which can be induced during a Valsalva manoeuvre) or atrial fibrillation (due to sudden increases in blood pressure).

These patients require cardiac review, particularly of their cardiovascular risk factors and medication, and they may require specialist referral and further investigations.

Giving advice about sexual activity in primary care

It is helpful if someone in the practice is interested in and able to discuss these matters with patients and their partners, who are often too embarrassed to initiate the discussion directly.

There are few hospital-based specialists, particularly with an understanding of the cardiac aspects of the problem, in the UK. There remains a need for trained personnel to provide an integrated service in this field. Sexual matters for patients, particularly for those with cardiac conditions, are as important as other lifestyle issues and should be given equal consideration and care.

Their treatment and cardiovascular risk factors should be reviewed, and patients with angina and/or heart failure may need specialist review.

Both the patient and his partner may feel understandably anxious about the possible dangers of sexual intercourse, and may ask for advice directly or hint at it during the consultation. Primary care clinicians should be willing to discuss this openly, sympathetically and constructively, as with any clinical problem. It is important that after the cause of erectile dysfunction has been identified, primary care staff try to enhance and restore the emotional well-being and quality of life of the patient. Coexisting depression should be managed appropriately. These matters may also be discussed in conjunction with secondary prevention and lifestyle modification in a cardiac rehabilitation clinic.

Patients and their partners often want to know when it is safe to resume sexual relationships after a heart attack, angioplasty or heart surgery. It is difficult to generalise, and it depends on a number of factors, including the age of the patient and his partner, the haemodynamic status of the patient and the presence or absence of ischaemia. Patients at low risk are generally young, with normal or near normal left ventricular function and no reversible ischaemia more than two weeks after an uncomplicated infarct. Patients with significant left ventricular impairment and/or known coronary artery disease should be referred to a cardiologist for assessment, including an exercise test. The GP should be prepared to discuss sexual practice with those patients who want further detailed advice.

Drug-induced erectile dysfunction

This is common and well recognised with β-blockers and thiazide diuretics, and less commonly with statins. Patients may feel convinced that they became impotent only after they started a certain drug. The side-effects of the drug should be researched. If there are no reports that impotence is a recognised adverse effect, it may be necessary to withdraw the incriminated drug and ask the patient whether their symptoms have improved after a week or so. If their sexual function has improved and they are willing, they should be rechallenged with the drug. Recurrent symptoms suggest a drug side-effect, which is generally related to the class of drug rather than idiosyncratic reactions.

Drug withdrawal and rechallenge is probably not necessary if the problem started before taking β-blockers. Drug withdrawal may be necessary when patients with heart failure or hypertension are on ACE inhibitors (which are known to cause erectile dysfunction) or angiotensin II antagonists which are an important component of their treatment and for which there are no other classes of drug with similar benefits.

Phosphodiesterase type 5 (PDE5) inhibitors in erectile dysfunction

These drugs inhibit the breakdown of cyclic GMP and improve the rigidity and duration of erections. So long as they are prescribed and used according to the manufacturer's recommendations, they are safe in patients with stable coronary artery disease. They are successful in over 80% of cases.

PDE5 inhibitors are contraindicated in patients who are taking nitrates or nicorandil (because of the risk of potentiating important hypotension) and in those in whom sexual activity is inadvisable. They should be used with caution in patients who are taking doxazocin. Around 80% of patients with cardiovascular disease who are taking PDE5 inhibitors are at low cardiac risk and therefore unlikely to be taking long-acting nitrates.

PDE5 inhibitors may be given together with β-blockers and ACE inhibitors.

Sildenafil (Viagra)

A full review of the cause of the patient's erectile dysfunction and medication is required before starting sildenafil. It is otherwise safe for the vast majority of patients with cardiovascular disease. It is not indicated for use in women.

This drug has had a major impact in the treatment of erectile dysfunction, and is generally safe in most cardiac and hypertensive patients. It is a vasodilator and results in a reduction in blood pressure. There are no other important interactions, and it is not contraindicated with antihypertensive drugs. The most common side-effects are headache and facial flushing in around 10% of patients.

The recommended dose is 50 mg (25 mg in the elderly) to be taken one hour before sexual activity. It is effective 30 minutes after taking it and lasts for 4–6 hours. The recommended maximum dose is 100 mg. Further information can be found on the drug data sheet.

Other newer compounds

Tadalafil and vardenafil are similar in structure to sildenafil, and the trial data show them to be as safe as placebo, with no excess cardiovascular mortality compared with age-matched controls or placebo.

The duration of onset, action and efficacy of vardenafil are similar to those of sildenafil. Tadalafil has a longer half-life, and its action may last for over 36 hours.

Advice for patients

✧ We consider that your sexual health is as important as any other aspect of your health, so please do not feel embarrassed or uncomfortable about discussing this with us. If there is a particular doctor or nurse you would like to discuss this with, please let us know.
✧ Impotence in men may be a sign of heart disease, and we may need to do some tests.
✧ Adopting a healthy lifestyle may help people with impotence.
✧ Viagra and other drugs like it are effective in the majority of patients with impotence.
✧ If you or your partner are worried that having sex might be dangerous to you, come and talk to us. Usually sex is not dangerous except in people with very severe heart problems.
✧ There are several causes of impotence, including stress and anxiety, which can make it worse. All potential factors need to be considered, and we are happy to help.

Answers to questions about clinical cases

1. It is important to be sure of this patient's precise symptoms. If he is impotent, there are several possible causes. He might require more than one consultation, but will need time, sympathy and understanding and possibly psychological and marital counselling. It is important to exclude angina and heart failure, possibly with further cardiac tests, and to review his cardiovascular risk factors and medication, and optimise his secondary prevention. If he is taking β-blockers these may need to be stopped or the dose reduced.
2. If the husband has no erectile dysfunction and no cardiac problem, he is at low risk of having a cardiac problem during sexual activity. If necessary, he could be prescribed Viagra.
3. This patient will need a full medical assessment and should be referred to a urologist to exclude a primary urological problem.

FURTHER READING

Carrier S, Brock G, Kour NW *et al.* Pathophysiology of erectile dysfunction. *Urology*. 1993; **42:** 468–81.

DeBusk R, Drory Y, Goldstein I *et al.* Management of sexual dysfunction in patients with cardiovascular disease: recommendations of the Princeton Consensus Panel. *Am J Cardiol.* 2000; **86:** 175–81.

Lue TF. Erectile dysfunction. *NEJM.* 2000; **342:** 1802–13.

Congenital heart disease

FIFTEEN

Clinical cases

1. You hear a systolic murmur in a previously fit teenage boy with a chest infection. What do you do?
2. A woman who is pregnant for the first time comes to see you for a routine prenatal check at 16 weeks. She is concerned that her sister gave birth to a baby with congenital heart disease, and wants reassurance. What do you do?
3. A 47-year-old woman who had an atrial septal defect successfully repaired 10 years previously forgot to ask her gynaecologist whether she needed antibiotics before a D & C. What do you advise her to do?
4. A 53-year-old woman comes to see you complaining of chest pain, which you feel is not related to her heart, but you hear a loud systolic murmur. She was told that she was born with a hole in the heart but did not have an operation. What do you do?
5. A 19-year-old woman with a ventricular septal defect presents with tiredness and a fever. What do you do?

Prevalence and diagnosis of congenital heart disease

The prevalence of congenital heart disease overall is eight per 1000 live births. Ventricular septal defects account for 30% of all cases, atrial septal defects account for 10% and patent ductus arteriosus accounts for 10%. The other common forms of congenital heart disease are aortic stenosis, pulmonary stenosis, coarctation of the aorta, and tetralogy of Fallot. Other cardiac malformations occur infrequently and will be seen only rarely in primary care. Mitral valve prolapse is considered to be a variant of normal mitral valve anatomy and not a form of congenital heart disease.

Not all affected babies survive to infancy, so there would be less than 80 patients with congenital heart disease in a general practice with 8000 patients. Due to the success of paediatric cardiology and cardiac surgery over the last 30 years, there will soon be more adults than children with congenital heart disease.

Prenatal diagnosis of congenital heart disease

Fetal echocardiography (at 16–18 weeks), magnetic resonance imaging and computerised tomography are used alone or in combination to diagnose affected babies in mothers at risk during pregnancy. Mothers with babies at risk from Down's syndrome should be investigated with amniocentesis. Some congenital heart defects may be corrected *in utero*, while others are corrected in the neonatal period.

Optimal long-term survival and quality of life are achieved by early diagnosis and intervention for patients with simple shunt lesions or single obstructive valvular lesions.

Genetic counselling

The risk of congenital heart disease in a baby born to a couple where one of the partners has a congenital heart defect is in the range 2–50%. Genetic counselling should be offered to couples, and this is available in specialised centres. Single-gene disorders (Marfan's syndrome and congenital forms of hypertrophic cardiomyopathy) have the highest recurrence rates.

Drugs with teratogenic effects include ACE inhibitors, angiotensin II receptor antagonists, warfarin and amiodarone. Drugs should be avoided in pregnancy unless they are absolutely necessary.

Organisation of care

Some patients are appropriately managed with care shared between a paediatric cardiologist and the GP. The management and follow-up of patients with complex congenital heart disease demand the skills and experience of regional paediatric cardiological centres and grown-up congenital heart disease units. There are also centres that specialise in the care of patients over 16 years of age, an increasingly large group known as Grown-Up Congenital Heart Disease (GUCH). These are regional centres, staffed by multi-disciplinary teams, which have facilities for invasive diagnosis, intervention and cardiac surgery, and some centres provide heart transplantation.

Patients with known congenital heart disease should, depending on their age, be referred to the relevant centre for long-term monitoring. Similarly, patients with suspected undiagnosed congenital heart disease should be referred for evaluation. All patients with significant congenital heart disease will be followed up by a major centre. Most GPs in the UK would have no more than one or two patients with congenital heart disease on their lists.

Educational role of primary care clinicians in the management of patients with congenital heart disease

Primary care physicians should educate and remind patients with congenital heart disease about their condition and their future prospects. Patients should be reminded about the importance of excellent dental and oral hygiene, regular visits to a dentist, and antibiotic prophylaxis before undergoing potentially septic procedures. The *British National Formulary* provides this information, and where there is doubt GPs should contact the patient's consultant cardiologist. Antibiotic prophylaxis is recommended for all patients with congenital heart disease except those with isolated secundum atrial septal defect, and after successful repaired atrial and ventricular septal defects and patent ductus arteriosus.

Patients may also need to know about insurance issues. Those with small atrial and ventricular septal defects, repaired ventricular septal defects, and correction of pulmonary stenosis should be insurable at normal rates. Insurance premiums may be higher or unobtainable for patients with more complex forms of congenital heart disease (e.g. tetralogy of Fallot), and after surgery for correction of transposition of the great arteries.

Patients with cyanotic congenital heart disease should be educated about the dangers of dehydration, and advised that they have a tendency to bleed due to a reduced platelet count, and that the coagulation pathways may be abnormal. They are at risk from infection, commonly in adolescence from acne, and good gum and dental hygiene is important. They should have an annual flu jab and vaccination against pneumonia.

Contraception

The risk of pregnancy must be weighed against the risk of contraception. The patient should choose her personally preferred method.

Barrier methods are preferred for compliant couples under 35 years of age.

The low-dose-oestrogen combined oral contraceptive is effective, but is contraindicated if there is an appreciable risk of paradoxical embolisation (cyanosis, atrial fibrillation/flutter).

Medroxyprogesterone, levonorgestrel or progesterone-only pills are less effective than the combined oral contraceptive, and are associated with fluid retention, depression and breakthrough bleeding.

There are risks associated with surgical sterilisation, but this may be the method of choice.

Antibiotics should be given at the time of insertion of intrauterine devices. They are not the method of choice in women who have not been pregnant.

Risk factors for congenital heart disease

The causes of congenital heart disease are unclear, but are thought to involve genetic and environmental factors during formation of the heart, including:

◇ maternal rubella
◇ alcohol abuse
◇ lithium
◇ certain drugs
◇ radiation
◇ congenital heart disease in the mother
◇ congenital heart disease in a previous pregnancy or in a first-degree relative.

Congenital heart disease in infancy

Causes

The principal causes of heart failure in infancy are age related:

◇ newborn small preterm – persistent patent ductus arteriosus
◇ full-term newborn – hypoplastic left heart, coarctation of the aorta
◇ over two weeks – ventricular and atrial septal defects.

Presentation

Feeding difficulties, failure to put on weight, a fast pulse rate and a fast respiratory rate are serious signs, and the infant should be referred urgently to hospital.

Ventricular septal defect

This is the most common congenital cardiac abnormality in infants and children, account-ing for 30% of all cases of congenital heart disease and occurring equally frequently in boys and girls. A large proportion of defects close spontaneously, completely or partially, within the first year of life, leaving the patient symptom-free but with a loud systolic murmur and a risk of endocarditis, for which they should receive prophylactic antibiotics.

Closure of the defect in patients with an insignificant shunt is not necessary, and their prognosis is good because there is a minimal increase in pulmonary blood flow. Follow-up is advisable.

Patients with a persistent significant ventricular septal defect present in the first year of life with congestive heart failure and a harsh systolic murmur, which necessitates recognition and urgent referral to a specialist centre where echocardiography will provide the diagnosis. Closure of the defect by either surgical repair or a double umbrella device is necessary to avoid the risk of pulmonary hypertension, which reverses the shunt (Eisenmenger's syndrome).

Atrial septal defect

This accounts for one-third of cases of congenital heart disease in adults, and is three times more common in females. It may occur with other cardiac abnormalities, particularly mitral valve prolapse and mitral regurgitation. It usually presents either in childhood or in adults, and is commonly associated with Down's syndrome.

Symptoms depend on the size of the defect and its haemodynamic consequences. The left to right shunt across the interatrial septum results in increased pulmonary blood flow with gradually progressive pulmonary hypertension, dilatation of the atria, right ventricle and pulmonary arteries, right heart failure and atrial fibrillation. It is an uncommon cause of palpitation, breathlessness or unexplained stroke in young adults.

The diagnosis may not be made until adulthood because most patients remain symptom free until their thirties. Affected individuals are vulnerable to heart failure and stroke by their fifties. Atrial septal defect is diagnosed by clinical findings of fixed splitting of the second heart sound, chest X-ray showing large pulmonary vessels, ECG and echocardiography.

Uncomplicated atrial septal defects should ideally be diagnosed and closed in childhood, or before adulthood if possible, percutaneously with an umbrella device in a specialist centre. Surgical closure is otherwise effective and carries a low risk of around 1%. Successful closure before the development of pulmonary hypertension results in a normal life expectancy. Surgical closure of atrial septal defects in symptomatic adults over the age of 40 years with significant left to right shunts results in a better survival and exercise tolerance compared to medical treatment, but does not reduce the risk of stroke or the risk of development or persistence of atrial fibrillation. Patients with symptomatic atrial flutter or fibrillation should be managed as discussed in Chapter 11. Closure is too late once pulmonary hypertension occurs. The decision to close atrial septal defects in symptom-free adults is controversial, but with advances in low-risk, percutaneous umbrella-device closure, many specialist units believe that this will prevent symptomatic deterioration in the long term. Long-term cardiological follow-up is recommended for patients with unclosed atrial septal defects, and for those patients in whom closure was performed in adulthood. Antibiotic prophylaxis against infective endocarditis is not recommended for patients with atrial septal defect (repaired or unrepaired) unless there is an associated valve abnormality.

Patent foramen ovale

This is found in 25% of the normal population. Approximately 10–40% of strokes have no obvious cause, and 50% of these are thought to be due to a patent foramen ovale. It is diagnosed by transoesophageal echocardiogram. Although it is not yet clear whether all of these lesions should be closed, the safety and ease of percutaneous closure provide an attractive method of reducing the risk of stroke. In the UK, this procedure is mainly performed by paediatric interventional cardiologists.

Patent ductus arteriosus

The ductus arteriosus connects the descending aorta, distal to the origin of the left subclavian artery, to the main pulmonary artery trunk at the origin of the left pulmonary artery. In the fetus, it allows arterial blood to bypass the unexpanded lungs and enter the descending aorta for oxygenation in the placenta.

Normally, it closes spontaneously shortly after birth. Non-closure of a patent ductus accounts for 10% of cases of congenital heart disease. The persistent left to right shunt leads to pulmonary hypertension, right heart failure and a high mortality in the first year of life.

Most patients should be diagnosed shortly after birth with echocardiography. The classical sign is a systolic and diastolic 'machinery murmur'. The duct can be closed using percutaneous catheter techniques, or ligated in infancy conferring a normal prognosis. A patent ductus is diagnosed rarely in adults. Closure is recommended in adults with a murmur, because of the risks of endarteritis and heart failure. Closure is not recommended in patients without a murmur, because the patient may have already developed Eisenmenger's syndrome or the shunt may be too small and pose a negligible risk of endarteritis and heart failure.

Life expectancy is normal with a small patent ductus, but carries a risk of endocarditis. Large shunts may lead to left ventricular failure and flow reversal. Survival is possible without closure, but patients experience breathlessness and palpitation in adulthood, and are at risk of developing infective endarteritis and endocarditis and heart failure in adulthood. Death occurs in one-third of patients with a persistent ductus by the age of 40 years, and in two-thirds by the age of 60 years.

Therefore, closure or ligation is recommended for even a small patent ductus.

Eisenmenger's syndrome

Originally described by the German physician Victor Eisenmenger in 1897, Eisenmenger's syndrome signifies obstruction to blood flow in the lungs, with shunting of deoxygenated blood into the systemic circulation. It develops in a variety of types of congenital heart disease, including atrial septal and ventricular septal defects, patent ductus arteriosus, nearly 50% of patients with Down's syndrome, and less common congenital heart conditions. Initially and until childhood, oxygenated blood flows from the left side of the circulation into the lung arteries. After several years, the resistance in the lung arteries increases as the small vessels in the lungs get thicker and the very small lung arteries block off. As the resistance in the lung circulation increases, this causes increasing pressure in the lung arteries. The right ventricle, which unlike the left ventricle is not able to cope with high pressures, soon fails. This causes a fall in cardiac output, and the patient dies soon after the right ventricle begins to decompensate. The flow of blood is reversed from the left to the right when the vascular resistance in the lungs exceeds that in the systemic arteries. With reversal of the blood flow (shunting from right to left), the patient becomes cyanosed and develops finger clubbing.

At rest and particularly with exertion, patients become breathless, tired, and more cyanosed and hypoxic. Although gentle exercise is recommended, vigorous exercise can be dangerous. The increased blood flow to the arm and leg muscles reduces the systemic vascular resistance, and increases the cardiac output and the right ventricular pressure. This may result in sudden right ventricular failure with a sudden and catastrophic fall in cardiac output.

Complications of Eisenmenger's syndrome include bleeding disorders, atrial fibrillation, syncope, stroke, transient ischaemic attacks, renal dysfunction and angina. Such complications usually affect patients after the age of 30 years. Congestive heart failure is a serious, usually end-stage complication that occurs in patients in their forties. Around 40% of patients survive into their forties. Most patients die suddenly as a result of a sudden fall in cardiac output, which may be induced by ventricular fibrillation related to hypoxia.

Chronic cyanosis causes increased red blood cell metabolism and calcium bilirubinate gallstones. Gout is common, due to raised uric acid levels. Hyperviscosity of the blood causes blurred vision, headaches, myalgia and fatigue.

Surgical correction and transplantation are of little value. The aim of management is to educate the patient and their family to reduce risk. Influenza vaccination is important.

Phlebotomy is not necessary (in contrast to the situation in polycythaemia rubra vera) unless patients have symptoms due to hyperviscosity.

The principles of management of patients with Eisenmenger's syndrome are as follows:

✧ Avoid dehydration.
✧ Avoid iron deficiency from 'routine' phlebotomy, which does not prevent transient ischaemic attacks or stroke.
✧ Any form of surgery and general anaesthesia is high risk.

✧ Prevent and treat chest infections.
✧ Pregnancy is high risk. Contraception should be offered and discussed.

Heart–lung transplantation is rarely performed because of the lack of donor organs. Less than 50% of the patients who have lung transplantation and repair of the heart malformation survive for four years after surgery. The one- and 10-year survival rates after heart and lung transplantation are 70% and 30%, respectively.

Pregnancy and general anaesthesia for all but life-saving operations are hazardous and contraindicated. All infections should be treated vigorously, and patients should be referred to hospital for all but minor coughs and colds, which respond quickly to antibiotics.

Bosentan, the non-selective endothelin antagonist used in pulmonary arterial hypertension, has been shown to improve haemodynamics and exercise performance by reducing pulmonary vascular resistance. This drug can only be prescribed in special centres. There are other drugs (other endothelin antagonists, phosphodiesterase-5 inhibitors and prostanoids), which can be used in combination, which may improve symptoms and slow down the progression of this condition.

Coarctation of the aorta

This is a fibro-muscular narrowing of the descending aorta in the region of the ductus distal to the left subclavian artery. It occurs in 0.4 per 1000 live births, and is much more common in males. It is associated with a bicuspid aortic valve, patent ductus arteriosus, ventricular septal defect, Turner's syndrome and aneurysms of the circle of Willis.

The presentation and prognosis vary according to age. Neonates, even after repair, have a worse prognosis than children and adults. Coarctation of the aorta may be detected in the first week of life in a breathless, pale neonate with a history of poor feeding and absent foot pulses due to reduced or absent blood flow through the coarct. Urgent referral is necessary because the coarct restricts blood flow down the aorta, leading to increased left ventricular afterload and heart failure. Prostaglandin infusion to re-establish patency of the ductus may be life-saving. Even with prompt intervention and repair of the coarct using either angioplasty or surgical intervention, patients remain at risk from premature atherosclerosis, hypertension and premature death.

The older child or adult may be symptom-free with upper limb hypertension and leg claudication with absent or diminished foot pulses. The 25-year survival rate is 80% when the coarct is repaired in childhood.

In adults, coarctation may present as hypertension, aortic dissection, heart failure, aortic stenosis, infective endocarditis, and premature coronary artery and cerebrovascular disease. Pregnant women with aortic coarctation are at high risk of aortic dissection.

The ECG may be normal and the chest X-ray abnormal in severe cases. Doppler echocardiography, CT scanning and magnetic resonance imaging of the aorta provide information on its location and severity. Long-term survival is optimised with repair performed in childhood. Hypertension persists in 50% of patients if repair is performed after the age of 40 years, when the 15-year survival rate is only 50%.

Surgical repair is performed if the transcoarct gradient exceeds 30 mmHg, but restenosis occurs in 30% of adults after surgical resection. Restenosis and aortic aneurysm repair are more frequent after angioplasty, which is currently used mainly for restenosis occurring after surgery.

After repair of the coarct, patients remain at risk from complications of hypertension, which may be difficult to control, and should have long-term follow-up to monitor blood pressure and signs of heart failure. Two-thirds of patients over the age of 40 years with uncorrected coarctation have heart failure. Around 75% die by the age of 50 years, and 90% die by the age of 60 years.

Advice for patients

✧ Congenital heart disease means that the affected person was born with an abnormality in the way their heart is formed. This may, for example, be a hole in the heart that connects the two collecting chambers or the two pumping chambers, a narrowed or leaking heart valve, or a problem with the main vessels that come out of the heart.

✧ Heart defects occur in eight per 1000 deliveries. Half of these have a mild abnormality which usually does not need surgery or medical treatment.

✧ The cause of congenital heart disease remains unclear. Congenital heart disease is more common in babies whose mother or close family relative has congenital heart disease, or has taken anticonvulsants, lithium, cocaine or excessive alcohol, or had rubella, HIV or toxoplasmosis during pregnancy.

✧ Advances in prenatal diagnosis, keyhole surgery and corrective surgery have improved the outcome of babies born with heart defects.

✧ Congenital heart disease may be diagnosed before birth by ultrasound examination of the baby's heart in the womb (fetal echocardiography).

✧ Babies with congenital heart disease are usually referred and, depending on the condition, followed up by a cardiologist who specialises in congenital heart disease.

Answers to questions about clinical cases

1. The murmur may be innocent and/or related to the chest infection. Other possibilities include congenital aortic stenosis, ventricular septal defect, mitral valve prolapse and other structural congenital heart disease. The boy and his parents should be advised that an echocardiogram may be necessary if the murmur is still present when he is re-examined after the chest infection has resolved.

2. This patient is at risk and should be referred to a paediatric cardiac unit for assessment, including fetal echocardiography.

3. Antibiotic prophylaxis is not necessary after successful closure of an atrial septal defect.

4. It would be helpful to have all of this patient's previous notes. If she has been generally fit and well, the murmur is most probably due to a small, restrictive, residual and harmless ventricular septal defect, and she has a good prognosis. She should have antibiotic prophylaxis. An echocardiogram should be performed if this has not been done within a year, to confirm the diagnosis and exclude associated valve abnormalities.

5. The history and examination are important. If there is any suspicion that this patient could have infective endocarditis, she should have two sets of blood cultures before antibiotics are given. If she is unwell, she should be referred to her cardiac centre for evaluation. You should speak to the cardiologist and the infectious disease team. Most defects put patients at lifelong risk of endocarditis. Low-risk defects include secundum atrial septal defect, ventricular septal defect after closure, pulmonary valve stenosis or a small patent ductus arteriosus.

FURTHER READING

Deanfield J, Hoffman A, Kaemmerer H *et al.* ESC guidelines on the management of grown-up congenital heart disease. *Eur Heart J.* 2003; **24:** 1035–84.

Heart disease in the elderly

SIXTEEN

Clinical cases

1. A 79-year-old man had a myocardial infarction four years ago. He had a total cholesterol level of 5.3 mmol/l and an LDL-cholesterol level of 2.9 mmol/l. His wife has told him that he should take a statin, but he is not keen to do so. What do you advise him?
2. An 85-year-old woman has been falling and has swollen ankles. She cannot remember why she falls, but her carer tells you that she is 'not with it' for several minutes after the fall. What do you do?
3. A 69-year-old man has claudication. He smokes and cannot stop. He is getting rest pain. What do you do?
4. An 87-year-old woman asks you to visit her at home because recently she has been unable to get out of bed and has been confused. What are the likely causes?
5. A 76-year-old man whom you have not seen for a year and who has had severe hip and back pain comes to see you. He is unwell, and the blood tests show that he has an estimated glomerular filtration rate (eGFR) of 28. What do you do?

What is old age?

With an increasing proportion of the population living and working for longer, and hoping and expecting that their retirement years will be enjoyable and active, primary care clinicians need to understand how increasing age affects the cardiovascular system and how medical advances can be applied appropriately and safely to benefit elderly patients.

> Old age should not be defined simply by a number, but by the individual's biological and psychological state, which determines their prognosis, lifestyle and view of their future.

There is no general agreement on an age watershed that identifies an elderly patient. Thirty years ago, people over 65 years of age were categorised as 'geriatric.' In some hospitals they were often excluded from major surgery and were rarely admitted to the intensive-care unit. Nowadays, cardiac surgery, particularly aortic valve replacement and complex, high-risk coronary artery surgery, is performed in patients aged over 80 years. Cardiovascular prevention is relevant and appropriate in all but the very elderly.

The current medical literature categorises people over 80 years of age as elderly. The proportion of the population aged over 80 years is increasing rapidly, and represents the fastest-growing segment of the population, accounting for 11% of those over 60 years of age worldwide. An 80-year-old has a life expectancy of approximately eight years.

General principles of cardiology management in the elderly

The most appropriate clinical management necessitates a comprehensive evaluation of the patient's clinical state, an accurate diagnosis of all their medical conditions, and an understanding of their social circumstances.

Interventions are undertaken mainly for symptomatic reasons in the elderly. The history is therefore of great importance, but is not always easy (and is sometimes impossible) to obtain.

The investigation and treatment of common symptoms (breathlessness, chest discomfort, dizzy turns, falls, loss of consciousness, feeling light-headed, and palpitations) depend largely on the cause of the problem and the impact that it has on the patient's life and their ability to do what they would like to do.

The management of nearly all cardiac conditions in the elderly is similar to that for younger adults. The risk–benefit ratio is more finely balanced, particularly in prevention. Operative procedures (angioplasty, cardiac surgery, and ablation of arrhythmias) are technically more difficult and risky in the elderly because of co-morbidities (e.g. atherosclerosis, renal impairment, cerebrovascular disease, diabetes) and less robust tissue. Drug side-effects are more likely due to reduced renal excretion and impaired gastrointestinal and hepatic function.

Our patients are getting older, so primary care clinicians and cardiologists need to learn how best to manage the 'whole patient', taking into consideration their general health, lifestyle, and their own wishes and those of their family.

> Increasing age should not be a barrier to investigation and treatment. All potential risks and benefits of all medical and surgical interventions should be carefully considered and discussed with the patient and their family.
> Drugs should be started at low doses and increased slowly with careful monitoring, because of reduced renal function.

Cardiovascular prevention in the elderly

Most major coronary events and coronary deaths occur after the age of 65 years. Around 50% of men aged over 65 years will have at least a 20% 10-year risk of a cardiovascular event. This risk is much higher in patients aged over 80 years. Therefore, the elderly have a lot to gain, both symptomatically and (depending on the condition) prognostically, from prevention and treatment of cardiac conditions. This also applies to smoking cessation and treatment of hypertension.

Statins, aspirin and treatment of hypertension improve symptoms of angina and also improve the prognosis in some patients.

There is little evidence for statins in primary prevention in the elderly, because it is unlikely that lipid lowering alone would significantly increase the lifespan of a 90-year-old person. However, by stabilising an ulcerated unstable atheromatous plaque, statins may theoretically improve the short-term prognosis of a 90-year-old patient with an acute coronary syndrome. There is less reticence about using statins in patients with vascular disease or multiple risk factors. In general, statins and other preventive treatments are underused in the elderly.

The patient's perspective in clinical management decisions

Each elderly patient will have a different and personal perspective of what they expect and hope to achieve from the remainder of their life. They know what they are willing to put up with in terms of disability and symptoms. When they are ill and in need of an operation or simply a tablet, they will have to decide whether their symptoms, and the impact that the condition has on their lifestyle, merit the risks and side-effects of the proposed intervention. Some patients may not want to stop smoking or change their diet even though they understand that changing their lifestyle might help them to live longer.

Communicating with the patient

Explaining clinical problems and the risks and benefits of treatments in simple terms, and in a way that the patient understands, is often difficult and sometimes impossible. Clear communication necessitates empathy, patience and an understanding of the patient's culture and background, as well as an understanding of the medical issues involved. Clinicians must appreciate and respect the patient's aspirations and wishes and, importantly, their whole clinical state and social and personal circumstances. Patients who find it difficult to understand and retain medical advice may need to be seen on more than one occasion. They should be invited to bring a family member or close friend with them to help to remind them and explain to them what they have been told.

For example, it is not easy to give advice on the pros and cons of aortic valve replacement to a 90-year-old who is keen to pursue an active life. The risks of surgery are high, and have to be balanced against the risks of death due to heart failure or sudden death. The GP may need to discuss the risks with the cardiac surgeon in order to answer any questions that the patient and their family may have. The GP should also know the potential problems that may occur when the patient leaves hospital.

Giving elderly patients advice based on clinical trials and registry data

Although observational clinical studies have reported on the outcome of certain interventions (cardiac surgery, valve replacement and coronary angioplasty) in elderly patients, randomised clinical trials to evaluate medical treatments have not included patients aged over 80 years, usually because drug trials have an arbitrary upper age limit for recruitment, and patients may be excluded if they are taking conflicting medication which cannot be stopped, or if they have co-morbidity. It is therefore difficult to provide patients with quantitative information about outcome and risk in certain areas of cardiology where trial results do not apply to the elderly. However, outcome data gleaned from personal or practice-based prospective databases, including prognostically useful clinical information, can provide the clinical team with relevant information to guide decision making.

Risk–benefit analysis in cardiological treatments

Risk–benefit analysis is particularly important in the elderly. Advice should be tailored to the patient, based on a detailed and comprehensive knowledge of the clinical, social and psychological circumstances, put in the context of patients with a similar risk profile who have undergone a similar intervention.

This is a particularly difficult aspect of clinical care in elderly patients. The prevalence of nearly every cardiac condition becomes higher with increasing age. In the absence of guidelines specifically written for elderly patients, clinicians have to rely on their clinical judgement and experience when recommending certain interventions with a finely balanced risk–benefit ratio. Important examples include deciding whether to start long-term anticoagulation to prevent thromboembolism in atrial fibrillation, or as treatment for pulmonary emboli, and whether to start or stop aspirin in patients with vascular disease. These long-term treatments may need to be stopped if complications occur which increase the risk–benefit ratio.

Certain interventions (e.g. thrombolysis or primary coronary angioplasty for acute myocardial infarction) carry greater risks in elderly patients but have a correspondingly greater potential benefit.

It is very important to take into account the views of the patient and their family.

Stopping treatment in patients when they reach the age of 80 years

Treatment for cardiovascular prevention (e.g. antihypertensive drugs, lipid-lowering tablets) should not be stopped in the elderly simply because there is no evidence from controlled trials that these treatments are beneficial in this age group. Increasing age is an important cardiovascular risk factor. Effective treatment of risk factors may be particularly beneficial in the short and medium term in the elderly. Long-term prognostic benefits are not generally expected.

- The principles of management in the elderly are similar to those for younger patients.
- All drugs should be prescribed with an understanding of their altered pharmacokinetics in the elderly.
- An understanding of the patient's clinical profile, social situation, personal perspective of their condition, and the benefits and risks of investigation and treatment is crucial for reducing treatment-related problems.
- Advice given to elderly patients must be individualised.

Age-related medical changes

The following conditions are increasingly common with advancing age, and complicate the medical management of elderly patients.

General medical and social conditions

- ✧ Renal impairment – increasing serum creatinine levels and a decrease in eGFR.
- ✧ Urinary and faecal incontinence.
- ✧ Decrease in bone density, leading to a loss of mechanical strength and increased vulnerability to fracture.
- ✧ Cerebrovascular disease.
- ✧ Impaired mental state due to dementia.
- ✧ Lack of social interaction, leading to introspection, isolation and depression.
- ✧ Neurological and musculoskeletal conditions, and impaired mobility.
- ✧ Difficulty opening bottles and packets of drugs.
- ✧ Visual problems, macular degeneration.
- ✧ Thyroid abnormalities.
- ✧ Liver impairment.
- ✧ Diabetes.
- ✧ Prostatism in men.

Cardiovascular conditions and changes in the elderly

- ✧ Coronary artery disease and acute myocardial infarction.
- ✧ Hypertension (most commonly, low renin and isolated systolic hypertension).
- ✧ Systolic and diastolic heart failure due to left ventricular wall thickening with amyloid deposition.
- ✧ The heart valves become fibrosed and calcified, resulting in mitral valve regurgitation and aortic stenosis.
- ✧ Hypertension may lead to aortic wall dilatation, thoracic and abdominal aortic aneurysms and aortic regurgitation.
- ✧ Sinus node and conducting tissue disease leading to bradycardia, atrial arrhythmias (particularly atrial fibrillation) and heart block.
- ✧ Infective endocarditis presenting with non-specific features.

✧ Arteries become thicker, more tortuous and calcified. This increases the risks associated with invasive arterial investigations and coronary intervention.

✧ There is an increasing incidence of atheromatous disease, affecting the brain, coronary and leg arteries.

> In the elderly, myocardial infarction may be silent or it may present atypically with confusion and other non-specific symptoms, rather than typical chest pain.

Multiple morbidities and the 'domino effect'

Because elderly people have a reduced physiological and anatomical tolerance of any form of physical or emotional stress, they are vulnerable to a 'domino effect' of illnesses once a clinical problem occurs. For example, a female patient with cardiovascular disease and visual impairment may trip and fall. Osteoporosis predisposes her to a fractured hip, which requires surgery. This puts her at high peri-operative risk of myocardial infarction due to underlying coronary heart disease and heart failure, and stroke. Her poor mobility increases the risk of deep vein thrombosis and pulmonary embolism. This explains the high mortality among elderly patients who are admitted to hospital with a hip fracture.

Rehabilitation and return to independence are often difficult. Involvement of all the relevant medical and surgical specialties improves management and enables the team to predict and possibly prevent potential complications.

- A full general medical assessment should be made and coexisting conditions corrected where possible, particularly before any operation.
- Multiple morbidities and social problems are best managed by a multi-disciplinary team.
- Multiple morbidities multiply the risk.

Cost implications of treating the elderly

The cost implications of certain expensive interventions, such as cardiac surgery, must also be borne in mind, although this is a secondary consideration when deciding whether to offer a patient treatment. Pacing for complete heart block or symptomatic bradycardia is performed as a day case with local anaesthesia. It is cost-effective because it avoids the costs of treating falls and fractures in vulnerable people.

Clinical signs in the elderly

Isolated systolic hypertension with associated visible carotid artery and brachial artery pulsation is common. Systolic murmurs may be due to aortic valve thickening ('aortic sclerosis'), aortic stenosis or mitral regurgitation. A third heart sound due to a stiff, non-compliant left ventricle, and a fourth heart sound due to heart failure, are not uncommon in the elderly. It may be difficult to measure the jugular venous pressure because of tethering of the overlying skin and subcutaneous fascia. Elderly, immobile patients who sit for long periods may have swollen feet and ankles. This 'postural oedema' needs to be distinguished from venous hypertension due to right heart failure.

Prescribing principles and problems in the elderly
Pharmacokinetics
Elderly patients have reduced muscle mass, reduced liver and renal function and cerebrovascular disease. Starting additional cardiovascular medications may result in drug interactions, toxicity and adverse effects. Drug frequency and dosages for all medications may need to be reduced.

Depending on the drug and its toxicity and safety margin, renal function should be measured before starting the drug. This is not necessary for most drugs with a low side-effect profile. The risks of toxicity can be reduced by using low doses and increasing the interval between doses. Age-related changes in pharmacokinetics mean that smaller doses of nearly all drugs need to be used, and the doses increased gradually with careful monitoring of biochemistry and haematology. In patients with severe renal impairment, this applies to ACE inhibitors, β-blockers, angiotensin II receptor blockers, digoxin, eplerenone, spironolactone and other potassium-sparing diuretics, statins and anticoagulants.

Simple prescribing and administration
Only essential drugs should be prescribed. Multiple therapies are confusing. Compliance is likely to be better if a simple, once daily, all-at-one-time regime is devised. This may need to be supervised by the person who is living with or caring for the patient, or by a visiting nurse or the pharmacist.

Multiple treatments for multiple conditions increase the risk of interactions
Elderly patients are commonly taking treatment for non-cardiac conditions (e.g. diabetes, gastrointestinal problems, Parkinson's disease, musculoskeletal pain, depression, insomnia, osteoporosis). They may also be taking non-prescription, homeopathic or over-the-counter medications (e.g. non-steroidal anti-inflammatory agents and analgesics). In addition, they may have access to antibiotics and other medications from their family or friends, and some medications of dubious provenance can be obtained via the Internet.

> It is very important to know precisely what tablets and medications a patient is taking, not simply what they have been prescribed.

Non-compliance
Elderly patients may not take all of the medication they have been prescribed by their GP.
- They may not like taking tablets.
- They may find them difficult to swallow.
- They may forget to take them or forget where they have left them.
- They may not think they need them, and are too embarrassed to tell their GP.
- They may think that they will experience side-effects to a drug.
- The drug may cause unpleasant side-effects.

Patients are often persuaded by reading a drug data sheet that they have one of more of the listed adverse effects. Loop diuretics are commonly omitted by elderly patients because they cause embarrassing and upsetting urinary incontinence. The elderly may not consider it necessary or worthwhile to take tablets to treat cardiovascular risk factors.

Expanding role of pharmacists

Obtaining the advice and co-operation of a pharmacist is important for ensuring drug compliance. Putting tablets into easy-to-open, clearly labelled drug dispensers is helpful. Some pharmacists are licensed to prescribe certain medications, and it is likely that they will be licensed to provide more medical advice in the future. Some patients find this accessibility very helpful.

Cardiovascular disease prevention in the elderly: estimating risk

The risk of developing cardiovascular disease is estimated by combining several risk factors. Those used in the charts include age, gender, smoking habits, systolic blood pressure and the ratio of total to HDL-cholesterol. The risk is expressed as a probability (percentage chance) of developing cardiovascular disease over the next 10 years. A risk of 25% means that over the next 10 years, 25 out of 100 people of similar age and gender, with similar risk factors, will experience a cardiovascular event.

The risk factor charts overestimate the risk in people under 70 years of age and underestimate the risk in people aged over 70 years. The charts also underestimate risk in South Asians, those with a family history of premature cardiovascular disease (affected male relative under 55 years of age), individuals with raised triglyceride levels (> 1.7 mmol/l) and those who are overweight or who have a high-fat diet.

> Like all guidelines, the charts are intended to aid rather than to dictate clinical management. The advice and treatment given to patients should be tailored to the patient based on their clinical profile.

Currently, all individuals with a greater than 20% cardiovascular risk are considered to be at high risk and reach the threshold for treatment, whether they have symptoms or not. This 20% estimated risk threshold is largely based on cost-effectiveness.

Increasing age is probably the strongest risk factor for cardiovascular disease, so most elderly patients are at high risk. The Joint British Societies' cardiovascular risk prediction charts for primary prevention show that nearly all men aged over 60 years, whether they smoke or not, and irrespective of their blood pressure or lipid status, have at least a 20% cardiovascular risk (i.e. risk of non-fatal myocardial infarction and stroke, or death from myocardial infarction or stroke, or new angina). The risk in women of a similar age is slightly lower.

Principles of cardiovascular disease prevention

The current principles of cardiovascular disease prevention recommended by the Joint British Societies are as follows.

❖ All people aged over 40 years without cardiovascular disease or diabetes should have a cardiovascular disease risk assessment.
❖ Cardiovascular disease prevention should focus on all people at high risk.
❖ High-risk patients are those with established cardiovascular disease and/or diabetes (type 1 or 2), or those who have a greater than 20% risk of developing cardiovascular disease over the next 10 years.
❖ Statins and antihypertensive medication are appropriate for symptom-free patients with a 20% or greater 10-year cardiovascular risk.
❖ Patients with a risk of less than 20% should be given lifestyle advice.

All elderly people are at high risk of developing cardiovascular disease.

Patients with elevated single risk factors

Patients whose 10-year cardiovascular risk is less than 20% may need medication and other cardiovascular prevention measures because of the risk conferred by a single risk factor. These factors include:

✧ blood pressure > 160 mmHg systolic or > 100 mmHg diastolic, or lesser degrees of hypertension with target organ damage, left ventricular hypertrophy, grade 3 or 4 hypertensive retinopathy, or renal impairment (micro- or macroalbuminuria or proteinuria)
✧ a ratio of total cholesterol to HDL-cholesterol of > 6
✧ familial dyslipidaemias.

Goals for all high-risk patients include:

✧ smoking cessation
✧ a healthy, low-fat diet
✧ regular and preferably daily aerobic exercise
✧ weight loss (to a target waist circumference of < 102 cm in men and < 88 cm in women)
✧ body mass index (BMI) < 25 kg/m^2
✧ blood pressure < 130/80 mmHg
✧ total cholesterol level < 4.0 mmol/l or a 25% reduction, whichever is lower
✧ LDL-cholesterol level < 2.0 mmol/l or a 30% reduction, whichever is lower
✧ fasting glucose level < 6.0 mmol/l
✧ HbA$_{1c}$ < 6.5% (diabetics only)
✧ use of cardiovascular protective drug therapies where appropriate, including antithrombotic drugs (aspirin, clopidogrel) and drugs to lower blood pressure, cholesterol and glucose levels.

Hypertension

Several factors contribute to hypertension in the elderly. Isolated systolic hypertension, due to arterial atherosclerosis and loss of elasticity, is the most dominant factor. It is associated with increased cardiovascular risk. Increasing age is also associated with renal impairment and low levels of renin.

Currently, hypertension is classified as either 'high renin' or 'low renin.' People aged over 55 years and Afro-Caribbeans of any age tend to have low-renin hypertension. Young people and white people tend to have high-renin hypertension. Therefore, thiazide diuretics (D drugs) and calcium-channel blockers (C drugs), rather than ACE inhibitors and angiotensin-receptor antagonists (A drugs), are generally more effective and are preferred for initial blood pressure control in the elderly. β-blockers (B drugs) are now recommended as fourth-line treatment for both groups.

Most hypertensive patients need more than two drugs to control their blood pressure.

Antihypertensive treatment should be started in the elderly if the blood pressure is persistently higher than 160/90 mmHg over three to six months, despite non-pharmacological treatment.

Most elderly patients tolerate antihypertensive drugs well. Postural hypotension (a fall in systolic pressure of > 20 mmHg or a fall in diastolic pressure of > 10 mmHg) is infrequent with modern antihypertensive drugs. It can sometimes be managed by reducing the dose of tablets, and advising the patient not to stand up or get out of bed too quickly. Antihypertensive drugs rarely have to be stopped because of adverse effects. Dihydropyridine calcium-channel blockers may cause ankle swelling, and this adverse effect can be reduced by adding a thiazide diuretic. ACE inhibitors, angiotensin II receptor blockers and diuretics may cause renal and electrolyte disturbances.

✧ Effective treatment of hypertension reduces the incidence of cardiovascular events in patients up to the age of 80 years.

✧ The role of antihypertensive drugs in patients over the age of 80 years is being addressed in current trials.

✧ Diuretics are recommended as initial treatment.

✧ A calcium-channel blocker can be added or substituted if necessary.

Treatment of hypertension in the elderly should include dietary salt reduction to less than 2 g per day. This reduces blood pressure sufficiently in 40% of patients, making drugs unnecessary.

NICE guidelines for initial treatment of hypertension in the elderly

In 2004, the National Institute for Clinical Excellence (NICE) published its first guidelines for treating hypertension in the elderly. These guidelines recommended thiazide diuretics (D in the algorithm) for the initial treatment of hypertension, with β-blockers (B in the algorithm) as either first- or second-line treatment, or combination treatment, in the elderly.

Against a background of concerns about the comparative effectiveness of β-blockers in reducing stroke in the elderly, the fact that older patients tend to respond better to calcium-channel blockers or diuretics, and the publication of the primary prevention Anglo-Scandinavian Cardiac Outcomes Trial (ASCOT), NICE revised its guidelines in 2006.

- The 2006 NICE guidelines recommend that patients over 55 years of age, as well as black patients of any age, should be treated with a calcium-channel blocker (C in the algorithm) or a thiazide diuretic (D in the algorithm) as initial therapy.

- The second step is the addition of an ACE inhibitor (A), to give the combination of C + A or D + A.

- The third treatment step is the addition of either a diuretic or a calcium-channel blocker to give the combination of A + C + D.

- β-blockers are reserved for patients whose blood pressure is not controlled on A + C + D.

- Alpha-blockers, spironolactone or another diuretic can be added as a fourth step.

The ASCOT trial

The ASCOT trial found that, compared with atenolol (with or without bendroflumethiazide), amlodipine (with or without perindopril) was superior in controlling blood pressure, and in reducing stroke, cardiovascular death, all cardiovascular events and procedures, and new-onset diabetes.

The ASCOT trial also found that a statin (atorvastatin) reduced cardiovascular events in hypertensive patients who had 'normal' lipid levels as well as in those who had hypertension and diabetes.

Patients who were treated initially with a calcium-channel blocker (with or without an ACE inhibitor) and a statin had a 50% lower risk of stroke and myocardial infarction compared with patients who were treated with a β-blocker (with or without a thiazide diuretic) without a statin. Therefore patients with an estimated cardiovascular risk of more than 20% over 10 years benefit from a statin even if their cholesterol level is 'normal.'

Hypertensive patients of any age should be considered for a statin.

Role of β-blockers

Treatment need not be changed in patients whose hypertension is well controlled on β-blockers (with or without a thiazide) and who do not experience adverse effects. β-blockers are particularly useful in patients with hypertension who have angina, or as a secondary preventive drug in patients with myocardial infarction.

If a patient's blood pressure is well controlled on their current treatment, even if this does not conform to NICE guidelines, the treatment should be continued so long as the patient has no side-effects.

Hypertension and stroke in the elderly

Hypertension is the most important treatable risk factor for stroke. Effective treatment of hypertension reduces the risk of stroke. Around 80% of strokes are due to cerebral infarcts, 10% are due to cerebral haemorrhage, and the remainder are due to subarachnoid haemorrhage and other less common conditions. Around 20% of patients die within the first few months. A further 35% of patients lose their independence. Mortality after one year is due mainly to cardiovascular disease.

Around 50% of patients who have a stroke have hypertension. Controlling blood pressure at or below 130/80 mmHg reduces the risk of stroke recurrence and other cardiovascular events. Other cardiovascular risk factors should be treated.

Patients who have had a transient ischaemic attack (TIA) should be treated with a statin and aspirin (75 or 150 mg a day).

Dizzy turns or 'funny turns' in the elderly

These are common and difficult to diagnose. There are several causes of dizzy turns or 'funny turns.' The common causes in the elderly include:
⬧ cardiovascular causes:
  — postural hypotension, which may be due to drugs
  — cough or micturition syncope
  — intermittent or permanent complete heart block or severe bradycardia precipitated by β-blockers, verapamil or anti-arrhythmic drugs
  — ventricular tachycardia or uncontrolled atrial fibrillation with collapse. These arrhythmias require urgent treatment
⬧ labyrinthine and vestibular disorders:
  — Menière's disease
  — acute labyrinthitis
  — benign postural vertigo
  — ototoxicity from aminoglycosides

✧ brainstem disorders:
  — brainstem ischaemia or transient ischaemic attacks
  — excess alcohol.

Questioning patients with dizzy turns or 'funny turns'

The history is crucial for diagnosis, but this is often difficult because patients may not be able to remember or describe how they felt. The history may need to be sought from a witness.

✧ Was it loss of consciousness or near loss of consciousness, or a feeling of rotation (vertigo)?
✧ Were there any associated symptoms (e.g. nausea, vomiting, a preceding cold or infection, neurological symptoms)?
✧ Does the patient feel light-headed when they stand up or get out of bed, suggesting postural hypotension?

The examination may be unhelpful. Look for postural hypotension, signs of aortic stenosis, severe hypertension, bradycardia (heart rate less than 40 bpm), arrhythmia (frequent ectopic beats, atrial fibrillation), carotid bruits, signs of endocarditis, nystagmus, visual loss or neurological deficit.

Management of patients with dizzy turns

An ECG, haematology and biochemistry blood tests should be done. The patient should be referred to the most appropriate specialist. Very often the first port of call is the cardiologist to exclude bradycardia or another serious arrhythmia with ambulatory ECG recordings. When a cardiac cause has been excluded, referral may be necessary to exclude a peripheral vestibular or central neurological cause.

Peripheral vascular disease

The prevalence of peripheral vascular disease increases with age. It is associated with vascular disease in the neck and coronary arteries, and in the aorta. Most patients with peripheral vascular disease have coronary heart disease. Around 25% of patients who present with coronary heart disease have peripheral vascular disease. Patients may not have symptoms in all arterial territories.

> Apart from peripheral vascular disease, leg pain in the elderly may also be caused by lumbar canal stenosis or lumbar radiculopathy, or degenerative or malignant bone disease. Multiple pathology should be considered in patients with atypical symptoms.

Examination should include an assessment of all peripheral pulses, listening for bruits over the carotid and femoral arteries and feeling for an abdominal aortic aneurysm. Check the blood pressure in both arms to exclude dissection of the ascending aorta.

Management of peripheral vascular disease

The principles of management are similar for patients of all ages. Aggressive risk factor management, particularly smoking cessation, and daily exercise (walking and cycling) are very beneficial, and may make intervention and surgery unnecessary. Comfortable walking shoes, weight loss, control of diabetes and hypertension, and lipid lowering improve the prognosis. Statins reduce the five-year risk of vascular events by 20%.

Patients with peripheral vascular disease should have comprehensive cardiovascular and renal evaluation. Carotid imaging is indicated for transient ischaemic attacks.

Drugs

β-blockers should be stopped. ACE inhibitors should be used cautiously because of the likelihood of associated renovascular disease and renal artery stenosis.

Aspirin reduces the incidence of fatal myocardial infarction by 25%. All patients should take aspirin 75 mg a day if they can tolerate it. Clopidogrel may be more effective than aspirin, but is more expensive. It should be used in patients who cannot tolerate aspirin.

Several vasodilators have been used unsuccessfully to improve peripheral blood flow and symptoms.

Surgery and angioplasty for critical ischaemia

Surgical bypass is rarely needed. Patients with critical foot and leg ischaemia (ischaemic pain at rest, ulceration, gangrene) should be referred urgently to a vascular surgeon. Percutaneous angioplasty, endarterectomy and bypass surgery may be necessary, either individually or in combination. Limb amputation may be necessary for intractable pain and severe ischaemia when revascularisation is not feasible. The surgical risks are greater, and satisfactory prostheses and rehabilitation are more difficult, in elderly patients.

Patients with acute arterial thrombosis, which may be due to either thrombosis or embolism, should be sent as an emergency to a vascular unit with interventional radiology facilities. If the thrombosis is embolic, the source may be from the heart (thromboembolism due to atrial fibrillation or, less commonly, infective endocarditis), or fat emboli from the aorta after arterial catheterisation, known as 'trash leg'). Thrombolysis, with or without embolectomy, may be indicated for recent acute thrombosis.

Trauma (e.g. road traffic accidents, bad falls) may also cause arterial occlusion. Patients require a full surgical assessment with advanced arterial imaging.

Categorising renal impairment in the elderly: use of estimated glomerular filtration rate (eGFR)

Renal impairment increases with age. The creatinine level alone is an unreliable indicator of renal impairment because it is released from muscle, and muscle bulk decreases with age. Renal function is now measured using the estimated glomerular filtration rate (eGFR), which is calculated on the basis of serum creatinine concentration, age, gender and ethnic origin. There are five bands or categories of eGFR. Hospital laboratories now provide the eGFR result in addition to the urea and creatinine levels.

Management according to stage

Patients with even mild renal impairment have a high risk of cardiovascular events and mortality, rather than rapid deterioration in renal function. Minor renal impairment adversely affects both the outcome of patients with acute coronary syndromes and myocardial infarction, and the results of angioplasty and coronary artery surgery. Patients in stage 2 may be referred for a renal opinion if they have proteinuria, microalbuminuria or haematuria. They are likely to have widespread vascular disease.

Patients in stages 3 to 5 would be under the care of a nephrologist. They are at higher cardiovascular risk.

TABLE 16.1 Classification of chronic renal disease and prognosis

Stage	eGFR (ml/min/1.73m²)	Clinical state	5-year probability of dialysis (%)	5-year probability of death %
1	>90	No renal impairment	<1	<1
2	60–90	Mild impairment, microalbuminuria proteinuria haematuria	1	20
3	30–59	Moderate impairment, bone disease, anaemia, creatinine 150–300*	1.3	24
4	15–29	Advanced impairment, prepare for replacement, dialysis, creatinine 300–700*	18	46
5	<15	End-stage, creatinine >700*		>50

* Creatinine levels in µmol/l. Serum creatinine levels are only a rough guide of renal function.

Diet and salt intake in patients with renal disease and hypertension

Patients with hypertension and/or renal impairment should reduce their intake of salt. This is a complicated subject, and it will need to be explained to the patient in simple terms, and probably more than once. Salt is present in packaged and tinned foods, 'ready meals', snacks, crisps, nuts, convenience foods, sauces and condiments, ethnic foods and processed foods. Many elderly patients eat ready-prepared foods and may find it difficult to change the way they shop and eat.

Obesity is comparatively uncommon in people over 80 years of age, because the obese are less likely to have a long lifespan. All patients, particularly those with hypertension and dyslipidaemia, should try to achieve an optimal weight. This makes it easier to achieve blood pressure control.

Exercise

All patients should be encouraged and taught to exercise and stretch daily to improve their fitness, strength and mobility. Each individual should do as much as they are able. Physically able people should do at least 30 minutes of cardiovascular exercise each day.

> Retirement from work allows people more time to look after themselves and to take a greater interest in their health.

Exercise allows the elderly to remain more active and productive for longer. An individualised exercise programme is recommended, and this should include exercises to improve spinal flexibility as well as strength in the neck, arm and leg muscles. Exercise reduces stress and depression, which are common in the elderly, often due to social isolation. Exercise classes, or dance and music groups, offer both social interaction and exercise.

Hyperlipidaemia

Statins reduce the risk of secondary coronary events in people over 60 years of age, and also reduce the risk of stroke and transient ischaemic attacks. Because patients over 80 years of age have not been included in clinical trials of lipid lowering, there is no evidence that statins are beneficial in reducing cardiovascular events in this age group. However, this lack of evidence does not mean that statins should be withheld in the elderly, who are at high risk, and theoretically have much to gain from the varied effects of statins on vascular health.

The new General Medical Services contract has led to increased prescribing of statins to patients over 80 years of age.

Diabetes

The prevalence of type 2 diabetes is increasing in all age groups. It is common in people aged over 60 years, particularly in the overweight and obese.

Apart from the well recognised diabetic microvascular complications (including retinopathy, nephropathy and neuropathy) and the macrovascular complications (including coronary heart disease, stroke and peripheral artery disease), there are other less well recognised complications which have similarly devastating effects in the elderly. These include cognitive disorders and physical disability. These conditions have a major impact on the lifestyle of these patients, with loss of independence, and increased demands on carers and family. They constitute a major drain on social, manpower and financial resources.

Smoking

Older smokers are more likely to have smoked for longer than younger smokers, and are therefore more likely to have smoking-related illnesses. They may be less inclined to stop smoking, but should be told that quitting will reduce the risks of coronary events and fatal infarction. The benefits of stopping smoking occur at all ages, and are greatest in patients with vascular disease and others at high risk.

Primary care clinicians should not be reluctant or defeatist about encouraging the elderly to stop smoking. The elderly are at least as successful as younger patients in quitting smoking. Those who have had a heart attack will have a lower risk of another heart attack if they stop. Smoking cessation treatments should include one-to-one counselling or group therapy, with pharmacotherapy if necessary.

Heart failure in the elderly

Diastolic rather than systolic heart failure is the most common haemodynamic abnormality in the elderly. Around 70% of elderly patients with heart failure have preserved left ventricular systolic function.

The prognosis of elderly patients with heart failure remains worse than for those with some forms of cancer. The management of patients with end-stage disease demands considerable clinical and organisational skills in co-ordinating input from specialists, geriatricians, general physicians and experts in palliative care.

Causes of acute heart failure

Myocardial infarction (which may be silent), infection, uncontrolled hypertension, an arrhythmia (e.g. atrial fibrillation or bradycardia) or a valve problem (possibly due to endocarditis) may present as acute or compensated heart failure.

Severe low-output heart failure may result from pulmonary embolism, which is common and life-threatening in elderly, dehydrated, immobile people.

Acute heart failure may also develop in patients with compensated heart failure, due to non-compliance with treatment. Drugs which depress the contractility of heart muscle (e.g. β-blockers, verapamil, anti-arrhythmics, and drugs that cause salt and water retention, such as non-steroidal anti-inflammatory drugs, and steroids) may also precipitate heart failure in patients with impaired left ventricular function.

Acute or chronic heart failure: non-compliance

A large proportion of elderly patients with compensated heart failure may decompensate because they do not take their tablets, often because of confusion, or because they wish to avoid the inconvenient and embarrassing diuresis and urinary incontinence caused by loop diuretics. Patients should be told that if they omit a dose of diuretic because they are going out, they should take the tablet when they get home.

Clinical features of heart failure

Symptoms include breathlessness, tiredness, fatigue and ankle swelling. The signs may be non-specific, such as confusion, depression, falls, anorexia and weight loss or immobility.

Signs include cool, clammy hands, a high venous tone, tachycardia, irregularity of the pulse if the patient is in atrial fibrillation, a raised venous pressure and swelling of the legs.

> Ankle swelling is common in the elderly and may not be due to heart failure. Immobility and sitting in a chair for long periods, venous hypertension due to venous valve incompetence or venous thrombosis, oedema due to calcium antagonists (amlodipine and nifedipine used to treat hypertension), hypoproteinaemia (nephrotic syndrome) and, less commonly, lymphatic obstruction may cause ankle swelling.

There may be signs of valve abnormalities. Signs of infective endocarditis (fever, heart murmurs and emboli) should be looked for.

Severe anaemia or thyrotoxicosis can result in 'high-output' heart failure with warm extremities.

Investigations for heart failure

Troponins should be measured if there is a history of chest discomfort or sudden breathlessness.

Electrolytes, renal function, uric acid levels, liver function, glucose levels and haematology should be checked. Thyrotoxicosis should be excluded as a possible cause of atrial fibrillation. It may not give rise to symptoms, but may present as heart failure, dizzy turns or palpitations. Occasionally anaemia may contribute to symptoms of breathlessness and tiredness. The possibility of coexisting diabetes and renal impairment should be investigated.

An ECG will show the heart rhythm and rate, conduction abnormalities and signs of myocardial infarction. Atrial fibrillation is common in the elderly. Bradycardia due to complete heart block, sinus node disease or β-blockers may present as heart failure rather than as syncope or dizziness. Patients with permanent heart block require permanent pacing.

A chest X-ray is very helpful for showing signs of pulmonary oedema and a large heart shadow in patients with heart failure. It will also show lung shadowing in patients with pneumonia or lung cancer, which may present as breathlessness and tiredness.

Echocardiography is an essential investigation for assessing and characterising left ventricular function, size and wall thickness, valve structure and competence, and for assessing aortic valve stenosis.

The N-terminal brain natriuretic peptide (BNP) level is useful for diagnosing and excluding heart failure. This is a simple blood test that is available in most hospital laboratories, which have their own normal ranges. This blood test can be used to assess the response to treatment, and to monitor the condition.

Management of heart failure in the elderly
Home care
A domiciliary heart failure specialist nurse can decide whether continued treatment at home is appropriate, or whether the patient should be sent to hospital. It may be helpful to arrange a consultant domiciliary visit. If possible, the patient should be managed at home.

Patients should be assessed for oxygen treatment. Intravenous diuretics can be given at home.

Bed rest should be avoided because of the risks of venous thrombosis and embolism, chest infection, limb weakness and bedsores. Ideally, the patient should be advised to rest in a chair but to remain as mobile as they can without getting too breathless.

Patients who have been diagnosed and evaluated by a cardiologist or their GP can be managed at home by a nurse specialist who monitors their progress, assesses whether they are able to cope with normal daily activities (e.g. nutrition and diet, mobility, bathing) at home, records their weight, checks their electrolytes, renal function and other blood tests, ensures drug compliance and recommends changes to treatment when necessary. The patient's psychological state should also be monitored.

Patients with end-stage heart failure should receive palliative care. This is commonly provided in a hospice, but can be given at home in some cases, depending on the patient's social and personal circumstances. This is a difficult specialty and it requires the involvement of a team of experts. Frequent discussions with the patient and their family are essential.

Referral to hospital
Patients who are too ill to be treated at home, and those who cannot cope at home, need to be admitted to hospital for further investigation and intravenous diuretics.

Exercise as treatment for heart failure
Exercise is recommended as a component of treatment for heart failure, if the patient is well enough. It should be supervised initially and tailored to the patient. Supervision and active encouragement usually need to be continued.

All forms of exercise are helpful. Cardiovascular exercise (e.g. dancing, walking, cycling, Tai Chi) improves balance, flexibility, strength, confidence and cardiorespiratory fitness. These benefits reduce the number of falls in elderly people. Patients should be taught and encouraged to exercise while sitting or lying in bed. This strengthens their arms and legs and improves suppleness.

Medical treatment of heart failure
The aims of treating chronic heart failure are to relieve symptoms, improve exercise tolerance and reduce acute exacerbations and mortality.

Contributing conditions

Isolated systolic hypertension, myocardial ischaemia and arrhythmias should be evaluated and treated. Obesity puts a strain on the heart and is associated with metabolic conditions which contribute to morbidity and mortality.

Medical treatments

In most patients, oral loop diuretics are sufficient to treat pulmonary oedema and peripheral oedema. In resistant cases, the diuretic can be injected intravenously or combined with aldosterone antagonists (spironolactone or eplerenone) or intermittent short-term thiazides. This combination is very effective, and patients need careful clinical and biochemical monitoring of their electrolytes and renal function, uric acid levels (gout is common), and fluid status.

Potassium supplements should be stopped if potassium-sparing diuretics are prescribed. The combination of a loop diuretic and an aldosterone antagonist is less likely to be effective if the glomerular filtration rate is less than 40 ml/minute.

Intravenous diuretics will have to be used if the patient cannot swallow tablets, or cannot absorb the tablets due to gut wall oedema, which occurs in right heart failure (resistant oedema). All diuretics may result in incontinence and urinary retention, as well as electrolyte disturbances (most commonly hyponatraemia) and gout.

Digoxin is useful for controlling the ventricular rate in atrial fibrillation, and compared with other anti-arrhythmic drugs it is less likely to cause myocardial depression. Low doses (0.0625 mg a day) should be used in the elderly, and loading doses are not necessary. Digoxin does not decrease mortality. Toxicity is increased in patients with hypokalaemia, a low magnesium level or renal impairment. Digoxin is contraindicated in heart block. Side-effects that suggest toxicity include anorexia and nausea (which are common in liver congestion due to right heart failure), vomiting, visual disturbances and arrhythmias.

Subcutaneous fractionated heparin and compression stockings are used in immobile patients and those at high risk of venous thromboembolism.

Fluid restriction is no longer recommended. It makes patients very uncomfortable and can aggravate malnutrition. A low-salt diet is advised. 'Ready meals' and other processed foods usually contain high levels of salt, and should be avoided.

Hyperkalaemia may result from potassium-sparing diuretics and diuretics containing supplemental potassium, particularly when these types of diuretics are combined with ACE inhibitors. Renal function should be monitored in all patients.

Risks of drugs acting on the renin–angiotensin system: ACE inhibitors and angiotensin II receptor blockers

The risks are low in patients with chronic kidney disease stages 1 or 2, but are higher in the elderly because they are more likely to have vascular disease. Patients with peripheral vascular disease are likely to have renal artery stenosis affecting one or both kidneys. ACE inhibitors and angiotensin II blockers are contraindicated in patients with severe bilateral renal artery stenosis, as they are likely to cause severe and progressive renal failure. ACE inhibitors may be tolerated by patients with unilateral renal artery stenosis if the contralateral kidney function is normal, although the renal function in the affected kidney is likely to be further impaired.

Increases in creatinine levels to 200 μmol/l and increases in potassium levels to 5.9 mmol/l are acceptable. The ACE inhibitor should be stopped if there are excessive increases in creatinine and potassium levels, and specialist advice should be sought.

It is best to avoid both ACE inhibitors and angiotensin II blockers in patients with known significant renovascular disease and hypersensitivity to ACE inhibitors.

Renal function and electrolytes should be checked before starting ACE inhibitors, and should be monitored during treatment, particularly in the elderly. These groups of drugs will need to be stopped if significant renal impairment develops (eGFR < 30). The risks of renal damage are further increased in patients who are taking non-steroidal anti-inflammatory analgesics. Hyperkalaemia may occur in patients who are taking potassium-containing salt substitutes (to decrease their sodium intake in order to reduce the risk of hypertension) and potassium-sparing diuretics.

Starting ACE inhibitors

ACE inhibitors and angiotensin II receptor blockers may cause hypotension in patients who are taking large doses of diuretics (equivalent to furosemide 80 mg a day). Taking a small first dose at night reduces this risk. The dose should be increased slowly, if possible to the dose shown to be effective for that ACE inhibitor. A low blood pressure is acceptable if the patient does not have severe dizziness and can control or prevent postural hypotension by not getting up too quickly.

ACE inhibitors should be used with caution in patients with severe symptomatic aortic stenosis. Rarely, they may cause idiopathic angioedema.

In the absence of fluid retention, ACE inhibitors should be started before diuretics. They should also be used in patients with asymptomatic left ventricular systolic impairment.

Patients with an intolerable cough may need to be switched to angiotensin II receptor blockers. It is important to exclude pulmonary oedema as the cause of the cough with a chest X-ray. Both ACE inhibitors and angiotensin II receptor blockers may unmask renal artery stenosis. They should be given cautiously to patients with stage 3 renal disease and those taking non-steroidal anti-inflammatory drugs.

ACE inhibitors and angiotensin-receptor blockers can be used together in patients with heart failure. This combination in the elderly is more likely to result in renal impairment, so frequent blood tests should be performed.

β-blockers improve the prognosis in heart failure, and should be considered in the elderly. They should be started at a low dose, and the dose should be increased slowly every two weeks or so. They can be used with ACE inhibitors and angiotensin II receptor blockers.

β-blockers are contraindicated in patients with bundle branch block, bradycardia and obstructive airways disease. Tiredness, fatigue, bradycardia and hypotension may necessitate them being stopped.

A combination of hydralazine and isosorbide may be used in patients who cannot tolerate ACE inhibitors or angiotensin II blockers. This combination is particularly effective in black people.

Coronary artery disease and angina

Angina is a clinical diagnosis. Other causes of chest pain need to be excluded. Anginal symptoms in elderly patients are often atypical; breathlessness or difficulty walking is more common than chest tightness.

It may be argued that the lifestyle of patients who survive past the age of 80 years must be satisfactory, or they would not have reached that age. Nevertheless, conventional risk factors should be reviewed and treated when appropriate, even where there are areas of doubt or lack of evidence that intervention improves survival. These aspects are difficult to prove in this population of patients.

Isolated systolic hypertension may result in angina and should be controlled. Obesity in the elderly is uncommon, possibly because the obese are selected out of this population. Diabetes, smoking and hyperlipidaemia should be treated in the same way as in younger patients. A low-fat diet is recommended, although elderly patients may find it even more difficult to change their diet than younger patients.

Medical treatment for angina is the preferred option. Anti-anginal drugs should be added one at a time and with gradual dose increases. If it is tolerated, aspirin should be given to all patients. β-blockers, short- and long-acting nitrates (which may be given both orally and transdermally), calcium-channel blockers and potassium-channel-opening agents should be used, adding one class of drug at a time and starting with low doses.

Intolerable angina despite optimal medical treatment

Non-invasive ischaemia provocation tests (exercise stress tests) may be impractical. When the diagnosis of angina is clear, these tests do not provide further diagnostic information, but they do provide prognostic information and an indication of the patient's exercise performance and haemodynamic response. Patients who perform well on an exercise test and whose angina is acceptable to them may be treated medically. Those who perform badly and can manage less than four minutes of the Bruce treadmill protocol or the WHO cycle protocol, and whose angina is troublesome with attacks of angina at rest, preventing them from performing normal daily activities, should be considered for myocardial revascularisation. They should be referred for coronary angiography.

> Symptom severity is the main indication to perform coronary angiography and revascularisation.

Both stress echocardiography and nuclear tests can be open to observer bias, and may confirm myocardial ischaemia but add very little to clinical management decisions in the elderly patient with clear-cut angina whose pre-test likelihood of having coronary artery disease is over 95%.

Myocardial revascularisation

The risks of angiography and coronary angioplasty are higher in the elderly. They include myocardial infarction and death, renal impairment, stroke and peripheral vascular complications. Coronary angiography should be performed if angina is not controlled satisfactorily on medical treatment.

> Revascularisation should be performed in the elderly only for angina that is refractory to optimum medical treatment. All cardiovascular risk factors should be managed effectively.

Coronary angioplasty

Coronary angioplasty has a lower peri-operative risk compared with coronary artery bypass grafting. Drug-eluting stents reduce the risk of restenosis. Coronary angioplasty does not improve the prognosis in any patient subset. It is more effective than medical treatment in controlling anginal symptoms, but should only be performed if angina cannot be adequately controlled with medical treatment.

> Angioplasty is preferred over coronary artery surgery unless there are other compelling reasons for surgery (e.g. aortic valve replacement).

Coronary artery bypass surgery

There are no data from randomised trials including patients aged over 80 years comparing angioplasty and coronary surgery, so the choice of revascularisation has to be made on an individual basis. It is likely that surgery would confer survival benefits for patients with a critical stenosis of the left main coronary artery or three-vessel coronary artery disease, including a stenosis of the proximal left anterior descending coronary artery, at any age.

If the patient agrees, the management should be discussed with their family and the risks of treatment discussed and put in context, as far as possible, with a non-interventional, conservative strategy.

Treatment of myocardial infarction in the elderly

Patients aged over 75 years constitute around 30% of those with acute myocardial infarction and 50% of those who die acutely from their infarct. The 30-day mortality in elderly patients treated with thrombolysis for acute ST elevation myocardial infarction is around 20%, compared with 11% for patients under 80 years of age.

Thrombolysis

This is the most common form of reperfusion in the UK. Patients are now transported to hospital very quickly in urban centres. In certain parts of the country, thrombolysis is given by paramedics at the patient's home.

Thrombolysis is effective in restoring blood supply to the heart in 60% of patients. Survival and left ventricular function are improved if treatment is given within 12 hours and there is ST elevation. The sooner thrombolysis is given (ideally within four hours), the better the outcome. It is not given to patients with a normal ECG or if there is ST depression. It is not always possible to know precisely when the chest pain first occurred.

Primary coronary angioplasty and stenting

For suitable elderly patients who are being treated in major centres with experienced operators, primary coronary angioplasty is superior to thrombolysis in reducing mortality.

Compared with younger patients, who may have a ruptured plaque with minimal underlying stenosis, elderly patients with acute ST elevation myocardial infarction or symptoms and new left bundle branch block (the indications for primary coronary angioplasty) are more likely to have a plaque overlying an important calcified atheromatous stenosis, which would be suitable for coronary angioplasty and stenting. Primary angioplasty is also performed in patients with acute infarction where thrombolysis is contraindicated (e.g. due to recent stroke, surgery, internal bleeding, suspected aortic dissection, previous haemorrhagic stroke, or previous allergy to thrombolytic).

In order to salvage jeopardised myocardium as soon as possible by reperfusing it with blood, the 'door to balloon time' should be less than 60 minutes. The audit target in UK centres is less than 90 minutes. This service is only available in major centres in the UK.

Primary angioplasty is also performed after unsuccessful thrombolysis where patients have continuing or recurrent pain and ECG changes show failed reperfusion or recurrent infarction.

Streptokinase is associated with a lower risk of intracerebral bleeding and death compared with tissue plasminogen activator in the elderly. Allergic reactions and hypotension are more common with streptokinase than with recombinant tissue plasminogen activator (rtPA).

Thrombolysis is most effective in patients:

✧ with anterior (compared with inferior) infarcts
✧ aged > 75 years
✧ with impaired left ventricular function or left bundle branch block
✧ with hypotension (blood pressure < 100 mmHg)
✧ who present within one hour of pain.

Valve disease

Mitral valve regurgitation

This can be due to mitral annulus calcification (more common in women), papillary muscle dysfunction due to ischaemia or degeneration, or mitral valve leaflet prolapse. All of these conditions are common in people aged over 70 years.

Aortic stenosis and sclerosis

Senile calcific aortic stenosis is associated with cardiovascular risk factors and increasing age. It may progress rapidly, causing heart failure and sudden death within months of the onset of symptoms. Therefore, prompt diagnosis and quantification of its severity using echocardiography and Doppler examination are important.

Calcific aortic stenosis is a progressive disease. Patients do not develop symptoms until the valve has become very narrow. Patients who experience chest tightness, breathlessness, dizzy turns or loss of consciousness, particularly during exercise, may have aortic stenosis. Examination may show a slow or 'shuddery' upstroke of the carotid pulse, and a loud ejection systolic murmur radiating to the neck. Aortic murmurs can be heard all over the front of the chest.

Patients with suspected aortic stenosis should be referred for echocardiography and Doppler examination. Referral is essential for patients with significant aortic stenosis.

> All patients with aortic stenosis should have antibiotic prophylaxis.

Aortic valve replacement is performed primarily to relieve symptoms. It can prolong and improve the quality of life in the elderly patient, so age should not be a contraindication to surgery.

Surgery may also be appropriate in asymptomatic patients with severe aortic stenosis and impaired left ventricular function not due to another cause, in patients for whom serial echocardiography has shown rapid deterioration in the condition, and in patients who develop symptoms during exercise. The operative risk in patients over 70 years of age is 5–15%. Individuals at very high risk include the very elderly (over 90 years of age), women, and patients with associated co-morbidities, severe symptoms, emergency surgery, severe left ventricular impairment, pulmonary hypertension, coronary artery disease, and previous coronary or valve surgery.

Percutaneous aortic valve replacement is a new technique that is offered to patients who have been refused surgical aortic valve replacement. There is little information available about this procedure.

There is no consistent evidence that statins or ACE inhibitors are beneficial in aortic stenosis, despite the acceptance that hypercholesterolaemia and hypertension are risk factors.

Infective endocarditis

Infective endocarditis is uncommon, and is often difficult to diagnose due to its insidious nature and atypical presentation. Elderly patients may not have the classic features of fever, changing heart murmurs and signs of emboli. They may present with weight loss, anorexia and fatigue, with no fever. This leads to delayed diagnosis and a worse outcome, often in a patient with other medical problems and a reduced resistance to infection. In-hospital mortality is 25%, which is twice that of patients aged 50–70 years. The aortic and mitral valves are most commonly affected.

The digestive tract is the most frequent portal of entry, due to the higher incidence of colonic lesions. *Streptococcus bovis* is the predominant organism. In men, prostatic lesions are common. This highlights the importance of prophylactic antibiotics for gastroenterological and urological procedures in high-risk patients. Pacemaker endocarditis is also more common in the elderly.

⋄ It is important to suspect infective endocarditis in the generally unwell elderly patient with a heart murmur, whether they have a fever or not. They can be investigated in primary care.
⋄ Blood cultures should be taken. As well as haematological and biochemical tests, C-reactive protein levels should be checked. The ESR is diagnostically less helpful in the elderly because it is generally higher than in younger patients.

Transthoracic echocardiography may show vegetations, although the absence of a vegetation does not exclude the diagnosis of endocarditis.

Transoesophageal echocardiography is more sensitive than transthoracic echocardiography for detecting vegetations and abscesses, and is usually well tolerated.

If the diagnosis is suspected, treatment with appropriate antibiotics should be started as soon as possible, after consultation with a microbiologist and after blood cultures and other investigations have been performed. Attention to the general medical and haemodynamic state is important.

Surgery carries high risks in the elderly, but should be performed if a patient with severe valve problems which could be resolved by surgery (e.g. heart failure secondary to valve regurgitation, an unstable valve prosthesis, uncontrolled infection, or an aortic valve or root abscess) does not respond to antibiotics.

Cardiac surgery in the elderly

Elderly patients are being referred for cardiac surgery more frequently. In-hospital complications and mortality are higher, and hospital stays are longer due to coexisting cerebrovascular and peripheral artery disease, diabetes, pulmonary disease and renal impairment.

Difficult and common questions include the following:

⋄ Should surgery be performed at all or is there an alternative strategy?
⋄ How and when should surgery be performed?
⋄ In a patient with both valve disease and coronary artery disease, should coronary artery bypass surgery be performed at the same time as valve replacement because it increases the peri-operative risks?

There are also cost–benefit considerations.

TABLE 16.2: The outcomes of cardiac surgery in patients over 80 years of age

	CABG	AVR	CABG + AVR	MVR
Death (%)	10	9	27	25
Stroke (%)	3	3	4	8
5-year survival (%)	66	63	62	57

CABG, coronary artery bypass graft; AVR, aortic valve replacement; MVR, mitral valve replacement.

Cardiac surgery in patients over 80 years of age

✧ The overall operative mortality for these different and combined routine operations was 13%. Mortality is higher in emergency operations.
✧ Post-operative complications, including any one or more of the following – chest infections, pulmonary oedema, pulmonary embolism, arrhythmias (most commonly atrial fibrillation), stroke, renal failure requiring dialysis, and myocardial infarction – occur in approximately 60% of patients.
✧ The five-year survival rate is 63%, but this depends largely on the age of the patient at the time of surgery.
✧ Most patients (87%) believe that they made the right decision, but there are many factors which influence this type of retrospective quality-of-life assessment.

Predictors of death are New York Heart Association functional class and procedure time. Atheromatous aortic disease increases the risk of stroke. Pre-operative myocardial infarction increases the risk of late-out-of-hospital death. Cardiac surgery can be performed with an 'acceptable' risk in patients with near normal left ventricular function. 'Off-pump', beating-heart coronary surgery is now commonly performed.

With the increasing use of angioplasty, the number of patients having coronary artery surgery has fallen.

Atrial fibrillation in the elderly

Atrial fibrillation is the most common arrhythmia in clinical practice in patients of all ages, and is particularly common in people over 80 years of age. The prevalence of atrial fibrillation in the elderly is 10% in those aged over 75 years and 15% in those over 80 years. Hospital admissions for atrial fibrillation are increasing as the general population ages.

Atrial fibrillation increases the risk of death by nearly twofold in both men and women.

Common causes of atrial fibrillation in the elderly include:

✧ coronary heart disease and acute myocardial infarction
✧ hypertension
✧ rheumatic heart disease
✧ sinus node disease (sick sinus syndrome)
✧ acute infections in patients with sinus node disease
✧ electrolyte depletion
✧ lung cancer
✧ pulmonary embolism
✧ thyrotoxicosis
✧ following cardiac or thoracic surgery.

Lone atrial fibrillation

This is atrial fibrillation without structural heart disease, with no abnormal clinical findings, and normal echocardiography.

Clinically, it may be difficult to distinguish atrial fibrillation from frequent ectopic beats. An ECG recording is essential for diagnosis. Persistent atrial fibrillation is more likely than ectopic beats to cause heart failure.

Both chronic persistent and intermittent paroxysmal atrial fibrillation are often detected during routine examination, or on a 24-hour ECG performed during the investigation of dizzy turns. It is important to characterise the type of atrial fibrillation that is present.

Most patients with atrial fibrillation can be managed in primary care.

Clinical features

Atrial fibrillation may be discovered during examination for an unrelated condition, or in a patient with a stroke. Elderly patients in atrial fibrillation often do not have palpitations or any other symptoms. They may have tiredness, fatigue or signs of congestive heart failure, or only slight ankle swelling.

Symptoms and signs depend on the ventricular response and rate, the underlying state of the coronary arteries, and left ventricular function. For example, the loss of atrial contraction in a patient with heart failure results in a low cardiac output, leading to breathlessness, dizziness, and occasionally loss of consciousness. Compared with young patients, elderly patients, because of the stiffening of the heart associated with ageing, are more likely to go into heart failure. Stasis of blood in the enlarged atria predisposes to a fivefold increased risk of stroke, transient ischaemic episodes and emboli. At least 25% of strokes in the elderly are due to atrial fibrillation. Cardiovascular risk factors and peripheral arterial disease increase their vulnerability to peripheral arterial or mesenteric emboli.

Atrial fibrillation leads to a reduction in exercise tolerance, mental acuity and quality of life.

Signs include a completely irregular pulse, discrepancy between the atrial and radial rates, and fibrillary waves in the jugular venous pulse.

Principles of management of atrial fibrillation

These are as follows:
- assessment and treatment of heart failure
- control of unpleasant palpitations with control of heart rate
- evaluation of possible angina due to uncontrolled tachycardia
- antithrombotic treatment to prevent thromboembolism.

In primary care:
- all patients with an irregular pulse should have an ECG
- most patients will be treated with rate control (β-blockers, or digoxin or verapamil)
- the risk of stroke should be assessed. Most patients will be suitable for warfarin.

Anticoagulants

Most elderly patients except those at low risk should be on warfarin, unless there are contraindications.

Warfarin

Anticoagulants antagonise the effects of vitamin K. They take 24–48 hours to become effective. Warfarin is the most commonly used anticoagulant in the UK. Phenindione is rarely used. Coumadin is used in the USA.

An increasing number of patients are having their warfarin monitored and prescribed in primary care. This is safe and more convenient for patients.

Some patients buy their own INR monitoring machine for use at home, and can be taught to measure their INR and control their dose of warfarin with minimal supervision.

Warfarin is believed to be underused in general, and particularly in the elderly, for the prevention of thromboembolic disease complicating atrial fibrillation. Warfarin should be taken in the evening to allow time for the drug to be distributed throughout the body. If it is taken shortly before the INR blood test, there may be a spuriously high blood and INR level.

Deciding which patients should have warfarin based on their thromboembolic risk

Patients can be categorised as high, medium or low risk according to the presence of one or more risk factors.

High risk

- Previous ischaemic stroke, transient ischaemic attack or thromboembolic event (any of these increases the risk of stroke by threefold).
- Age > 75 years, with hypertension, diabetes or vascular disease.
- Valve disease (mitral stenosis or prosthetic heart valve), heart failure, impaired left ventricular function, or large left atrium on echocardiography.

Medium risk

- Age > 65 years with no high-risk factors.
- Age < 75 years with hypertension, diabetes or vascular disease.

Low risk

- Age < 65 years with no moderate- or high-risk factors.

Antithrombotic treatment for atrial fibrillation according to risk of emboli

- Patients at *high risk* should have warfarin with an INR of 2–3, unless there are contraindications.
- Patients at *low risk* should have aspirin 75 mg per day if there are no contra-indications.
- The treatment decision in patients at *medium risk* should be individualised. This group of patients may be treated with either aspirin or warfarin, and if in doubt, the patient should be referred. Warfarin may be preferred in patients with a heart size at the upper limit of normal, the more elderly and those with two or more moderate-risk factors.

> Patients over 75 years of age (except those with lone atrial fibrillation) should have warfarin unless there are contraindications. These include a greater risk of bleeding (e.g. very low platelet count), recent gastrointestinal bleeding or surgery, severe liver disease with raised INR, practical or logistic problems in monitoring the INR, or non-compliance.

Warfarin dosage

In the elderly, depending on their body weight, the initial doses can be 5 mg and the INR checked within 1 week and the dose altered to maintain the INR between 2 and 3.

In younger and larger patients, a loading dose of 10 mg can be given and then doses of 5 mg given. The INR should be checked within seven days. Because of the higher risks of bleeding and its complications in the elderly, monitoring of the INR in these older patients should be performed more frequently – for example, every six weeks, and in some patients, depending on their clinical condition, more frequently. Warfarin is available in 1 mg, 3 mg and 5 mg tablets.

It is important that the patient and their family understand why they have been advised to take warfarin and for how long, how it is monitored and why the dose may need to be adjusted.

The INR is affected by a wide range of drugs, as well as alcohol and some foods, including salads and vegetables (e.g. spinach).

TABLE 16.3: Indications for warfarin and recommended INR

Indication	Recommended INR
Atrial fibrillation	2–3
Recurrent above-knee deep vein thrombosis	2–3
Pulmonary embolism	3–4
Mechanical prosthetic aortic heart valve	3–4
Mechanical prosthetic mitral heart valve	3.5–4

There are rarely absolute contraindications to warfarin, and treatment has to be individualised. The risk–benefit ratio must be judged carefully for each patient, taking into account the risk factors for left atrial thrombosis and embolisation. Patients with a structurally normal heart and no vascular risk factors are at low risk and do not necessarily need warfarin. Patients with a dilated heart, mitral regurgitation, hypertension and diabetes are at high risk and should be anticoagulated.

There are no guidelines regarding the upper age limit at which warfarin in contraindicated, or when it should be stopped because of the risks of gastrointestinal bleeding or stroke.

Contraindications and cautions when prescribing warfarin

There are no contraindications based on age, but most clinicians would feel that for almost all conditions the benefits of warfarin are outweighed by the risks in patients over 90 years of age.

General contraindications

✧ Mental impairment.
✧ Non-co-operation.
✧ Alcoholism.

Cardiovascular contraindications

✧ Uncontrolled hypertension.
✧ Neurological conditions.
✧ Recent stroke, neurological surgery or trauma to the central nervous system.

Gastrointestinal contraindications

✧ Uncompensated cirrhosis.
✧ Recent gastrointestinal bleed.

Haematological contraindications

✧ Pre-existing haemostatic defect.

Bleeding due to a high INR

This is an important and potentially serious but uncommon complication of warfarin. It may be due to too high a dose being prescribed, but is often due to the patient's confusion about dosage.

Management of haemorrhage in patients who are taking warfarin

Major bleeding

The patient should be sent to hospital as an emergency. Stop the warfarin, and give vitamin K (phytomenadione), 5–10 mg by slow intravenous injection. Give prothrombin complex concentrate (factors II, VII, IX and X), 30–50 units/kg, or fresh frozen plasma. The haemoglobin should be checked, and a blood transfusion may be necessary if the haemoglobin concentration is less than 8.0 g/dl.

INR > 8, but no haemorrhage

The patient does not need to be referred immediately to hospital. The warfarin should be stopped, and it should only be restarted when the INR is < 5.0. Phytomenadione should be given if there are other risk factors for bleeding.

Aspirin in atrial fibrillation

This is recommended in patients with atrial fibrillation and no risk factors, and in patients at moderate risk, or where there are contraindications to warfarin. The dose is 75–300 mg a day. Compared with warfarin, it is less effective in preventing emboli, but less liable to result in major bleeding complications. Concomitant use of a proton pump inhibitor to reduce the risk of gastrointestinal bleeding is advisable.

An enlarged left atrium (> 50 mm), left ventricular enlargement on echocardiography, and the time spent in atrial fibrillation are used to predict the risk of stroke.

The main interventions in atrial fibrillation are:

✧ anticoagulation or antithrombotic therapy to reduce the risk of thromboembolism in patients at risk
✧ anti-arrhythmic drugs to control the rate and rhythm
✧ electrical cardioversion when anti-arrhythmic therapy is inadequate
✧ radio-frequency ablation for patients who are severely symptomatic despite anti-arrhythmic drugs.

Symptoms determine management

Patients who have deteriorated quickly may have acute-onset (new) atrial fibrillation against a background of severe left ventricular impairment. If they have symptoms of breathlessness, hypotension or angina, they may need urgent cardioversion. This may be possible medically, or it may require electrical cardioversion.

Elderly patients with haemodynamic compromise or sustained fast heart rates (ventricular rate of more than 120 bpm) should be referred to hospital as an emergency.

Patients *without* symptoms or signs of heart failure can be managed, at least initially, in primary care. They may need anticoagulation and heart rate control. Those with persistent atrial fibrillation can be managed medically with anticoagulation and rate control. Those who do not tolerate atrial fibrillation should be considered for cardioversion, and may require long-term anti-arrhythmic therapy.

Pulmonary vein isolation and radio-frequency ablation

Atrial fibrillation ablation is performed occasionally in elderly patients who have recurrent attacks of paroxysmal atrial fibrillation and disabling symptoms, after all medical treatments have been shown to be unsatisfactory. It is more useful in young patients and those with 'lone' atrial fibrillation. It is also theoretically most helpful in patients whose atrial fibrillation is caused by ectopics originating from a focus in one or more of the pulmonary veins. This can only be ascertained during invasive electrophysiological study.

Patients with disabling symptoms, in whom further investigation or intervention is considered, should be referred to a cardiologist.

History and examination

The nature of the symptoms, type of atrial fibrillation, date of onset, frequency, duration, response to previous therapy and the presence of underlying heart disease should be sought. Hypertension, diabetes, contraindications to aspirin or anticoagulation, previous stroke, transient ischaemic attack, recent myocardial infarction and heart failure increase the risk of stroke.

Infection, infarction and heart failure should be excluded. Other predisposing conditions include hyperthyroidism, overuse of or sensitivity to β-agonists, alcohol, hypokalaemia (from diuretics) and chronic obstructive lung disease.

ECG diagnosis

Confirm atrial fibrillation and look for signs of myocardial infarction, heart block, bundle branch block and pericarditis.

Echocardiography

Look for signs of valvular disease, atrial size (increased atrial size reduces the likelihood of successful cardioversion), left ventricular size and function, intracardiac clot and pericardial disease.

Blood tests

Check full blood count and renal, liver and thyroid function. Investigate for infection where appropriate in the chest, urinary tract or bloodstream. Measure the patient's troponin levels if myocardial infarction is suspected.

Chest X-ray

Look for signs of infection, cancer and cardiac enlargement.

Heart rate control in atrial fibrillation

It is important to control the ventricular rate in order to reduce the likelihood of heart failure. Diltiazem, verapamil and β-blockers may be used, depending on the clinical state of the patient and coexisting conditions. Digoxin is less effective than these drugs for controlling the heart rate during exercise, but can be combined with amiodarone.

Amiodarone is the drug least likely to impair left ventricular function, but it is more likely to cause side-effects (photosensitivity, lung fibrosis, polyneuropathy, gastrointestinal upset, hepatic toxicity, thyroid dysfunction and eye complications), which necessitate drug withdrawal in around 20% of patients. Low doses should be used in the elderly. When taken orally, it has a slow onset of action.

Sotalol and other β-blockers can be used in patients with no or only minimal heart disease, and those with angina.

Sinus node disease and atrial fibrillation

Atrial fibrillation in the elderly may be part of sinus node disease. Because of the risk of inducing bradycardia, all anti-arrhythmic drugs that are used for rate control may precipitate severe bradycardia and loss of consciousness, so should be used cautiously, particularly in combination. The advice of a cardiologist should be sought. Some patients with sinus node disease ('tachy-brady syndrome') may present with atrial fibrillation or other atrial arrhythmias, rather than with bradycardia. A pacemaker will be necessary for patients who develop bradycardia, with or without symptoms, when treated with anti-arrhythmic drugs.

Cardioversion

This may have no advantage over rate control and anticoagulation in the elderly, unless the patient has recent atrial fibrillation and haemodynamic compromise due to diastolic dysfunction. Sinus rhythm is maintained in only 30–60% of patients, but this can be very advantageous by making long-term anticoagulation unnecessary. Aspirin may be recommended for patients with long episodes of paroxysmal atrial fibrillation.

The decision to attempt cardioversion in the elderly has to be individualised. In elderly patients there is an increased risk of bleeding with warfarin and of drug interactions with warfarin, the cardioversion requires a general anaesthetic, and there is possibly an increased risk of stroke at the time of cardioversion.

> In younger patients, rhythm control for atrial fibrillation has no clear advantage over rate control, and this also applies to the elderly.

The use of anti-arrhythmic drugs, including flecainide, amiodarone, propafenone and sotalol, may help to maintain sinus rhythm.

If atrial fibrillation has been present for more than 24 hours, the patient should be anticoagulated before cardioversion. Although there is no convincing evidence for this, amiodarone is sometimes given to increase the likelihood of successful cardioversion. Amiodarone increases the INR, so the dose of warfarin may need to be lowered.

Long QT syndrome and torsade de pointes

Long QT syndrome presents as syncope or, less commonly, as sudden death, due to a form of ventricular tachycardia known as torsade de pointes. It is defined as a QT interval longer than 460 ms (more than 12 small ECG squares).

In children and young adults it is caused by a genetic problem that leads to prolonged depolarisation of the heart muscle cells.

In adults and the elderly it may be caused by nearly all anti-arrhythmic drugs, and also by antimicrobial drugs (e.g. macrolide antibiotics, antifungal agents), antihistamines and antidepressants. Other causes include hypokalaemia, hypomagnesaemia, hypocalcaemia and severe bradycardia. Anti-arrhythmic drugs may cause prolongation of the QT interval, which results in ventricular tachycardia (torsade de pointes) and ventricular fibrillation. Patients at risk should be monitored clinically and with ECGs when starting an anti-arrhythmic drug.

Atrioventricular node ablation and pacemaker implantation

This should be considered for patients with resistant and haemodynamically compromising atrial fibrillation. It is most useful for patients with both atrial fibrillation and bradycardia due to sinus node disease and conduction tissue disease.

Pacing for bradycardia

Pacemakers are indicated for patients with symptomatic bradycardia and heart block, which becomes increasingly common with advancing age, due to degeneration of the sinus node and cardiac conducting tissue in the His-Purkinje system. This leads to sinus bradycardia, sinus pauses, atrial fibrillation, bundle branch block and complete heart block. Elderly patients with sinus node disease commonly present with intermittent paroxysmal atrial fibrillation, which then becomes established. Drugs that are used to slow the heart rate response may unmask bradycardia or complete heart block. These patients should be paced, and episodes of tachycardia can then be safely controlled with β-blockers or other bradycardic drugs.

Pacing is a cost-effective procedure because it corrects bradycardia and syncope, which results in falls and fractures. It is often performed as a day case, under local anaesthesia and usually mild sedation, and takes approximately one hour.

Ventricular tachycardia

This is underdiagnosed. It should be suspected in patients with left ventricular hypertrophy, most commonly due to hypertensive heart disease. A myocardial scar due to myocardial infarction may also be a substrate for ventricular tachycardia, which should be considered in the differential diagnosis of dizzy turns, syncope and breathlessness.

Ventricular tachycardia may be diagnosed with an ECG recorded during an attack, or more usually by ambulatory electrocardiography showing a broad complex tachycardia with independent atrial and ventricular activity. It can be difficult to distinguish from a supraventricular tachycardia with bundle branch block. 'Slow' ventricular tachycardia can sometimes be tolerated without symptoms.

Ventricular tachycardia is a medical emergency, and the patient should be sent to hospital immediately. Oral medication is of little use, due to the length of time that it takes to act.

If ventricular tachycardia is suspected, the patient should be urgently referred to a cardiologist.

Treatment is with one or a combination of:
 ✧ anti-arrhythmic drugs (amiodarone, sotalol)
 ✧ devices (automatic implantable cardiac defibrillators)
 ✧ ablation
 ✧ surgery
 ✧ myocardial revascularisation.

Ablation of ventricular arrhythmias is indicated in:
 ✧ patients who are at low risk of sudden cardiac death and have sustained monomorphic ventricular tachycardia that is drug resistant, or who are drug intolerant, or who do not want to take drugs

✧ bundle branch re-entrant ventricular tachycardia
✧ patients who continue to have ventricular tachycardia despite having an automatic implantable cardiac defibrillator
✧ patients with Wolff–Parkinson–White syndrome and rapid conduction down the accessory pathway.

Answers to questions about clinical cases

1. This patient is at high risk because he has vascular disease, and he should be advised to take a statin. He should undergo a comprehensive clinical evaluation, and all risk factors should be identified and treated in line with current guidelines.
2. There are several possible causes, including heart block, serious cardiac arrhythmias, transient cerebral ischaemia, epilepsy, and falls due to a variety of other causes. It is important to exclude a cardiac cause. Examine the patient, and if possible record an ECG and check her blood tests. Depending on the duration and character of these episodes, she may need an urgent cardiology outpatient appointment. If you are worried, you could discuss this with the cardiology team at your preferred hospital. Complete heart block and other serious arrhythmias should be excluded and treated urgently.
3. This patient should be told that he could well lose his leg if he does not stop smoking, and that he may lose it even if he does stop. He is at high risk of cardiovascular events (heart attack and stroke). However hopeless the situation may appear, you and your colleagues should do everything you can to help the patient stop smoking, and attend to all of his cardiovascular risk factors. If he has rest pain, he should be referred for an urgent hospital assessment and imaging. He should be on aspirin and a statin, and if he is on a β-blocker for hypertension, this should be stopped and, if necessary, another drug (e.g. amlodipine) substituted.
4. This patient may have an infection, or she may have had a stroke or a heart attack. Visit her, and talk to her carer or other people who see her regularly. Infection and myocardial infarction may present non-specifically and should be excluded. She will probably need specialist assessment at hospital for investigations, possibly preceded by a domiciliary visit. Discuss her case with your preferred care-of-the-elderly physician. Causes include high drug levels (e.g. hypnotics, sedatives, opiates), excess alcohol, metabolic causes (e.g. electrolyte imbalance, renal or liver failure, anaemia), intracranial lesions (e.g. tumour, meningitis, subdural haematoma) and nutritional deficiency (e.g. vitamin B_{12}, nicotinic acid).
5. This patient has severe renal failure, possibly related to non-steroidal anti-inflammatory tablets that he has been taking for his back pain. He will probably need renal replacement therapy, at least in the short term. He should be seen urgently by a nephrologist, and he should not take any nephrotoxic drugs.

FURTHER READING

Hypertension

Dahlöf B, Sever PS, Poulter NR *et al*. Prevention of cardiovascular events with an antihypertensive regimen of amlodipine adding perindopril as required versus atenolol adding bendroflumethiazide as required, in the Anglo-Scandinavian Cardiac Outcomes Trial – Blood Pressure Lowering Arm (ASCOT-BPLA): a multicentre randomized controlled trial. *Lancet*. 2005; **366:** 895–906.

Joint British Societies. 2: Joint British Societies' guidelines on prevention of cardiovascular disease in clinical practice. *Heart*. 2005; **91 (Suppl. V):** 1–52.

National Institute for Health and Clinical Excellence. *Full Guidance on the Management of Hypertension in Primary Care;* www.nice.org.uk/page.aspx?o=CG034fullguideline.

SHEP Cooperative Research Group. Prevention of stroke by antihypertensive drug treatment in older persons with isolated systolic hypertension. *JAMA*. 1991; **265:** 3255–64.

Staessen JA, Fagard R, Thijs L *et al.* Morbidity and mortality in the placebo-controlled European trial on isolated systolic hypertension (Syst-Eur) in the elderly. *Lancet*. 1997; **350:** 757–64.

Heart failure

American College of Cardiology and American Heart Association. *Guideline Update for the Diagnosis and Management of Chronic Heart Failure in the Adult;* www.acc.org/qualityandscience/clinical/guidelines/failure/HFPrimer.pdf.

Lewis EF, Lamas GA, O'Meara E *et al.* Characterization of health-related quality of life in heart failure patients with preserved versus low ejection fraction in CHARM. *Eur Heart J*. 2007; **9:** 83–91.

Cardiac surgery

Glower DD, Christopher TD, Milano CA *et al.* Performance status and outcome after coronary artery bypass grafting in persons aged 80 to 93 years. *Am J Cardiol*. 1992; **70:** 567–71.

Kohl P, Kerzmann A, Lahaye L *et al.* Cardiac surgery in octogenarians: peri-operative outcome and long-term results. *Eur Heart J*. 2001; **22:** 1235–43.

Infective endocarditis in the elderly

Di Salvo G, Thuny F, Rosenberg V *et al.* Endocarditis in the elderly: clinical, echocardiographic and prognostic features. *Eur Heart J*. 2003; **24:** 1576–83.

Hoen B, Alla F, Selton-Suty CH *et al.* Changing profile of infective endocarditis. Results of a 1-year follow-up in France. *JAMA*. 2002; **288:** 75–81.

Atrial fibrillation

American College of Cardiology, American Heart Association and European Society of Cardiology. Guidelines for the management of patients with atrial fibrillation: executive summary. *Eur Heart J*. 2006; **27:** 1979–2030.

National Institute for Clinical Excellence. *Clinical Guideline 36*. London: National Institute for Clinical Excellence; 2006.

Peri-operative risk assessment in cardiac patients

Clinical cases

1. An 80-year-old man presents with an acute ascending aortic dissection. He has a chest infection and is hypertensive. What do you do?
2. A fit 68-year-old man who had coronary artery surgery four years ago and has no cardiac symptoms is scheduled for a total hip replacement. What pre-operative assessment does he need?
3. A 75-year-old hypertensive man, who is unable to walk more than 100 yards on the flat due to breathlessness, has diabetes and mild angina and needs a prostatectomy. What pre-operative assessment should he have?
4. An 84-year-old woman is admitted for a gastroscopy and is found to be diabetic and in atrial fibrillation. What do you do?
5. A 68-year-old woman with a previous myocardial infarction and decompensated heart failure is admitted for peripheral arterial surgery. She has moderate renal impairment. What do you do?

Role of the primary care team in explaining risk of surgery to patients with heart disease

The primary care team has an integral role in the risk assessment of patients undergoing non-cardiac surgery. They are part of a multi-disciplinary team that includes the surgeon, anaesthetist, cardiologist, intensivist, nurses, physiotherapists and technicians and other specialists.

> The risks of non-cardiac surgery are most frequently due to coronary artery disease and impaired cardiac function, as well as other medical conditions. Peri-operative risks can be eliminated or reduced if they are predicted pre-operatively and appropriate measures taken. This necessitates a comprehensive and detailed knowledge of the patient's clinical risk profile.

Good communication between all members of the team and documentation of relevant previous medical conditions are important. Because the GP is very often the clinician responsible for making the diagnosis and recommending referral for a surgical opinion, the patient may want to consult their GP after their specialist consultation to seek further advice and reassurance that the proposed operation is really necessary, is safe and will improve their quality of life – questions that some patients may feel reticent about asking the surgeon.

Explaining the risks of non-cardiac surgery to patients with heart disease is difficult, and demands an understanding of the patient's clinical profile and how this affects their risk from the proposed operation. This aspect of the work for primary care clinicians will probably become increasingly important, because the likelihood of co-morbidity and of patients needing surgery increases as people live longer.

SEVENTEEN

Aims of risk assessment and its effect on clinical management

The aim of risk assessment is to prevent or reduce peri-operative risk. Some risk factors may be correctable. For example, myocardial ischaemia may be corrected by revascularisation and anaemia may be corrected by blood transfusion. Hypertension and diabetes can be controlled. Age is a major predictor of risk, but is not correctable. The problems posed by other conditions, such as recent (less than four weeks old) myocardial infarction, can be reduced by delaying the operation and assessing cardiac function and residual ischaemia, improving cardiovascular risk factors and starting appropriate treatment for left ventricular impairment. Temporary cardiac pacing may be necessary for patients with symptomatic bradycardia and for those at risk of heart block.

Identifying patients at high risk who need further investigation is a skill that is gained from experience. The surgeon and the relevant specialists have to weigh up the risks of surgery against the risks of not operating. The views of the patient must also be taken into consideration.

Peri-operative risk depends on the:
✧ type of procedure to be performed
✧ patient's risk profile
✧ experience and quality of the medical team and hospital facilities (which will not be discussed here).

Classification of risk according to the operation
High risk (risk of death and non-fatal infarction > 5%)
✧ Urgent major operations in the elderly.
✧ Aortic and other major vascular surgery.
✧ Peripheral vascular surgery.
✧ Prolonged abdominal operations.

Intermediate risk (risk of death and non-fatal infarction < 5%)
✧ Intraperitoneal and intrathoracic surgery.
✧ Carotid endarterectomy.
✧ Head and neck surgery.
✧ Orthopaedic surgery.
✧ Prostate surgery.

Low risk (cardiac risk < 1%)
✧ Endoscopic procedure.
✧ Superficial procedures.
✧ Cataract surgery.
✧ Breast surgery.

Assessing the patient's risk profile
A thorough clinical history and examination is important, and provides a fairly accurate estimation of peri-operative risk.

Clinical evaluation
All patients with known or suspected heart disease should be evaluated for the presence of heart failure, coronary artery disease, arrhythmia and previous myocardial infarction.

The following factors help to determine risk:
✧ age

✧ functional capacity. This is an important predictor of risk. Patients with a very restricted functional capacity and who are breathless at rest may have underlying heart failure with significant cardiac impairment and structural heart disease, myocardial ischaemia, lung disease and/or other medical conditions. They are at high risk and require a comprehensive pre-operative evaluation. Patients who can walk up two flights of stairs quickly without breathlessness or angina would generally have an acceptable functional capacity and be at low peri-operative risk

✧ co-morbid conditions (diabetes, peripheral vascular disease, renal impairment, chronic lung disease)

✧ type of surgery to be performed.

The features listed below provide useful information for risk assessment.

Major clinical predictors of increased peri-operative risk
✧ Heart failure with breathlessness at rest.
✧ Unstable coronary syndromes (myocardial infarction within four weeks, unstable angina, or new or severe angina).
✧ Ischaemia induced within three minutes of the Bruce treadmill protocol.
✧ Heart block.
✧ Important ventricular arrhythmias.
✧ Uncontrolled supraventricular arrhythmias.
✧ Severe valvular disease.

Pre-operative evaluation of high-risk patients
✧ Specialist cardiology assessment.
✧ ECG.
✧ Chest X-ray.
✧ Blood tests (renal function, blood count, glucose).
✧ Echocardiography.
✧ Test(s) for ischaemia.
✧ Coronary angiography for patients with symptomatic or objective features of significant ischaemia if not done within one year.

Predictors of intermediate and low increased peri-operative risk
Most cardiac patients will be in this category.
✧ Advanced age (> 80 years).
✧ Inability to climb one flight of stairs without symptoms.
✧ Mild angina.
✧ Co-morbid conditions (diabetes, peripheral vascular disease, renal impairment, chronic lung disease).
✧ History of myocardial infarction.
✧ Compensated heart failure.
✧ Controlled atrial fibrillation.
✧ Left bundle branch block.
✧ History of stroke.
✧ Uncontrolled hypertension.
✧ Renal impairment.
✧ Poor functional capacity (restricted to light gardening or housework, and able to walk only slowly on the flat).

Note: No ischaemia and an exercise tolerance of 12 minutes on the Bruce treadmill protocol predict low risk.

Pre-operative evaluation of patients at intermediate risk

✧ Specialist cardiology referral.
✧ ECG.
✧ Chest X-ray for patients who experience breathlessness when walking on the flat.
✧ Echocardiography.
✧ Exercise testing (or other test for ischaemia) for patients who are breathless when walking and also for patients who are to have a high risk procedure.
✧ Patients who can walk up two flights of stairs quickly with no symptoms, and who are to have a low-risk procedure do not need exercise testing or echocardiography.
✧ Hypertension should be controlled.

Quantification of the risk

The doctor's perspective

This remains difficult, and only approximate percentage risks can be given. A number of risk indices have been formulated for weighting and scoring risk factors, but these are not widely used. Better pre-operative assessments, anaesthesia and an improved understanding and treatment of risk factors have reduced the peri-operative risks. Quantitation of peri-operative risk has to be individualised, and may be obtained from the surgeon's personal results for the procedure performed in patients with a similar risk profile to the patient under consideration.

The patient's perspective

In general, patients understand the implications of the terms 'high risk' and 'low risk', but assume that surgery would be performed only if it was necessary and if there was an acceptable risk. Attempts to quantitate risk are inaccurate because there are many variables which interact in a complex and inconsistent way in different patients. Ultimately it is the decision of the surgeon to explain the operative risks to the patient. A risk prediction of 20% is very high, but only if the patient is one of the 20%!

Urgent or emergency surgery

In certain circumstances surgery has to be performed as an emergency, so only a post-operative evaluation can be made.

Who should be referred to a cardiologist?

The aim is to identify patients at high and intermediate risk of cardiac problems.

Patients with known heart failure, angina and coronary artery disease, previous infarction, myocardial revascularisation, valvular disease or significant conduction tissue disease, and those with a poor functional capacity or major clinical markers of risk, should be referred to a cardiologist for assessment. Specialist referral is advisable for those with other medical conditions which increase the peri-operative risk.

Patients with major predictors of risk and those at intermediate risk who are to have high-risk surgery should be referred and investigated.

Patients with a poor functional capacity and more than one minor predictor of risk may also be considered for further testing prior to arterial surgery.

Cardiac investigations

The indications for invasive and non-invasive testing are similar to those in the non-operative setting. Patients with coronary artery disease, renal impairment, diabetes or a poor functional capacity, and those who are to have a high-risk surgical procedure, should have cardiac testing.

Patients for whom cardiac testing is not necessary

- ✧ Those who have a high functional capacity, no evidence of heart or vascular disease, or who have had a full cardiac and medical assessment within the last year.
- ✧ Those known to have coronary artery disease but who are symptom free and have no evidence of ischaemia on an exercise test performed within the last year.

When surgery should be delayed or cancelled

- ✧ If one or more *major* predictors of risk are present.
- ✧ If the patient or their family do not want to proceed with surgery, or want a second opinion.

Evaluation of cardiac function
Echocardiography

This is a useful, widely available method for evaluating left and right ventricular function and valve structure. Patients with a resting left ventricular ejection fraction of less than 35%, those with severe diastolic dysfunction, those with uncompensated heart failure and those with important valve disease are at high risk.

Twelve-lead ECG

This is recommended for patients with a history of coronary artery disease and for patients undergoing a high- or intermediate-risk procedure, patients with diabetes and those aged over 50 years with more than one cardiovascular risk factor.

Reversible myocardial ischaemia

The main indications for tests to assess myocardial ischaemia are:
- ✧ patients with an intermediate pre-test probability of coronary artery disease
- ✧ prognostic assessment of patients with known or suspected coronary artery disease or a significant change in their clinical status
- ✧ documentation of reversible myocardial ischaemia
- ✧ assessment of patients after an acute coronary syndrome
- ✧ evaluation of exercise performance when subjective assessment is unreliable.

Exercise testing

Treadmill or cycle exercise testing is widely available, and is useful for quantifying exercise tolerance and haemodynamic responses and for diagnosing ischaemia. These variables can accurately identify patients who are at low risk for cardiac events and who probably do not need coronary angiography. Patients with ischaemia should undergo coronary angiography. Failure to exercise to 85% of the age-predicted heart rate confers a high risk of peri-operative cardiac events (around 25%). In patients with previous myocardial infarction or angina, exercise testing provides no additional diagnostic information, and coronary angiography should be performed.

Alternative tests to assess myocardial ischaemia

When exercise testing cannot be performed because the patient cannot walk or cycle due to arthritis, claudication or lung disease, or if the patient has other conditions which make interpretation of the exercise test result difficult, stress echocardiography and nuclear perfusion imaging may be used to identify patients at high and low peri-operative risk.

Pharmacological stress testing

This is useful for patients who are unable or unwilling to perform an exercise test. Dobutamine echocardiography performed by an experienced operator provides useful diagnostic and prognostic information, is safe, and allows the examination of resting right and left ventricular function, valve structure and function, and the effects of dobutamine on regional and global left ventricular function.

Nuclear perfusion imaging

This may be used instead of exercise testing in patients with bundle branch block, but it does not offer any significant advantages over exercise testing in predicting peri-operative complications or long-term outcomes. It is significantly more expensive than exercise testing, and because of its limitations is performed in only a few centres in the UK. The dose of radioactivity is not inconsiderable, although probably not clinically significant for a single isolated test.

On the basis of current information, there is no justification for the use of either dobutamine echocardiography or nuclear perfusion imaging as a screening test in low-risk populations.

Medical management of angina

Patients may need to stop aspirin and other antithrombotic treatments before certain types of operation.

Patients with angina or hypertension, those with asymptomatic coronary artery disease and those with major cardiovascular risk factors should take β-blockers, which have been shown to reduce peri-operative ischaemia and cardiac events in high-risk patients.

Coronary angiography

Coronary angiography provides anatomical rather than physiological information, and also the opportunity to improve myocardial blood supply with angioplasty performed at the same time.

Coronary angiography is appropriate for patients:
✧ at high risk
✧ at intermediate risk prior to a high-risk procedure (e.g. vascular reconstruction), without preliminary non-invasive testing
✧ with angina at rest or on minimal exertion
✧ with equivocal non-invasive test results
✧ with recent myocardial infarction who need urgent surgery.

Myocardial revascularisation prior to non-cardiac surgery

Coronary artery surgery and/or angioplasty may need to be performed in patients with angina and those with prognostically significant coronary artery disease (left main stem, proximal three-vessel coronary artery disease and severe left ventricular impairment).

Surgery should be delayed for one week after plain angioplasty and for four weeks after coronary stent implantation to allow for endothelialisation of the stent. Clopidogrel is recommended as long-term antithrombotic treatment in patients with coated stents, and the decision to stop this drug must be individualised. In patients with drug eluting stents, stopping clopidogrel before completing one year of treatment, increases the risk of stent thrombosis and myocardial infarction.

Management of hypertension prior to surgery

This is a common clinical management problem. Patients may have well controlled hypertension during normal activities, but their blood pressure rises to a high level when they are admitted to hospital. These patients should be referred to a cardiologist, and their blood pressure must be controlled prior to surgery. Surgery should only be undertaken in patients with uncontrolled hypertension when it has to be performed as an emergency, and in these circumstances the blood pressure can be controlled with intravenous agents, including nitrates, labetalol and nitroprusside (*see* Chapter 5). Sometimes the high blood pressure may be due to anxiety and a pronounced 'white coat syndrome', in which case anxiolytics and sedation may be effective in the short term. Patients should be restarted on oral antihypertensive treatment as soon as possible after surgery.

Valvular heart disease
Dental care and antibiotic prophylaxis

Depending on the procedure to be performed, all patients should be considered for appropriate antibiotic prophylaxis, and some patients may need a dental assessment and treatment before surgery. Pulmonary valve lesions are rare and usually do not require antibiotic prophylaxis.

Stenotic valvular lesions

These patients should be referred to a cardiologist before surgery. Surgery in patients with symptomatic aortic and mitral valve stenosis may precipitate heart failure and pulmonary oedema. A comprehensive physical examination, echocardiography and, where appropriate, cardiac catheterisation and angiography should be performed. Patients in whom valvuloplasty or valve replacement is required will need to be transferred to a cardiac surgical centre, and non-cardiac surgery will have to be delayed.

Regurgitant valvular lesions

Aortic and mitral regurgitation are usually well tolerated, but patients should be referred to a cardiologist for a full assessment and appropriate investigations.

Cardiomyopathy

Patients with both dilated and hypertrophic cardiomyopathy should be referred to a cardiologist for assessment of functional capacity, cardiac function and (in patients with symptomatic arrhythmias) vulnerability to serious arrhythmia (by Holter monitoring).

Management when the patient returns home

When they return home, patients should be reviewed from the surgical and cardiovascular viewpoints. Cardiovascular and heart failure risk factors and all treatments should be reviewed. In particular, treatment of smoking, hypertension, diabetes and lipid status should be optimised. Symptoms of heart failure, angina and breathlessness may be more noticeable to patients after orthopaedic and peripheral vascular surgery because of an improvement in their mobility. Despite careful pre-operative risk assessment, some patients may develop peri-operative cardiovascular problems, and these individuals will need further cardiac review and investigation.

Advice for patients

⬦ The risks of surgery depend on the operation, your age, the state of your heart muscle, the heart arteries and other arteries, your kidney function and other factors. People with lung disease, smokers and those who are overweight are at greater risk of developing lung infections. Before you have an operation, the surgeon will usually arrange with colleagues for you to be assessed so that any risks are minimised.

⬦ It may be necessary for you to have some heart tests to make sure that your heart is strong enough.

⬦ If you smoke, you should stop.

⬦ If you are overweight, you should try to lose weight.

⬦ If you have a bad chest, you may benefit from seeing a physiotherapist to learn some breathing exercises.

⬦ You should try to get as fit as possible before the operation.

Answers to questions about clinical cases

1. Repair of the aortic dissection is an emergency and should be performed without delay. All of the relevant specialists should be advised about the procedure and consulted.

2. This patient needs only a pre-operative assessment by the anaesthetist and an ECG, and can then proceed to surgery without any further cardiac investigations, because he is at low risk and is to have an intermediate-risk procedure.

3. This patient has a poor functional capacity and a number of intermediate predictors of peri-operative risk, and needs a cardiology opinion and further cardiac testing before surgery. If he can exercise, he should have an exercise test to assess his exercise capacity and the severity of reversible myocardial ischaemia. If he cannot exercise sufficiently to 85% of his age-predicted maximal heart rate, he should have a dobutamine stress echocardiogram to look at his cardiac structure and function at rest and during pharmacological stress. If there are signs of significant reversible ischaemia or underlying left ventricular dysfunction at rest or during stress, he should have a coronary angiogram and revascularisation if necessary.

4. This patient should be referred to a cardiologist and assessed prior to gastroscopy, which is a low-risk procedure that is performed under light sedation. Her atrial fibrillation will need to be controlled, and her diabetes may need to be reviewed by a diabetologist both peri-operatively and in the long term. If she is generally fit and active, she would not need further cardiac tests apart from an ECG. After her gastroscopy she should be reviewed and, depending on the result and her other risk factors for embolisation (*see* Chapter 11), she should be considered for rate control and anticoagulation.

5. This patient has major predictors of risk and is scheduled to have a high-risk operation, which should be postponed until she has been fully assessed by a cardiologist and other relevant specialists. Before surgery is performed she will need investigation with an ECG, chest X-ray, echocardiography and, if there is evidence of residual ischaemia, coronary angiography in view of her previous myocardial infarction. She will require

treatment for her heart failure, and her renal function and blood count will need to be reviewed. If there is a compelling need to operate urgently, she must be treated as an emergency and the peri-operative risks minimised as much as possible.

FURTHER READING

Eagle KA, Berger PB, Calkins H *et al.* ACC/AHA guideline update for perioperative cardiovascular evaluation for non-cardiac surgery: executive summary. A report of the American College of Cardiology/American Heart Association Task Force on Practice Guidelines (Committee to Update the 1996 Guidelines on Perioperative Cardiovascular Evaluation for Noncardiac Surgery). *J Am Coll Cardiol.* 2002; **39:** 542–53.

Cardiac tests and procedures

EIGHTEEN

Clinical cases

1. A 55-year-old hypertensive man who smoked cigarettes until one year ago complains of intermittent chest pain related to exercise. What do you do?
2. An 82-year-old woman who was diagnosed with aortic valve disease 15 years ago, but has not been back to hospital since, feels unwell, has lost her appetite and has lost 7 lbs in weight over the last three months. What are the likely causes of her symptoms and what do you do?
3. A 78-year-old woman has had one or two dizzy turns without loss of consciousness. What do you do?
4. The physiotherapist in your practice is treating one of your patients, who has a coronary stent, for sciatica. Is the patient suitable for an MRI scan?

Using cardiac tests in primary care

Cardiac tests are increasingly being performed in primary care because a larger proportion of patients with cardiovascular disorders are being diagnosed, treated and monitored by primary care clinicians. ECGs, echocardiography, 24-hour ambulatory blood pressure recording, 24-hour ambulatory ECG recording, and exercise testing are performed in primary care, and these tests may become more accessible with changes in service provision. However, it is important that tests are performed to the highest standards by appropriately trained personnel, and that the results are reported correctly and are relevant to the patient's clinical condition. GPs who have completed training courses in performing and interpreting these investigations are able to provide these services. Continual updating of skills and equipment is essential. There are funding implications and issues. Complex patients may need to be referred to a cardiac centre.

Explaining tests to patients

Patients may often prefer to ask their GP about a cardiac test, rather than ask the hospital specialist. They will want to know why the test is being performed, what it entails for them, what the risks are, what the result means and how it might affect their treatment. Several new imaging and physiological tests are now used in patients with cardiovascular disorders, and it is important that GPs understand what the tests are for, what they involve for the patient, and how the results influence management.

Open-access investigations

GPs have open access at their local hospital for non-invasive cardiac tests apart from magnetic resonance imaging and computerised tomographic scanning. The rationale is that open-access investigations reduce the length of time for which patients need to wait to be investigated. This may increase waiting times to see a specialist, because the test requested may reveal unexpected or irrelevant findings which the GP feels obliged to refer for clarification and reassurance. Inappropriate investigations may lead to further inappropriate and expensive tests, patient and doctor anxiety, and inappropriate, expensive and potentially dangerous treatment. An example is atherosclerosis imaging and screening with Electron Beam Computed Axial Tomography (EBCAT) scanning in low-risk individuals.

It is therefore essential that all tests are requested and performed with knowledge of the value and limitations of the test in the patient's individual clinical situation, and with an understanding of the possible implications of the result and how that result will influence clinical management.

It is helpful to discuss the clinical case with the consultant cardiologist or a senior medical member of the team if there is doubt about any aspect of a patient's investigations.

The clinical value of the test report depends on the information provided on the request form.

An abnormal test result does not necessarily indicate that the patient's diagnosis is only due to the reported abnormality (e.g. breathlessness may be due to both heart failure and lung disease). This emphasises the importance of the clinical examination and a comprehensive evaluation of the patient.

The cost implications of an investigation and the effects that the test and its result may have on the general well-being and psychological state of the patient should also be considered before requesting the test.

Test interpretation and blind management advice

An intrinsic limitation of most open-access investigations is that the result may be interpreted by the reporting physician in the absence of detailed knowledge of the patient's clinical background. In some cases it is difficult for management advice included in the report to be relevant to the patient. For example, a specialist consultation would not be necessary in the management of a young woman whose echocardiogram report confirms a clinical diagnosis of a mitral valve prolapse. However, a specialist referral is required for an elderly man with echocardiographic evidence of significant aortic stenosis. In addition, the test may be interpreted in the absence of detailed clinical information, and the reporting physician may not have had the opportunity to interpret the test result knowing the patient's clinical background. An exercise test showing ST depression in a patient with a low probability of having coronary artery disease will probably be a false-positive result, and this may lead to confusion and anxiety, and often further inappropriate testing.

GPs need to understand the value and limitations of the more commonly used cardiac tests so that these are used appropriately and efficiently. Primary care clinicians need to be able to explain to patients why the test has been requested, how the test helps in their management, what it involves and what the implications are.

Test result quality

The information obtained from a test depends on factors relating to the equipment, how the test is performed, the patient and the reporting physician. For example, a high-quality ECG recording depends on a properly maintained and calibrated ECG machine, good-quality electrodes and paper, correct skin preparation to obtain a satisfactory electrical signal, and a relaxed patient. Physicians who report test results will need to be provided with adequate clinical information.

Variability in the interpretation of test results

All cardiac tests involve interpretation, and are not a purely objective measurement like a blood test. There is a well-recognised inter- and intra-observer variability in test result interpretation. There is also a patient component in result variability in exercise testing, but this is not clinically important.

Questions to ask before requesting or performing a test

The value of any test result depends on a number of factors, and the following points should be considered before requesting a cardiac test.

✧ What is the most likely clinical diagnosis?
✧ Do I need to perform an investigation at all in order to confirm the diagnosis, provide prognostic information or help me to decide the best management for the patient, or can I rely solely on my clinical assessment?
✧ Will the test result influence clinical management? If so, in what way will it do so?
✧ What is the most appropriate and efficient way to investigate the problem?
✧ Is the patient willing and able to be subjected to the test?
✧ What do I need to tell the patient about the test and what it involves?
✧ What will I need to do if the test result is unhelpful or does not explain the clinical problem?

Chest X-ray

This is invaluable in the assessment of patients who present with breathlessness due to either cardiac or lung disease. Despite having been in use for over a century as the oldest method of imaging the heart, it remains a useful investigation mainly for imaging the lungs. Other imaging techniques provide more detailed and accurate anatomical and physiological information about the heart.

Value and limitations

A plain chest X-ray will show pulmonary oedema but not necessarily the cause. The heart shadow may appear spuriously enlarged due to projectional problems, a depressed sternum (pectus excavatum), or fluid or fat around the heart. Echocardiography provides more accurate information about cardiac chamber dimensions and wall thickness without these potential interpretational problems and without any radiological risks.

The test

Patients are familiar with X-rays, and understand that they are not a risky investigation unless they are repeated many times.

The report

Chest X-rays are usually reported by a consultant radiologist, who may advise on further imaging, depending on the question asked.

Electrocardiography (ECG)

This is the most widely used and available cardiac test, and it is now commonly performed in primary care by both GPs and practice nurses. It records the electrical activity of the heart over a period of several seconds.

Value and limitations

It is very helpful for excluding myocardial infarction as a cause of chest pain. However, ECG signs of infarction may develop several hours after infarction and may not be apparent on an ECG recorded during ischaemic chest pain. If myocardial infarction is suspected, the patient should be referred urgently to hospital.

A normal ECG has a high specificity in excluding heart failure, myocardial infarction and arrhythmia as a cause of palpitation during the test.

Indications

⬦ Suspected myocardial infarction.
⬦ Heart failure as a cause of breathlessness.
⬦ Palpitation.
⬦ Bradycardia.
⬦ Syncope and dizzy turns.
⬦ Screening before major surgery in patients aged over 50 years, or in younger patients with a history of cardiac problems.

The test

The patient lies down flat and as relaxed as possible. The ECG will show muscle tremor in patients who shiver, move, or have muscle movement due to Parkinson's disease, and this may make the ECG uninterpretable. A high-quality ECG trace depends on good electrode contact with a hairless and greaseless skin. Accurate electrode placement is important. The skin should be wiped with alcohol and, if necessary, shaved and then abraded with very fine sandpaper. No other preparations are necessary. The patient feels no discomfort other than the cold sensation of an alcohol skin wipe. The test carries no risk, and can be completed within a few minutes.

The report

Electrocardiographs may provide computer-interpreted reports, but these require confirmation by an experienced physician. These reports generally have a high negative predictive accuracy in excluding arrhythmia and infarction in healthy people, but have a relatively lower accuracy in diagnosing abnormalities.

Management of abnormal test results

If there is a clinical or computer-generated report that suggests myocardial infarction, the ECG and/or the patient should be referred for a specialist opinion, and this should be done urgently if clinically indicated.

Patients with newly diagnosed atrial fibrillation or benign ectopic beats who are clinically stable may be managed in primary care. Patients who feel distressed or who have chest pain, breathlessness or significant arrhythmias should be referred to hospital.

Exercise testing

This is the most widely used and useful method of investigating patients with known or suspected coronary heart disease, and it can be performed in primary care. The purpose of exercise testing is to assess reversible myocardial ischaemia. The test result provides both diagnostic and prognostic information. Resuscitation equipment must be available, although the risk of complications is very small. Patients are usually asked to sign a consent form, although the risk of death (one in 100 000), infarction or ventricular arrhythmia requiring treatment is very low. A profound vagal response is also uncommon, and resolves quickly when the patient lies down or, if necessary, is given atropine.

An understanding of probability analysis and Bayes' theorem is crucial when requesting and interpreting exercise test results.

Physiological responses to exercise

Normally, during exercise, the systolic blood pressure increases due to increased cardiac work, and the diastolic pressure decreases due to peripheral vasodilatation. The aim of exercise testing is to stress the heart and detect impaired blood supply to the heart muscle due to coronary artery disease. The most important factor determining myocardial oxygen demand is the heart rate. The higher the heart rate, the more oxygen and blood are required by the heart muscle. Patients should reach at least 70% of their age-predicted maximal heart rate (calculated as 220 minus the patient's age). Shortness of breath and fatigue are the usual reasons why healthy individuals have to stop exercise. Patients with coronary artery disease may experience angina and/or ST depression.

An inadequate heart rate response is a sign of sinus node disease, and would support the decision to proceed with pacemaker implantation assuming there are other indications. An exaggerated systolic blood pressure response (>200 mm Hg) is consistent with hypertension. An inadequate blood pressure response (failure of the systolic blood pressure to increase to a level higher than the resting pressure, or a fall in pressure during exercise) suggests impaired left ventricular function due to a weak heart muscle or reduced blood supply.

Markers of a poor prognosis

Any of the following features suggest left ventricular impairment and/or significant coronary artery disease and therefore a poor prognosis:

❖ a poor exercise time (less than 10 minutes on the Bruce treadmill or WHO cycle protocol)
❖ failure of the systolic blood pressure or heart rate to increase during exercise
❖ ischaemia (angina and/or ST depression) at a low heart rate and workload
❖ frequent ventricular ectopic beats or ventricular tachycardia during or after exercise
❖ ST elevation in Q-wave-bearing leads after infarction
❖ slow resolution of ST depression and heart rate after exercise.

Markers of a good prognosis

The absence of markers of a poor prognosis indicates a low probability of coronary artery disease and a good prognosis.

The test

Patients are exercised on either a cycle or a treadmill. Many patients prefer a cycle and feel more secure using this method. Only the resistance increases on a cycle, but the inclination and speed increase as well on a treadmill, and patients may feel unsteady and uncomfortable. Cycles are smaller, take up less space, are quieter and, because there is less upper body movement, the ECG quality may be superior. Cycles may not be suitable for patients who find cycling difficult.

Although anti-anginal medication, including β-blockers, may slightly decrease the sensitivity of exercise testing, most cardiologists do not advise patients to stop taking these drugs before the test, because of logistics and the small risk of withdrawal.

Recording the ECG

The skin preparation and electrode positions are similar to those for a resting ECG, but for exercise testing the arm leads are placed below the clavicles and the leg leads are placed above the iliac crests. In order to minimise noise, the electrodes and cables are taped to the skin. A resting blood pressure and ECG are recorded.

Exercise endpoints

The patient is usually exercised to their maximum tolerance. The test is stopped if the patient cannot continue due to fatigue, breathlessness, claudication or dizziness, or if they develop angina, ST depression or important arrhythmias, or their heart rate or systolic blood pressure fail to increase appropriately.

The patient then lies down or sits down until they and their heart rate and blood pressure have recovered and the ECG changes have resolved. Glyceryl trinitrate (GTN) may be given to patients who develop angina.

Analysis of the results

All exercise test variables are analysed. It is helpful for the physician to observe and talk to the patient during the test to ask them about their symptoms.

The Duke Treadmill Score is used in a few centres. It may improve the accuracy of an exercise test result. The formula takes into account the degree of angina, the extent of ST depression and the exercise duration. The test is of limited prognostic value in patients over 75 years of age and in women.

Value and limitations of the test

The test is of most diagnostic use in patients at intermediate risk of coronary heart disease. A 'negative' test result will probably be a false-negative result in a patient with a high probability of coronary heart disease. A 'positive' test result will probably be a false-positive result in a patient with a low probability of coronary heart disease.

Exercise testing adds no diagnostic information about the likelihood of the presence of coronary heart disease in patients with previous myocardial infarction, those with previous revascularisation and those with angina. However, it does provide prognostic information. It is commonly used to assess recurrent or new symptoms in patients who have had angioplasty or coronary artery surgery. An exercise test result that shows no ischaemic or haemodynamic abnormalities has a high negative predictive accuracy in a patient with a low risk of having coronary heart disease.

It provides an objective assessment of fitness and exercise capacity and is helpful in the evaluation of patients who complain of undiagnosed breathlessness.

It has a lower predictive accuracy in women, although the reason for this is not clear. The ST response to exercise is the objective hallmark of myocardial ischaemia, but this cannot be interpreted in patients with an abnormal ST segment at rest. This includes patients with bundle branch block and pre-excitation syndromes. Nevertheless, exercise tolerance, vulnerability to exercise-induced arrhythmia and symptoms can be evaluated.

Indications

⬦ Evaluation of patients with an intermediate risk of having coronary artery disease.
⬦ Prognostic evaluation of patients with known coronary artery disease and after myocardial infarction.
⬦ Serial evaluation of patients after revascularisation.
⬦ Evaluation of heart rate response in patients with suspected chronotropic incompetence.
⬦ Evaluation of blood pressure response in patients with hypertension.
⬦ Evaluation of response to anti-anginal treatment.
⬦ Evaluation of exercise capacity and response to treatment in patients with known or suspected heart failure and/or breathlessness.

Contraindications

⬦ Unstable angina at rest.
⬦ Physical disability that precludes exercise.
⬦ Severe aortic stenosis.
⬦ Uncompensated heart failure.
⬦ Severe uncontrolled hypertension.

The report

The report should include the protocol used, the exercise duration, the reason(s) why the patient stopped, whether they experienced angina, breathlessness or leg fatigue, the resting and peak heart rate, the resting and peak blood pressure, the heart rate recovery time (normally the heart rate should decrease by > 20 bpm in the first minute after stopping exercise), and whether any important arrhythmias occurred during exercise. Ectopic beats, ventricular couplets or ventricular tachycardia occurring during exercise suggest a bad prognosis. Ectopic beats that disappear during exercise are usually benign.

Treatment and management recommendations (e.g. no treatment and no further tests *or* drugs and coronary angiography) should be included.

Nuclear cardiac imaging

This is of limited clinical value in a small number of clinical situations, and accordingly is only available in a few hospitals in the UK. The widespread availability of open-access exercise testing to assess myocardial ischaemia, transthoracic echocardiography to assess left ventricular function and cardiac anatomy, stress echocardiography to assess myocardial ischaemia and hibernating myocardium, and the availability of and short waiting times for coronary angiography in most district general hospitals have relegated nuclear perfusion imaging to a test restricted to a small minority of patients. There are several problems with nuclear imaging.

Principles of nuclear perfusion imaging

The uptake of radioactive chemical into the left ventricular muscle depends on the blood supply. No radionuclide will be taken up into dead heart muscle, and less will be taken up into an area of heart muscle supplied by a narrowed coronary artery compared with an area of normal heart muscle supplied by a normal artery. These differences become apparent only when the heart is subjected to stress using exercise or drugs.

The test

Most tests are done to assess myocardial ischaemia, and are similar to an exercise stress test on a cycle or treadmill. In addition, a radioactive nuclear chemical (usually thallium) is injected into an arm or hand vein at peak exercise. The patient then lies down under a gamma camera and the uptake of radionuclide is imaged in different projections. Further images are taken after around four hours to investigate reperfusion. The report is subjective.

Indications

Nuclear perfusion imaging may be used to investigate reversible ischaemia in patients with resting ECG abnormalities (pre-excitation, left bundle branch block), which complicate interpretation of ST-segment changes. The sensitivity and specificity of nuclear perfusion imaging are not significantly different from those of an exercise test or superior to stress echocardiography.

Value and limitations

The accuracy of the test is affected by many factors. False-negative scans occur with inadequate stress, patients on anti-ischaemic medication, collateral circulation, poor quality imaging and breast attenuation. False-positive scans occur in patients with conduction abnormalities, cardiomyopathies and technical problems. Nuclear material if used repeatedly carries a risk. The test is invasive, costly and time consuming. Although a single dose of radiopharmaceutical used is probably not very dangerous, patients may be reluctant to have an injection of these substances when much less hazardous, cheaper and quicker alternative tests are available.

The report

This should indicate the probability of coronary heart disease. Identifying the location of coronary artery disease is difficult and often unreliable in view of relative perfusion. For example, a patient with severe triple-vessel coronary artery disease and homogenous reduced myocardial blood supply may have no relative perfusion defect identified, and the scan may be reported as 'normal.' There is also variability in coronary arterial blood supply to the inferior wall of the left ventricle from either or both the right and circumflex arteries, so attempts to localise coronary artery disease with nuclear perfusion imaging are often inaccurate. Interpretation of the scans is open to observer error.

Echocardiography

This is the most powerful diagnostic non-invasive cardiac imaging test for assessing valve anatomy and physiological disorders. It is widely available, cheap and completely safe, and is performed by GPs as part of the clinical examination in primary care. Echocardiography is usually combined with Doppler measurements of blood flow across diseased valves and septal defects. Small laptop-computer-sized machines are now affordable for primary care services, and have acceptable diagnostic quality.

Value and limitations

Echocardiography provides important anatomical and functional information about the heart muscle, chamber sizes, ventricular wall thickness, valves and intracardiac connections. The pericardial space and pericardium may be visualised easily, and this is useful as part of the evaluation of breathlessness in patients with chest or breast malignancy.

A normal echocardiogram excludes heart failure, indicates that a heart murmur is probably due to turbulence of blood in a normal heart and not due to an underlying structural heart abnormality, and excludes pathological enlargement of the heart (cardiomegaly), a question that is commonly raised as an incidental finding on a chest X-ray.

Images may not be of diagnostic quality in obese patients and those with chronic airways disease. Interpretation of left ventricular function is subjective, but is made more objective by measurements of left ventricular end-systolic and end-diastolic dimensions.

Indications for echocardiography

* Left and right ventricular function and size in suspected heart failure of any cause.
* Diagnosis and severity of valve abnormalities and septal defects in patients with murmurs.
* Ventricular wall thickness in patients with hypertension, cardiomyopathy and aortic valve stenosis.
* Mechanical complications of acute myocardial infarction.
* Intracardiac connections in patients with congenital heart disease.

The severity of heart valve conditions is assessed by examining the anatomical appearance of the valve, the flow characteristics with Doppler examination, and the haemodynamic consequences of the valve lesion for left ventricular function, dimensions and wall thickness. Intervention for heart valve conditions should be undertaken before left ventricular impairment occurs.

The severity of heart failure is assessed by examining right and/or left ventricular wall movement (pumping action of the ventricles) and thickening (the normal ventricular wall thickens in systole), and chamber dimensions.

The following common cardiac conditions may be diagnosed by echocardiography:

- heart failure
- aortic stenosis and gradient. Significant left ventricular impairment will result in a spuriously low aortic valve peak systolic gradient
- aortic regurgitation
- mitral stenosis and valve area (which determines severity and need for intervention)
- mitral valve prolapse
- mitral regurgitation
- hypertensive heart muscle disease
- left ventricular impairment due to infarction
- dilated cardiomyopathy
- hypertrophic cardiomyopathy.

Serial echocardiography is useful for monitoring the progression of valvular heart disease in order to decide on the timing of valve surgery and its effects on left ventricular dimensions and function, to assess the effects of antihypertensive treatment on left ventricular wall thickness, and after myocardial infarction to investigate recovery and resolution of left ventricular impairment.

The test

The test is completely harmless and carries no risk in pregnant women. The investigation is performed in a darkened room so that the heart images can be seen more easily on the monitor. The patient is asked to take off their outer clothing and lie at an angle of around 45° on their left side. Ultrasound jelly is then applied to the transducer, which is pressed firmly over the chest and moved in order to find a satisfactory echo-window in an intercostal space. The transducer is angled and rotated so as to obtain several views of the heart. The patient will hear a 'whooshing' noise, which represents the electronic Doppler signal denoting blood flow. The test can be completed within a few minutes depending on the question being asked and the echogenicity of the patient.

The report

This should provide both anatomical and physiological information. Colour flow Doppler examination may show physiological mitral and/or tricuspid regurgitation. Heart failure is excluded if left ventricular function is normal.

Transoesophageal echocardiography

This is complementary to transthoracic echocardiography. It is performed in outpatients in cardiac units, and often in very ill patients in the intensive-care unit. Transoesophageal echocardiography produces clearer images of the heart than transthoracic echocardiography because the probe is closer to the heart and the echo signals only have to pass through the posterior wall of the oesophagus, so are not attenuated by the chest wall and lungs.

The test

The procedure is similar to upper gastrointestinal endoscopy. Patients should fast for at least four hours before the test, and must sign a consent form. Some patients are unable to swallow the probe and find the procedure unpleasant, but with satisfactory preparation, explanation, sedation and pharyngeal anaesthesia, and in the hands of an experienced physician, most patients tolerate the procedure well. Antibiotic prophylaxis is not routinely given even in patients with prosthetic valves unless intubation is traumatic. The test is contraindicated in patients with dysphagia, oesophageal problems, respiratory disease or severe coagulopathy, and in those who are unable to cooperate. The patient's ECG, oxygen saturation and blood pressure are monitored during the procedure, because probe passage down the oesophagus may cause hypertension. The procedure takes around 30 minutes.

Complications are rare, occurring in 0.3% of patients, and include oesophageal perforation, arrhythmia, heart failure and laryngeal spasm. Mortality is reported to be one in 10 000, but the risk is principally in very ill patients.

Indications for transoesophageal echocardiography

- ⬥ Inadequate transthoracic echocardiography:
  - — airways disease
  - — obesity
  - — breast implants.
- ⬥ Atrial thrombus/myxoma:
  - — prior to cardioversion
  - — radio-frequency ablation
  - — closure of atrial septal defect.
- ⬥ Prosthetic heart valve:
  - — function
  - — thrombus
  - — vegetation.
- ⬥ Aortic disease:
  - — suspected dissection.
- ⬥ Endocarditis on a native or prosthetic valve:
  - — vegetations
  - — abscess.
- ⬥ Congenital heart disease:
  - — cardiac anatomy.
- ⬥ Atrial septum:
  - — patent foramen
  - — septal defect.
- ⬥ Unexplained stroke in young people:
  - — intracardiac thrombus/myxoma
  - — patent foramen
  - — atrial septal defect
  - — aortic/mitral vegetations.

Value and limitations of transoesophageal echocardiography

This procedure provides very clear anatomical information about the cardiac structures, but involves oesophageal intubation, which carries a small risk of complications.

It permits echocardiographic investigation in patients who are anaesthetised and unconscious in the intensive-care unit, and in those with chest wall problems or dressings that prevent adequate transthoracic study.

Stress echocardiography

This is a specialised extension of echocardiography, which is performed in specialist units and not in primary care. It may be used as an alternative to an exercise test to induce myocardial ischaemia and diagnose or exclude coronary artery disease. Increasing the heart rate and blood pressure leads to an increase in cardiovascular stress. If the blood supply to the heart is normal, there should be normal left ventricular wall thickening and contraction. If the blood supply to the heart is reduced, the segment supplied by a narrowed or blocked coronary artery will not thicken or contract normally in systole.

Stress echocardiography can distinguish between 'viable' myocardium (areas of heart muscle which may improve with revascularisation) and 'dead' muscle. The heart can be stressed using either dobutamine or dipyridamole, or exercise with a treadmill or cycle. Exercise is less practical and accurate because imaging is difficult if the patient is moving. The delay in imaging after exercise may result in a false-negative test result if the wall movement abnormality has resolved before imaging is performed.

The test

A conventional echocardiogram is performed first, and the images are stored as a baseline. Dobutamine, a β-agonist that increases heart rate and contractility, is then infused intravenously. In a normal heart, this results in an increase in left ventricular wall contraction and thickness. Dead heart muscle does not respond to dobutamine, whereas viable myocardium does.

Value and limitations of stress echocardiography

These are similar to those for echocardiography. Interpretation of the images is subjective, and the diagnostic quality of the test depends largely on the experience of the reporting physician.

The sensitivity and specificity of stress echocardiography are similar to those for exercise testing. It is more accurate than exercise testing in women, and in patients with an abnormal ECG at rest (left ventricular hypertrophy, bundle branch block and left ventricular hypertrophy – conditions that decrease the diagnostic accuracy of exercise testing).

Infusion of dobutamine may result in chest pain, dizziness, palpitations and arrhythmia, breathlessness and headache.

Indications

The presence or absence of viable myocardium helps to decide whether revascularisation is appropriate. Revascularising 'dead' (infarcted) heart muscle would not be expected to improve either symptoms or prognosis. 'Dead' myocardium is seen as an area of the left ventricular wall which does not move or thicken. Contraction or thickening of previously 'dead' myocardium during dobutamine infusion suggests viability. The rationale for revascularising these 'viable' areas of muscle is that their function might improve left ventricular function and prognosis. Viability is not an issue when considering revascularisation for patients with angina and narrowed coronary arteries supplying normal myocardium.

Indications for stress echocardiograpy include the following:
⋄ patients who cannot exercise
⋄ when the ECG response to exercise cannot be interpreted
⋄ evaluation of patients with known or suspected coronary artery disease
⋄ evaluation of viable myocardium.

24-hour ambulatory (Holter) ECG recording

First described by the physician Norman Jeff Holter in 1949, this test records a patient's heart rhythm and rate, usually over a 24-hour period. It enables the effects of exercise, sleep, emotion and other daily activities to be evaluated in patients who complain of intermittent palpitations, giddy turns or loss of consciousness. The commonly recorded arrhythmias are ectopic beats and atrial fibrillation.

Patients are given a diary card on which to record the time, duration and nature of their symptoms, so that these may be correlated with arrhythmias timed on the recorder.

Ambulatory devices also record the ST segment, and are occasionally used in the evaluation of patients with coronary heart disease and 'silent ischaemia.'

Magnetic tapes are still used in hospitals, and are the most widely used in all patients and yield most information in patients with frequent daily symptoms. Recently, solid-state and neural-network technology devices have enabled GPs to perform and print their own recordings, and computer software provides a reliable diagnosis.

Long-term ECG recording devices

For patients with less frequent symptoms, event recorders enable the patient to trigger the recorder, which is placed against the chest wall during an attack; some patients find these devices difficult to use. Loop recorders similar in size to a small pacemaker, which are implanted under the skin of the chest wall, record continuously for several months and are designed to capture arrhythmias responsible for elusive and occasional symptoms.

Arrhythmias in healthy people

It is important for GPs to appreciate the range of arrhythmias that may be recorded in healthy people, so that they can explain and reassure patients that not all arrhythmias indicate heart disease (*see* Table 18.1). Bradycardia and heart block are more common in young people. Ventricular ectopic beats and paroxysmal atrial fibrillation are not uncommon in older people, but may not result in symptoms.

TABLE 18.1: Ambulatory ECG findings in 'normal' subjects

Heart rate Range (bpm)	Heart rate sleep (bpm)	Ectopics (% pts)	VT (% pts)	SVT (% pts)	Sinus pause >2.0s (% pts)	Mobitz I (% pts)
37–180	45	10–25	2	5–30	2	2

VT: ventricular tachycardia; SVT: supraventricular tachycardia

Value and limitations of 24-hour ambulatory ECG recording

The quality of the ECG depends on good skin preparation, the absence of interference due to cable movement, and correct calibration. Tape slippage is a potential problem with conventional tape recorders. Reliable computer algorithms improve the diagnostic accuracy.

Symptoms and arrhythmias

A symptom occurring simultaneously with a significant arrhythmia provides important diagnostic information that the patient's symptoms are due to an arrhythmia. Conversely, a cardiac arrhythmia as a cause of symptoms is excluded if symptoms occur in the absence of an arrhythmia. It is difficult to reach a conclusive diagnosis if the patient is symptom-free, particularly if symptoms are infrequent. However, patients may not always experience symptoms with ectopic beats and short runs of paroxysmal atrial fibrillation. Unsustained ventricular tachycardia is less common, but may not result in symptoms. If the history is consistent with these arrhythmias, it is likely that an arrhythmia is responsible.

Indications

⬦ Patients with symptoms consistent with a cardiac arrhythmia.
⬦ Patients with palpitations, giddy turns, loss of consciousness or transient ischaemic attacks.

✧ To assess the response to medical treatment.
✧ To assess the prognosis in patients with arrhythmias after myocardial infarction.
✧ To assess symptoms after pacing for either bradycardia or tachycardia.

Cardiac catheterisation and angiography

The main purpose of this test is to obtain anatomical information on the location and severity of coronary artery disease and haemodynamic data. It provides superior information compared with non-invasive coronary artery imaging, and it also provides the opportunity to perform angioplasty at the same time. It is now widely available in district general hospitals as well as in major teaching centres, although coronary angioplasty is mainly performed in centres with on-site cardiac surgery facilities.

The test

This test is performed by cardiologists as a day case. Using local anaesthesia (and in some patients, light sedation), small-lumen tubes are passed sequentially through a sheath inserted most commonly into the right femoral artery. The sheath is used to allow easy access to the artery and prevents forward flow of blood through the sheath, although blood can still flow to the foot outside the sheath. The left femoral, right radial and brachial arteries are also occasionally used in patients with difficult arterial access. Different-shaped catheters are used to intubate and inject radio-opaque contrast into the left ventricle and the right and left coronary arteries. Another catheter may be used to measure pressures in the pulmonary artery and right heart chambers in patients with valvular disease or septal defects, and in the uncommon cases where cardiac transplantation is being considered.

The test is most commonly performed in patients with known or suspected coronary artery disease, when only the left ventricle and coronary arteries are catheterised. Fluoroscopy is used to position the catheters, and cine pictures are taken during contrast injection and opacification of the left ventricle and both coronary arteries (and bypass grafts in patients investigated after coronary artery surgery) in multiple views to obtain an accurate three-dimensional impression of each coronary artery narrowing.

A pigtail-shaped catheter is introduced into the left ventricle under fluoroscopy and the pressure is measured. This may be increased in patients with impaired left ventricular function. Contrast is then injected and pictures are taken to record left ventricular function. Mitral regurgitation is diagnosed by seeing reflux of contrast back into the left atrium. The pigtail catheter is then removed while any pressure gradient across the aortic valve (as may be seen in aortic stenosis) is recorded. Specially shaped catheters are next inserted in turn to inject the right and left coronary arteries. The catheters and the sheath are removed and digital pressure is applied over the femoral artery until the bleeding stops. Collagen plugs and other sealing devices are commonly used to allow patients to mobilise earlier and leave hospital after two hours of bed rest. Patients are able to get up sooner if the catheterisation is performed from the arm.

Patient information

Some patients find the test uncomfortable, but most are anxious about the implications of a result showing obstructive coronary artery disease. Injection of local anaesthetic into the skin over the femoral artery may sting, and injection of contrast into the left ventricle may cause a feeling of flushing and occasionally nausea. Passage of a catheter in the aorta is painless unless the aorta is dissected by the catheter tip, which is very rare. The patient should be warned by the operator about the recognised complications (one in a 1000 risk of stroke, myocardial infarction and death), which are more common in patients with atheromatous disease in the aorta. The result and the probable management plan should be explained to the patient before they go home, although the final management plan is often decided at a later department cardiothoracic meeting. The patient should not drive, cycle or participate in sports for at least 24 hours after the angiogram, in order to avoid the risk of bleeding.

Indications

⋄ Angina that is not controlled adequately with medical treatment.
⋄ Unstable angina.
⋄ Significant reversible ischaemia on exercise testing or other non-invasive testing.
⋄ In patients who cannot exercise, or when the exercise test is unhelpful.
⋄ Continuing angina, ischaemia or haemodynamic impairment after myocardial infarction.
⋄ After successful resuscitation from cardiac arrest or ventricular tachycardia.
⋄ Prior to aortic or mitral valve intervention in patients with angina or cardiovascular risk factors or endocarditis.
⋄ Certain types of congenital heart disease.
⋄ To assess the possibility of revascularisation in heart failure.

Value and limitations

Coronary angiography is the 'gold standard' test for investigating anatomical coronary artery disease, but it does not provide physiological information.

The percentage risks of coronary angiography in low-risk patients are small. Most complications occur in older patients with atheromatous vascular disease, which is the main indication for performing the investigation.

TABLE 18.2: Frequency (%) of complications of coronary angiography

Death	0.10
Myocardial infarction	0.08
Stroke	0.08
Transient ischaemic attack	0.10
Arrhythmia	0.50
Vascular complications	0.50
Other	0.50

The most common femoral artery vascular complications occur in patients with a wide pulse pressure (e.g. in hypertension and aortic regurgitation), and include haematoma or, less commonly, a false aneurysm of the femoral artery. These present as a painful, swollen and spreading bruise over the puncture site, and are diagnosed with duplex ultrasound. All patients with a painful, swollen, pulsatile mass over the puncture site should be referred back to the cardiologist for assessment. False aneurysms may close up and heal spontaneously if there is low flow between the main femoral artery and the sac of the aneurysm. Closure of an occlusion of the false aneurysm sac may be achieved by injection of thrombin into the sac of the aneurysm, duplex ultrasound-guided manual compression over the neck of the false aneurysm or, rarely, surgical repair may be required.

The report

A stenosis obstructing more than 50% of the arterial lumen would be expected to result in reduced flow down the artery and angina, whereas a short lesion less than 50% of the diameter of the arterial lumen would not be considered flow-limiting. Stenoses are therefore graded as a percentage narrowing or classified as mild (50–75%), moderate (76–90%), severe (91–99%) or blocked (100%) according to a visual examination ('eyeballing') of the angiogram.

The cardiologist should write back with the angiogram report including information about left ventricular function and other relevant information, including coexisting valve abnormalities. There should be a management plan with suggestions for medical and secondary prevention treatment and a decision with regard to revascularisation.

Coronary artery disease and symptoms

Surprisingly, there is a poor correlation between symptoms and coronary artery disease. A patient with severe triple-vessel coronary artery disease may be symptom free until the occurrence of a myocardial infarct. Conversely, a patient with very mild disease may have very troublesome angina. This paradox highlights the importance of treating the patient in conjunction with the angiographic result and other clinical and investigative information, rather than only the angiogram.

Possible treatment strategies

Medical treatment is advised when there is no need for revascularisation based on symptoms or coronary angiographic findings, or in the uncommon situation when revascularisation by either angioplasty or coronary artery surgery is not feasible or is too risky.

Coronary artery bypass surgery is generally advised in patients who are unsuitable for coronary angioplasty, which is equally effective in relieving angina. Repeat revascularisation is more likely to be required in patients who have had angioplasty, because of the risks of restenosis, which are lower with the use of stents and particularly coated stents. Coronary artery surgery is preferred to angioplasty in patients with severe triple-vessel coronary artery disease and left ventricular impairment, because it confers the added advantage of improving prognosis as well as symptoms. In patients for whom no prognostic benefit is expected and in whom coronary artery surgery is considered too high a risk or is refused, coronary angioplasty is considered. All patients with coronary artery disease should have cardiovascular risk factor evaluation and treatment.

Magnetic resonance imaging (MRI)

This is available in only a few centres in the UK, and it is expensive. Its diagnostic role in imaging the heart, pericardium, aorta and pulmonary vessels is developing, and remains unclear. It is occasionally used to provide anatomical information that cannnot be adequately obtained by echocardiography.

The test

Magnetic resonance imaging produces information about cardiac anatomy, valve disease, intracardiac and intravascular blood flow, cardiac chamber contraction and filling, and tissue perfusion. Because of cardiac and respiratory movement, the technique is currently most suited to the cardiovascular structures with least movement. These include the aorta, pericardium and pulmonary vessels. It is not yet as accurate as coronary angiography for imaging coronary arteries, although technological advances show promise in this area.

The patient has to lie within the magnet in a narrow, dark tunnel, and many find this intolerably claustrophobic, despite sedation. Open scanners are less claustrophobic. The test takes 20 minutes.

Indications and contraindications

This test is safe, non-invasive and does not require ionising radiation. It is therefore useful in the serial assessment of patients with congenital heart disease, valvular disease, intracardiac tumours and thrombus, cardiomyopathies and pericardial disease.

Magnetic resonance imaging is contraindicated in patients with pacemakers, cardiac defibrillators, cerebral aneurysm clips or cochlear implants. It is not contraindicated in patients with metallic prosthetic heart valves, coronary artery stents or metallic sternal wires inserted after cardiac surgery.

Conditions where magnetic resonance imaging is useful

✧ Acute aortic dissection.
✧ Characterisation of cardiomyopathies.
✧ Imaging of the pericardium.

Advice for patients

✧ Electrocardiograms (ECGs) are safe and harmless and you won't feel anything. No special preparations are necessary. Men may need to have some of their chest hair shaved. The test takes a few minutes and tells us about the rhythm of your heart, but only during the few seconds for which the test is recorded. It is also useful if you are having chest pain. It is not a perfect test – it may show an 'abnormality' when there is nothing to worry about, and it may not detect heart disease when there is something wrong. Nevertheless, like any test, it is useful if it is interpreted with a knowledge of your clinical condition.

✧ An exercise test or stress test is used to assess the blood supply to your heart muscle. It also tests your fitness and strength, the state of your heart muscle, and your blood pressure response to exercise. It is used to test a variety of different conditions and is very useful and safe – we exercise patients within a day or two of a heart attack. Wear a tracksuit or similar light, comfortable clothes and shoes. Men may need to have their chest hair shaved. Women should wear a comfortable bra and bring a loose-fitting shirt because electrode pads are stuck on the chest and connected to an ECG machine. You will be exercised on either a cycle or a treadmill. Some cardiologists suggest that you stop some of your tablets (e.g. β-blockers) before the test, but others don't. Do your best and let the technician or doctor know whether you want to stop or if you get chest ache or tightness or breathlessness. During the test your ECG and blood pressure will be recorded. The cardiologist will see you in clinic or one of the team will see you after the test to explain the result and tell you whether any other tests are necessary.

✧ A 24-hour ECG recording is made in order to find out whether you have any irregularities in your heart rhythm or rate. It is used to investigate the cause of palpitation in patients with fairly frequent episodes, occurring perhaps at least once a day. Sticky electrodes are put on your chest, secured with tape and connected to a small box which is strapped around your waist. Men may need to shave off some of their chest hair. You cannot bathe or have a shower during the recording, but you can do almost anything else. You will have to return the recorder the next day. Either our doctors at the surgery or the hospital cardiology team will see you or write to you with the result and let you know what, if anything, needs to be done. If you get any palpitation, you will be asked to record when it occurred and for how long. The recorder has a clock on it so that we know whether there was any rhythm abnormality at the same time. Some people have palpitation simply due to being aware of a normal but stronger heart beat. This is quite normal and is often caused by anxiety or exercise. Extra or missed beats are also normal in most people, and the tape may pick these up even in people who don't feel them. The tape may record very slow heart rates, and sometimes this may provide evidence that the patient needs a pacemaker. The test is harmless and is not interfered with by microwaves or X-rays. It is also safe during pregnancy.

❖ Echocardiography is an ultrasound examination of the heart. It is the same test as ultrasound done in pregnancy, and is completely harmless and painless. The test provides useful information about the structure and strength of the heart muscle, the heart valves and the size of the heart chambers. It is useful in all age groups. It tells us if your heart is weak and whether you might benefit from certain tablets. You will be asked to lie fairly flat on a couch, and some ultrasound jelly will be put on your chest. A probe is then pressed fairly hard on the chest wall and ultrasound pictures are displayed on a TV screen. If you hear a 'whooshing' noise, this is due to a Doppler test being done at the same time, which provides useful information about the flow of blood through the heart valves. It tells us whether the valves are working properly or if they are narrowed or leaky. The test does not usually take longer than 10 to 15 minutes. You can eat and drink normally before and after the test.

❖ Transoesophageal (through the gullet) echocardiography is a newer test in which the probe is passed into your stomach. It sounds difficult, but it is quite straightforward. The probe and cable are the width of a pen. The doctor will spray the back of your throat with local anaesthetic and you will be asked to swallow the probe, which should pass easily. The pictures obtained with transoesophageal echocardiography are clearer than those obtained with transthoracic echocardiography because the probe is closer to the heart, and the pictures of the heart are not obscured by the overlying lung.

❖ 24-hour blood pressure monitoring is used to record the blood pressure in people who may possibly have poorly controlled high blood pressure and already be taking tablets, and in those whose blood pressure is 'up and down' and who may need tablets. You will need to wear a cuff around your arm, and the cuff is connected by a tube to a box which you wear around your waist. The cuff inflates automatically every 30 minutes and even during the night. It can feel quite tight. It may inflate twice in succession if it does not get a good-quality recording. You will need to bring the recorder back to us or to the hospital. It will be analysed and then we will have a good idea of what your blood pressure is like over a 24-hour period.

Answers to questions about clinical cases

1. An exercise test would be the most appropriate test. This test evaluates reversible ischaemia, and it is important to know whether the patient experiences chest tightness, ST segment changes, and the exercise duration. Ask the patient to do his best and to exercise to his limit. Drugs do not need to be stopped, and his antihypertensive medication should be taken as usual.

2. Infective endocarditis is the most important diagnosis to consider. Examine the patient for signs of endocarditis, record her temperature, test her urine, do haematology, biochemistry, ESR and CRP tests, and send off two sets of blood cultures. Phone the microbiology laboratory and the hospital and ask to speak to one of the clinicians. If the patient is well, it is reasonable to wait for the blood culture results. If she is unwell, she should go to hospital, or you could start her on antibiotics after discussing this with the cardiologist and microbiologist.

3. Ask the patient about the attacks, and try to find out whether she had giddy turns with near syncope or rotational vertigo. Find out for how long she has had these dizzy turns, and make sure that she has not lost consciousness. Examine her for pulse rate and rhythm, lying and standing blood pressure, and signs of aortic stenosis, heart failure or infection. Perform an ECG for rate and rhythm, and look for conduction abnormalities. This patient will probably need a 24-hour ECG recording, and this can be done and analysed in some primary care clinics. Otherwise she should be referred to hospital. If a neurological cause is suspected, she should be examined and a CT brain scan arranged.

4. Magnetic resonance imaging is contraindicated in patients with pacemakers, cardiac defibrillators, cerebral aneurysm clips or cochlear implants. It is not contraindicated in patients with metallic prosthetic heart valves, coronary artery stents or metallic sternal wires inserted after cardiac surgery. Therefore, this patient is suitable for an MRI scan.

Index